Study Guide for

Essentials for Nursing Practice

Eighth edition

Patricia A. Castaldi, DNP, RN, ANEF
Director
Practical Nursing & Allied Health Programs
Union County College
Plainfield, New Jersey

ELSEVIER
MOSBY

3251 Riverport Lane
St. Louis, Missouri 63043

STUDY GUIDE FOR
ESSENTIALS FOR NURSING PRACTICE, EIGHTH EDITION

ISBN: 978-0-323-18778-7

Notices

Knowledge and best practice in this field are constantly changing. As new research and experience broaden our understanding, changes in research methods, professional practices, or medical treatment may become necessary.

Practitioners and researchers must always rely on their own experience and knowledge in evaluating and using any information, methods, compounds, or experiments described herein. In using such information or methods they should be mindful of their own safety and the safety of others, including parties for whom they have a professional responsibility.

With respect to any drug or pharmaceutical products identified, readers are advised to check the most current information provided (i) on procedures featured or (ii) by the manufacturer of each product to be administered, to verify the recommended dose or formula, the method and duration of administration, and contraindications. It is the responsibility of practitioners, relying on their own experience and knowledge of their patients, to make diagnoses, to determine dosages and the best treatment for each individual patient, and to take all appropriate safety precautions.

To the fullest extent of the law, neither the Publisher nor the authors, contributors, or editors, assume any liability for any injury and/or damage to persons or property as a matter of products liability, negligence or otherwise, or from any use or operation of any methods, products, instructions, or ideas contained in the material herein.

Executive Content Strategist: Tamara Myers
Senior Content Development Specialist: Tina Kaemmerer
Book Production Team Leader: Deepthi Unni
Senior Project Manager: Divya Krish
Cover Designer: Gopalakrishnan Venkatram

Printed in the United States

Last digit is the print number: 9 8 7 6 5 4 3

To John and Dan for all of your love and support.
To the faculty, students, and all of my colleagues who have inspired me throughout the years.

Patricia A. Castaldi

Introduction and Preface

This guide is designed to correspond, chapter by chapter, to *Essentials for Nursing Practice* (eighth edition). Each chapter in this guide contains study aids to assist in learning and applying the theoretical concepts from the text.

The comprehensive chapter review sections allow you the opportunity to evaluate your own level of comprehension after reading the text. Use of the study group questions with fellow students may help in your overall understanding of the nursing content as well as provide a way to further evaluate your familiarity with that content. There are also short-answer, priority order, and multiple-response questions to promote your preparation for classroom examinations and the alternate-format items on the NCLEX® examination. You may find that there are questions that require you to apply information from other chapters or use other reference sources to answer them.

General study tips to use while reading, taking classroom notes, and preparing for and taking examinations are also included in this guide. Other students have found these ideas to be helpful in their nursing course experiences.

Answers for all of the questions and activities can be found at the end of the study guide.

STUDY CHARTS

While reading through the chapters in the text, you may create study charts to assist you to organize the material that is covered. The charts allow for a comparison of key concepts in the chapter. Suggestions for creating charts are provided in the chapters of this text. An example follows.

Routes of Injection

The learning activities presented in this study guide should assist in your review of the text material and your application of the nursing concepts to classroom and clinical experiences.

Route	Angle of Insertion/Needle Size/Maximum Amount of Medication
Intradermal	
Subcutaneous	
Intramuscular	

General Study Tips

While Reading

- Read before the scheduled class: Highlight key points or outline content in the text that will be covered in the classroom. Don't highlight everything! Clarify with your instructor(s) what the expected readings are for your class. Tables and boxes in the text can help to summarize critical information.
- Look up definitions: Find the meanings of words you do not recognize while you are going through the text. It helps to have a medical dictionary and a regular dictionary handy!
- Make notes: Write down a list of topics that you do not understand while you are reading so that you may clarify them with the instructor.
- Compare notes: Use notes taken from the book and in class to create a complete picture of the content.
- Use study/comparison charts: Put facts and ideas in an organized form so that you can refer to them easily at a later point, such as when studying for an examination.
- Use references: Go back to texts and notes used in other courses (such as anatomy and physiology) to help in understanding new material.

In the Classroom

- Make notes: Do not try to write everything down. Note the essential information from the class. Use the margins of notebook paper or type in your mobile device any questions that you may have as you go along so that you remember to ask them at some point. Before the end of the class, note any areas that you need to clarify with the instructor.
- Ask questions: Remember to take advantage of the expertise of the instructor. Do not go away from the class without trying to clear up areas of confusion!
- Digital recordings/audiotape: Make recordings of classroom discussions, *only with instructor permission*, if
  1. There is time to listen to them at some point (such as in the car).
  2. There are positive results from this process, with better understanding of the material and improved examination grades.

On Your Own

- Use available resources: Take advantage of all of the resources at the school, such as the library, computer laboratory, and skill laboratory. Make time to practice nursing techniques, watch DVDs or videos, and complete computer learning programs.
- Join/create a study group: Get together with other students in your class to review material. Study groups offer an opportunity to share information, challenge one another, and provide mutual support.
- Use time management techniques: Use available time as efficiently as possible. For example, the time that is spent waiting for an appointment or riding on public transportation may be used to read over materials or complete assignments.

Before an Examination

- Try to remain calm: Easy to recommend, but hard to do! Learn and use relaxation skills. Do not jump immediately into the examination. Relax and get focused first, and then start the test.
- Be prepared: Check with the instructor to be sure you have covered the content that will be on the examination. Bring the right materials: pencils, pens, erasers, computer passwords, and so on. Leave enough time to get to the examination area to avoid last-minute "rushing in."

During the Examination

- Read the questions carefully: Determine what the question is asking. Stay focused on the actual question without reading into the situations. If allowed to mark on the examination paper, underline key words or cross out unnecessary information to assist in getting to the heart of the question.
- Do not keep changing your answers: Most of the time, the first answer selected is correct. Do not change an answer unless you have remembered the correct response.
- Stay focused: Take brief moments during the examination, if necessary, to stop and use relaxation techniques to compose yourself.
- For multiple response ("Select all that apply"), approach each answer as being true or false in relation to the question.
- When doing math of pharmacology, think about the answer that you obtain to see if it makes sense. How often would you give 10 tablets or 10 mL IM? If the answer does not seem realistic, recalculate!

General Suggestions for Classroom-Based and Online Courses

- Review the syllabus in advance to identify the course requirements and expectations.
- Make a calendar to keep track of dates for examinations, quizzes, and assignments.
- Schedule time to study or complete assignments, especially if you are working.
- Connect with other students in the course electronically, by telephone, or in person.

- Take advantage of all of the available resources, such as online or on-campus tutorial programs.
- If your study habits are leading to positive results in the class, then don't make major changes. If, however, you are finding that you are not passing or just getting by in the course, you should talk with an instructor about how to change your approach to be more successful. Don't wait until it is too late to make a difference in your grade!
- Keep in contact with the instructor! Do not forget to ask questions.
- Maintain professional behavior with your instructors and classmates.

Contents

The Nursing Profession

CASE STUDY

1. Mr. R., 24 years old, decides that he would like to become a nurse researcher.
   a. What formal education does Mr. R. need to reach this career goal?
   b. To maintain or enhance this role, what other education may be needed?

CHAPTER REVIEW

Match the description/definition in Column A with the correct term in Column B.

Column A		Column B
_c_	1. Demonstrate self-care activities.	a. Communicator
_d_	2. Act on behalf of the patient's interests.	b. Manager
_a_	3. Provide emotional support.	c. Educator
_b_	4. Coordinate members of the staff.	d. Advocate

Complete the following:

5. Identify the main purpose of the following nursing organizations:
   a. National League for Nursing (NLN)
   b. American Nurses Association (ANA)
   c. International Council of Nurses (ICN)

6. Identify four career paths that you can choose as a nurse.
   APRN, nurse ed, nurse ad, nurse research

7. Nurses and their professional organizations have lobbied on behalf of:

8. The three components of nursing care are:
   Care, cure, coordination

9. Select all of the accurate statements regarding Nurse Practice Acts in the United States.
   a. Regulate the scope of practice _____
   b. Determine ethical guidelines _____
   c. Use standards from the ANA _____
   d. Vary greatly from state to state _____
   e. Originate from federal legislation _____

10. Identify four core roles for the advanced practice nurse (APRN).
    CNS, CRNA, CNM, NP

11. Provide at least three examples of essential skills for nurses.
    therapeutic communication
    time management
    patient ed   Compassion

12. To become a nurse educator or advanced practice nurse, an individual needs what minimum level of formal education?
    masters or doctoral

13. What is the difference between continuing and in-service education?

Match the description/definition in Column A with the correct person in Column B.

	Column A	Column B
_____	14. Founder of the American Red Cross	a. Lillian Wald
_____	15. Began the Henry Street Settlement	b. Dorothea Dix
_____	16. First professor of nursing at Columbia University	c. Harriet Tubman
_____	17. Superintendent of the female nurses in the Union army	d. Mary Adelaide Nutting
_____	18. Active in the Underground Railroad movement	e. Mary Mahoney
_____	19. Founder of the Nurses' Associated Alumnae of the US and Canada	f. Clara Barton
_____	20. First professionally educated African-American nurse	g. Isabel Hampton Robb

21. Identify at least three external influences on the practice of nursing today. *health care reform, population change, nursing shortage, bioterrorism*

22. Provide examples of workplace hazards that are faced by nurses. *musculoskeletal injuries, back injuries, violence*

23. Nurses recognize that the use of genomics in health care allows providers to: *influence treatment decisions*

24. Select all of the examples of the QSEN competency for patient-centered care:
    a. Determining the patient's meal preferences _____
    b. Using a flow chart for the nursing care plan _____
    c. Identifying the cultural needs of the patient _____
    d. Documenting on the patient's electronic health record _____
    e. Resolving a staff conflict over vacation time _____
    f. Implementing a patient fall protocol _____

25. The ANA Standards of Professional Performance include which of the following areas? Select all that apply.
    a. Consultation _____
    b. Education _____
    c. Prescriptive authority _____
    d. Quality of practice _____
    e. Ethics _____
    f. Assessment _____
    g. Leadership _____

Select the best answer for each of the following questions:

26. The nurse is aware that a characteristic of today's health care system is:
    1. costs are decreasing.
    2. more services are hospital based.
    3. there are less underserved individuals.
    4. the population aged 65 and older is increasing.

27. An inaccurate statement regarding nursing and health care is:
    1. the majority of the public rank nurses highest among professionals for honesty.
    2. acting in a professional manner influences consumer perceptions of health care providers.
    3. public policy can be influenced by nursing involvement.
    4. there is less public access to health care information.

28. The nurse, in considering the difference between autonomy and accountability, recognizes that autonomy is:
    1. initiating nursing interventions that do not require medical orders.
    2. the legal responsibility for nursing interventions.
    3. incorporating values into practice.
    4. generating knowledge to support practice.

STUDY GROUP QUESTIONS

- How did the profession of nursing develop? Who were some of the founders of the profession?
- What are some of the major influences on nursing today?
- What is professionalism in relation to nursing? What are the characteristics of professional practice?
- How are the standards for nursing practice developed? What are the legal and ethical aspects of practice?
- What are the varied responsibilities and roles of nurses?
- How can individuals prepare to be nurses? What career opportunities are available?
- What professional nursing organizations exist and what are their goals/purposes?
- What are the current trends in nursing?

STUDY CHART

Create a study chart to compare the *different levels of nursing education* and the career roles that may be attained at each level.

2 Health and Wellness

CASE STUDIES

1. A personal friend has been experiencing severe stomach and intestinal distress for a few months. She is 35 years old and is employed as an advertisement salesperson for a local newspaper. During the past year, she has been pressured to create more income for her department. When you ask her if she has sought medical treatment, she responds, "I don't have the time to go to the doctor." In addition to her job responsibilities, she is a single parent of a grade school child who enjoys several after-school activities.
   a. What physical and lifestyle factors are present in this situation?
   b. What initial responses/interventions may be helpful for this individual?

2. Mr. G., 44 years old, has recently been diagnosed with diabetes mellitus. He requires a change in his diet and activity, and he will need to take insulin.
   a. Identify factors that could influence his coping with or managing of the disease.
   b. What illness behaviors could Mr. G. possibly demonstrate?
   c. What impact can this illness have on Mr. G.'s wife?
   d. How can the QSEN competency of safety be applied?

CHAPTER REVIEW

Match the description/definition in Column A with the correct term in Column B.

	Column A	Column B
e	1. A person's definition and interpretation of symptoms and use of the health care system	a. Health belief model
d	2. A belief that patients have the authority to be active participants in determining their health and well-being	b. Internal variables
g	3. Longer than 6 months' duration	c. Body image
c	4. A subjective concept of physical appearance	d. Holistic health
b	5. Developmental stage, intellectual background, emotional and spiritual factors	e. Illness behavior
f	6. Short term and severe	f. Acute illness
a	7. Addresses the relationship between a person's beliefs and behaviors	g. Chronic illness

Complete the following:

8. Health is the absence of disease.
   True _____ False __✗__

9. Identify at least one health promotion concern for older adults. maintain function + independence improve quality of life encourage physical activity

10. Identify Maslow's hierarchy of needs on the pyramid:

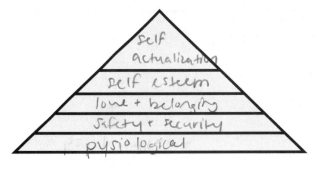

self actualization

self esteem

love + belonging

safety + security

physiological

11. Identify whether the following are internal or external variables that influence health beliefs and practices.
    a. Financial status _ex._
    b. Family health behaviors _ex._
    c. Cognitive abilities _in._
    d. Cultural values _ex._

12. What is an example of a positive health behavior?

    sleep, exercise, nutrition

13. What is an example of a negative health behavior?

    smoking, substance abuse

14. What are two goals of *Healthy People 2020*?

    health equality, quality of life

15. Identify all of the external variables that may influence a person's illness behaviors. Select all that apply.
    a. Visibility of symptoms _____
    b. Disruption of normal routine _____
    c. Accessibility of the health care system _____
    d. Acuity of the illness _____
    e. Cultural background _____
    f. Economics _____

Select the best answer for each of the following questions:

16. At the tertiary level of prevention, a nurse would prepare an educational program for a group requiring:
    1. chemotherapy.
    2. cardiac rehabilitation.
    3. genetic screening.
    4. sex education.

17. At the secondary level of prevention, what is the intervention with which a nurse expects to assist or provide instruction?
    1. Immunization
    2. Referral to outpatient therapy for monitoring
    3. Performance of a biopsy
    4. Parent bathing a newborn

18. A nurse is working with a patient who is experiencing chronic joint pain. To assist the patient to manage or reduce the pain, the nurse decides to use a holistic health approach. With this in mind, the nurse specifically elects to include:
    1. aroma therapy.
    2. wound care.
    3. hygienic care measures.
    4. analgesic medications.

19. A nurse is completing an assessment for a patient who has gone to a medical clinic. Variables that influence the patient's health beliefs and practices are being determined. The nurse is aware that an internal variable for this patient is the:
    1. way in which the patient celebrates family occasions.
    2. manner in which the patient deals with stress on the job and at home.
    3. frequency of the family's visit to the health care agency.
    4. amount of insurance coverage that is provided by the patient's employer.

20. A nurse recognizes that primary prevention is a critical aspect in health care. The target group for a program on hand hygiene for this level of prevention is:
    1. fourth grade children at the elementary school.
    2. patients in a cardiac rehabilitation program at the medical center.
    3. parents of a child with a congenital heart defect.
    4. patients with diabetes at the outpatient clinic.

21. A nurse is leading a group of community members who are trying to quit smoking. In the precontemplation phase of health behavior change, the nurse anticipates that the group members will respond by:
    1. discussing previous attempts at quitting.
    2. recognizing the benefits of not smoking.
    3. expressing irritation when the topic of quitting is introduced.
    4. requesting phone numbers of support people who have participated in the group.

22. A young adult student has gone to the university's health center for a physical examination. The nurse conducting the initial interview is looking for possible lifestyle risk factors. The nurse is specifically alerted to the student's:
    1. mild hypertension.
    2. mountain climbing hobby.
    3. family history of diabetes.
    4. part-time job at the auto factory.

23. According to Maslow's hierarchy of needs, a patient's priority should be:
    1. physical safety.
    2. psychological safety.
    3. self-esteem.
    4. adequate nutrition.

24. To determine a patient's stage in the process of changing behaviors in reponse to being diagnosed with diabetes, a nurse can conclude that the patient is in the maintenance stage on the basis of what response?
    1. "I don't believe I need injections because I feel okay."
    2. "I may need to adjust my diet a little."
    3. "I take my insulin daily as ordered."
    4. "I have been trying to learn the diet plan."

25. A nurse recognizes an environmental risk for illness upon learning that the patient:
    1. works in a chemical plant.
    2. has a history of heart disease.
    3. admits to intermittent substance abuse.
    4. is older than 65 years of age.

STUDY GROUP QUESTIONS

- What are the different health models and how can they be applied to different patient situations? What are the advantages and disadvantages of each model?

- What are the different internal and external variables that are present in health practices and illness behavior? Give specific examples of the different variables and possible nursing interventions.
- What behaviors may be observed in a patient during illness? What impact may the patient's illness have on the family and significant others?
- How do the levels of prevention relate to the nursing care of patients in different health care settings?

STUDY CHART

Create a study chart to compare the *Levels of Prevention* that identifies patient and nursing activities associated with each level.

3 The Health Care Delivery System

CASE STUDIES

1. An 80-year-old female patient has just been diagnosed with an inoperable cancerous growth in the brain. After being told of the poor prognosis, she opts to refuse chemotherapy.
   a. Where could this individual be referred for terminal care?

2. You are working as a unit manager on a busy medical unit in a hospital.
   a. What are some considerations that are involved in the management of care?
   b. How will you use the QSEN competency of teamwork and collaboration in the management of the unit?

CHAPTER REVIEW

Match the description/definition in Column A with the correct term in Column B.

Column A	Column B
_____ 1. Nationwide health insurance program that provides benefits to individuals older than 65 years of age	a. Medicaid
_____ 2. Integration of best knowledge, clinical expertise, and patient values	b. Capitation
_____ 3. Fixed amount of payment for services per enrollee	c. Globalization
_____ 4. Short-term relief for persons providing care to ill, disabled	d. Managed care
_____ 5. Income eligibility for coverage below the federal poverty level	e. Magnet status
_____ 6. Patient responses directly related to nursing care	f. Medicare
_____ 7. Administrative control over primary health care services practice for a defined patient population	g. Respite care
_____ 8. Worldwide in scope	h. Integrated delivery networks (IDNs)
_____ 9. A set of providers and services organized to deliver a coordinated continuum of care to the population of patients in a specific market	i. Nursing-sensitive outcomes
_____ 10. A program to recognize health care organizations that achieve excellence in nursing practice	j. Evidence-based

Complete the following:

11. A(n) _____ is a system of family-centered care designed to allow patients to live with dignity while dealing with a terminal illness.

12. In an acute care setting, when does discharge planning begin?

13. Technology influences health care delivery by:

14. The main purpose of a utilization review is to:

15. Match the appropriate health care service level for each of the following types of care (selections may be used more than once):

Well-baby care _____   a. Primary care
Intensive care treatment _____   b. Secondary acute care
Cardiac rehabilitation program _____   c. Preventive care
Visiting nurses _____
Adult day care center _____   d. Tertiary care
Immunizations _____   e. Restorative care
Family planning clinic _____
Mental health counseling _____   f. Continuing care
Appendectomy surgery _____
Assisted-living facility _____
CT scans _____
Sports medicine _____

16. a. The role of the case manager is to:

    b. The focus of case management is on:

17. An example of a vulnerable population is:

18. Based on the dimensions of patient-centered care, select all of the following that patients want specifically with regard to *access* to health care.
    a. To schedule appointments at convenient times without difficulty _____
    b. To have a setting that focuses on the quality of life _____
    c. To receive accurate and timely information _____
    d. To have an environment that is clean and comfortable _____
    e. To see a specialist when a referral is made _____
    f. To interact with a competent and caring staff _____
    g. To find transportation when going to different health care settings _____
    h. To have family members involved in the plan of care _____

19. What is involved in the process of patient referrals?

20. The Patient Protection and Affordable Care Act of 2010 focuses on:

21. Identify four areas that are part of the Minimum Data Set for Resident Assessment.

22. One of the biggest drawbacks of assisted-living facilities is:

23. Health care reform stimulated the development of these two systems:

24. What services does a nursing center provide? Select all that apply.
    a. 24-hour intermediate care _____
    b. Dietary management _____
    c. Acute care services _____
    d. An interdisciplinary approach _____
    e. Focus on a young adult patient population _____

25. Identify two ways that health care agencies demonstrate quality and safety:

26. Identify the characteristics of a critical access hospital: Select all that apply.
    a. It provides services during daytime hours only. _____
    b. Basic laboratory services are offered. _____
    c. There are usually more than 200 beds. _____
    d. Temporary care is provided for 96 hours or less. _____
    e. Staffing consists primarily of RNs and CNAs. _____

27. Identify three of the National Database of Nursing Quality Indicators (NDNQI).

28. How are globalization and nursing shortages related?

29. The National Priorities Partnership focuses on:

30. The purpose of a Professional Standards Review Organization (PSRO) is to:

Select the best answer for each of the following questions:

31. An older woman was recently diagnosed with Alzheimer's disease. Her daughter expresses her concern that, while she is at work, her mother has been found wandering around the neighborhood in a disoriented state. This family may benefit from the services of a(n):
    1. hospice.
    2. subacute care unit.
    3. adult day care center.
    4. residential community.

32. While working in the community health agency, a nurse visits an older adult patient who is having difficulty performing activities of daily living (ADLs) in her own home. The patient recognizes that she needs some supervision with medications. In discussions with this patient, the nurse refers the patient to a(n):
   1. subacute care unit.
   2. assisted-living facility.
   3. rehabilitation hospital.
   4. primary care institution.

33. A patient is discharged from a medical unit and requires more constant nursing care at a level above a nursing center or extended care facility. The nurse recognizes that this patient will be referred to a(n):
   1. subacute care unit.
   2. home health care agency.
   3. urgent care center.
   4. rural primary care facility.

34. A nurse's next-door neighbor has recently experienced some health problems. The neighbor visits the nurse to ask about Medicaid coverage. The nurse informs the neighbor that this program is:
   1. catastrophic long-term care coverage for older adults.
   2. a fee-for-service plan that provides preventive health care.
   3. a two-part federally funded health care program for older adults.
   4. a federally funded and state-regulated program for individuals of all ages with low income.

35. A graduate of a nursing program is interested in the occupational health field. The graduate nurse decides to pursue a position at:
   1. the local medical center.
   2. a car manufacturing plant.
   3. an urgent care center.
   4. a physician's office.

36. A patient is being discharged from the medical unit of the hospital. While working with the patient, the nurse identifies that intermittent supervision will be required. The patient will also need to rent durable medical equipment for use in the home. There is family support for the patient upon discharge. The nurse will refer this patient to:
   1. a subacute care unit.
   2. an extended care facility.
   3. a home health agency.
   4. an urgent care center.

37. The family of a patient has requested that the hospice agency become involved with the patient's care. The nurse recognizes that the services provided by hospice for this patient include:
   1. extensive rehabilitative measures.
   2. daytime coverage for the working caregivers.
   3. residential care with an emphasis on a return to functioning.
   4. provision of symptom management and comfort measures for the terminally ill.

38. Health care costs are generally reduced with:
   1. treatment in an outpatient facility.
   2. use of new technology.
   3. prescription medications.
   4. identification of acuity levels for hospitalized patients.

39. An individual has a type of managed care plan that limits an enrollee's choice to a list of "preferred" hospitals, physicians, and providers. An enrollee pays more out-of-pocket expenses for using a provider not on the list. The nurse recognizes that this individual is covered by a(n):
   1. managed care organization (MCO).
   2. preferred provider organization (PPO).
   3. exclusive provider organization (EPO).
   4. private insurance company.

STUDY GROUP QUESTIONS

- What types of health care financing are available, who is eligible, and what services are covered?
- What does managed care mean to patients and health care providers?
- According to the health care services levels, what health care agencies and services are available, and what are the usual roles for nurses in each agency?
- What are some of the key competencies required of nurses today?
- What processes are in place to measure health care agency quality, services, and patient satisfaction?

STUDY CHART

Create a study chart to compare the *Types of Health Care Delivery Agencies* that identifies the different health care services provided and the nursing roles and activities for each.

4 Community-Based Nursing Practice

CASE STUDIES

1. A nurse lives in a community that has had a steady increase in the number of older adult residents. The nurse has been approached by some of these residents and asked a variety of health-related questions. The nurse decides to investigate the needs of older adults and the resources available to this population.
   a. For the older adult, what problems and needs should the nurse anticipate?
   b. What kind of programs or services may be available or could be offered in this community for the older adult residents?

2. A 54-year-old patient was discharged from the medical center after being diagnosed with diabetes mellitus. The patient will be taking oral medication and needs to maintain dietary restrictions. Patient teaching was started during the brief stay in the medical center, but the discharge planning nurse has contacted the community health agency to follow up with the patient. You will be visiting this patient in his home today.
   a. What should you include in the assessment of the patient's home environment?
   b. What assessment data will you need to obtain from the patient?

CHAPTER REVIEW

Complete the following:

1. The focus of community-based care is to:

2. One challenge for community-based health care is:

3. The difference between public health and community health nursing is:

4. Identify a particular risk for individuals from the following vulnerable populations:
   a. Immigrant
   b. Poor and homeless
   c. Mentally ill
   d. Older adult

5. Identify the role of the nurse in community-based practice for each of the following examples:
   a. Coordinating the visits of physical and occupational therapists
   b. Demonstrating the use of an aerosol nebulizer
   c. Collecting and analyzing data to identify disease trends

6. What are the three components or parts of a community?

7. Identify three interventions for a family with a member who is dealing with substance abuse.

8. Specify four interventions for a patient with Alzheimer's disease.

9. Identify potential safety hazards in the photo(s) below:

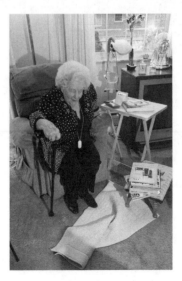

Select the best answer for each of the following questions:

10. A nurse is aware that the homeless population has a higher prevalence of:
    1. diabetes mellitus.
    2. heart disease.
    3. mental illness.
    4. asthma.

11. A nurse is working with a member of a vulnerable population within the community. What is the most appropriate intervention?
    1. Providing financial advice
    2. Setting priorities for the patient and family
    3. Focusing the assessment on only the needed information
    4. Considering the meaning of the patient's language and behavior

12. In completing an assessment of a community's social system, the nurse investigates the:
    1. schools.
    2. economy.
    3. educational level of the population.
    4. distribution of the population by age.

13. For an older adult with a cognitive impairment living in the community, a nurse should specifically plan to:
    1. provide a well-lighted, glare-free environment.
    2. promote activities that reinforce reality.
    3. make arrangements for a hearing evaluation.
    4. encourage the use of self-help groups.

STUDY GROUP QUESTIONS

- What are the essential functions of public and community health?
- How does the community health nurse care for the community?
- What competencies are required of a community health nurse?
- What roles are assumed by the community health nurse?
- What are the special needs of vulnerable populations?
- How does the nurse approach and care for vulnerable populations?
- What is included in the assessment of the community?

5 Legal Principles in Nursing

CASE STUDIES

1. In preparation for surgery, you are to have the patient sign the consent form for the procedure. During discussions about postoperative care, the patient does not appear to fully understand what will be done during the surgery.
   a. What are your responsibilities in this situation?

2. You are reviewing the doctor's orders for the medications to be given to the patient. One of the medication orders is very difficult to read. The nurse in charge tells you that she is sure it is Lasix 40 mg PO.
   a. What should you do in this circumstance?
   b. What legal implications may be involved if the order is incorrect?

3. A child arrives in the emergency department in critical condition. His parents are divorced.
   a. What issues concerning consent for treatment may be involved in this child's case?

4. You have been observing a nursing colleague on your unit, and she appears to be taking narcotics from the medication cart. There have been occasions where her behavior has been erratic.
   a. What, if any, are your legal responsibilities regarding this colleague's behavior?

5. You are looking at a popular social media site and notice that a staff member has posted photos of a patient without permission.
   a. What should you do?
   b. What are the possible consequences of the staff nurse's posting?

CHAPTER REVIEW

Match the descriptions/definitions in Column A with the correct term in Column B.

Column A	Column B
_____ 1. Completed when anything unusual happens that could potentially cause harm to a patient, visitor, or employee	a. Tort
_____ 2. Any willful attempt or threat to harm another person	b. Negligence
_____ 3. A civil wrong or injury for which remedy is in the form of money damages	c. Living wills
_____ 4. A crime of a serious nature that usually carries a penalty of imprisonment	d. Statutory law
_____ 5. Limitation of liability for health care professionals offering assistance at the scene of an accident	e. Good Samaritan law
_____ 6. Conduct that falls below the standard of care	f. Assault
_____ 7. Any intentional touching of another person's body without consent	g. Common law
_____ 8. A form of contemporary law created by elected legislative bodies	h. Battery
_____ 9. Documents instructing physicians to withhold or withdraw life-sustaining procedures	i. Incident report
_____ 10. A form of contemporary law created by judicial decisions in court when cases are decided	j. Felony

Complete the following:

11. The best way for a nurse to avoid being liable for negligence is to:

12. Two areas in which standards of care are defined are:

13. a. Informed consent requires that the patient:

    b. For informed consent, the nurse's role is to:

14. A 9-year-old boy arrives at the hospital after a fall from a tree. He will need emergency surgery. The 25-year-old brother who has brought him to the hospital may give legal consent.
    True _____ False _____

15. Professional negligence is termed:

16. Select all of the following correct statements regarding the Good Samaritan Law (1998):
    a. Health care providers are not liable for care provided during an emergency, even if they are not trained in the care they offer. _____
    b. In an emergency, nurses may treat minors without a parent's consent. _____
    c. Health care providers must follow through on care that is provided in an emergency, transferring the victim to EMTs or other emergency personnel. _____

17. A verbal or telephone order from a physician usually must be signed within _____ hours.

18. The two standards for determination of death are:

19. A "Do not resuscitate" (DNR) order may be given verbally by a physician.
    True _____ False _____

20. The elements of malpractice are:
    a. _____
    b. _____
    c. _____
    d. _____

21. The coroner is notified if the patient's death is:

22. Which of the following constitute a felony related to the Nurse Practice Act? Select all that apply.
    a. Giving the wrong medication to a patient _____
    b. Practicing without a license _____
    c. Misuse of controlled substances _____
    d. Not instituting safety protocols _____
    e. Sharing the patient's information with a co-worker _____

23. Advance directives act to:

24. Health care workers are required to report what incidents?

25. Provide an example of a preventable error.

26. A statute that encourages a health care provider to disclose patient care errors without admitting liability is called an:

27. Malpractice insurance carriers are required by law to report insurance settlements and verdicts to the:

28. Which of the following are examples of "never events"? Select all that apply.
    a. Patient falls _____
    b. Urinary tract infections _____
    c. Lost patient articles _____
    d. Omission of a drug dosage _____
    e. Intermittent catheterizations _____
    f. Pressure ulcers _____

29. Regulations specify that the use of physical or chemical restraint requires:

30. The Patient Self-Determination Act (1991) requires that health care institutions:

31. Place the following individuals in the order in which they will be approached for consent for organ donation:
    a. Guardian _____
    b. Adult son/daughter _____
    c. Spouse _____
    d. Parent _____
    e. Adult brother/sister _____
    f. Grandparent _____

32. The Health Insurance Portability and Accountability Act of 1996 (HIPAA) sets standards for:

33. Identify three common sources of negligence.

Select the best answer for each of the following questions:

34. A clinical experience is planned for an acute care facility. The student nurse recognizes that his or her liability for patient care includes:
    1. no individual responsibility for actions while being supervised.
    2. a shared responsibility with instructor, staff member(s), and health care agency.
    3. activities performed while working in another capacity, such as a nursing assistant.
    4. accountability for information and techniques that will be learned in the school.

35. There has been a serious flu epidemic among the staff at a medical center. Upon arriving to work on the medical unit, a nurse discovers that all other nursing staff members have called in sick and there are no other nurses available in the facility. In this situation, the nurse should:
    1. not accept the assignment and leave the unit.
    2. accept the assignment and identify the poor staffing in each patient's record.
    3. document the situation and provide a copy to nursing administration.
    4. inform the hospital administration that nursing responsibilities have been delegated to other personnel.

36. While a nurse is preparing to administer medication, the patient states that he or she refuses the medication. The nurse knows that the medication is important for the patient and proceeds with the injection of the medication. This is considered:
    1. invasion of privacy.
    2. negligence.
    3. assault.
    4. battery.

37. The urgent care center in town is busy this evening. There are many walk-in patients of different ages waiting for treatment. The nurse recognizes that in a non-emergency situation the individual who may give consent for a treatment is:
    1. a 16-year-old student.
    2. the grandparent of a minor.
    3. a teenage parent.
    4. the 14-year-old brother of a patient.

38. A nurse observes the following actions and recognizes that an invasion of patient privacy has occurred when another nurse:
    1. shares patient data with other agency personnel not involved in the patient's treatment.
    2. withholds the patient's diagnosis from the family members per the patient's request.
    3. provides details of a major scientific advancement to the public relations department.
    4. reports an incidence of an infectious disease to the health department.

39. A nurse enters the room of a patient and observes that an incident has already occurred. The situation is appropriately documented as follows:
    1. "Patient fell out of bed. Physician notified and x-rays ordered."
    2. "Patient found on floor. Laceration to forehead."
    3. "Patient given incorrect medication, became dizzy, and slid to the floor."
    4. "Patient got out of bed without assistance and appeared to have fallen."

40. While working as a receptionist in a physician's office, a student nurse is offered the opportunity to provide an injection to one of the patients. This individual's liability is based upon the:
    1. job description of a receptionist.
    2. educational level achieved in the nursing program.
    3. physician's willingness to accept responsibility for this individual.
    4. limits of the malpractice insurance held by the physician and this individual.

41. A nurse has administered a medication to a patient with a documented allergy to that medication. A standard of care is applied when:
    1. there is a determination of an injury to the patient.
    2. an amount of financial compensation is determined.
    3. criminal statutes from the federal government are investigated.
    4. the nurse's action is compared to that of another nurse in a similar circumstance.

42. Of the following actions, which one is considered to be assault?
    1. A nurse threatens to administer medication to a patient who refuses it.
    2. A surgeon operates on the wrong leg.
    3. A nurse fails to use aseptic technique.
    4. A nursing assistant restrains a confused patient.

43. The National Organ Transplant Act (1984) allows for or requires:
    1. health care agency removal of organs with the family's consent.
    2. donor transplant without the patient's consent.
    3. physicians who certify death to participate in organ removal and transplant.
    4. health care providers to ask family members to consider organ and tissue donation.

- Which individuals may give consent for treatment?
- What is the role of a nurse in obtaining consent?
- What is the role of a nurse in situations related to death and dying, employment contracts, and organ and tissue donation?
- How can a nurse minimize his/her liability?
- What situations require reporting by a nurse?
- How is the profession and practice of nursing influenced by legal issues?
- What are some of the legal concerns for nurses working in specialty areas, such as obstetrics?

STUDY GROUP QUESTIONS

- What are the sources and types of laws?
- What are intentional and unintentional torts?
- How may intentional torts be applied to nursing situations?
- What criteria are necessary for negligence/malpractice to occur?
- How are the standards of care defined and applied?

STUDY CHART

Create a study chart describing *How to Minimize Liability* that identifies the nursing actions that reduce possible liability for the following situations: short staffing, floating, patient occurrences, and reporting/recording.

6 Ethics

CASE STUDIES

1. You are the home care nurse for a 42-year-old male patient who has severe multiple sclerosis. He tells you on several occasions that he is tired of living this way, of not being able to do anything for himself. He says that he has read about individuals who have been "helped to die," and he asks if you can assist him in finding out more about this procedure.
   a. Apply the steps for processing an ethical dilemma to this situation.
   b. What is the role of the nurse in this situation?

2. The son of one of your patients asks you if he can look at his mother's medical record. He insists that he needs to know what is happening so that he and his sister can plan for the mother's care.
   a. What should you do in this circumstance?

CHAPTER REVIEW

Match the description/definition in Column A with the correct term in Column B.

	Column A	Column B
f	1. Supporting the patient's right to informed consent	a. Ethics
g	2. Considering the patient's best interest	b. Fidelity
h	3. Avoiding deliberate harm	c. Justice
b	4. Keeping promises	d. Morals
c	5. Determining the order in which patients should be treated	e. Bioethics
a	6. Consideration of standards of conduct	f. Autonomy
e	7. Ethics within the field of health care	g. Beneficence
d	8. Judgment about behavior	h. Nonmaleficence
i	9. Personal beliefs about the worth of an idea	i. Values or object

Complete the following:

10. According to the Health Insurance Portability and Accountability Act of 1996 (HIPAA), access to a patient's medical record by a family member requires:

11. Identify an end-of-life issue that has ethical implications for nurses.

12. Identify the ethical theory for each of the following descriptions:
    a. Proposes that actions are right or wrong based on the essence of right and wrong in the principles of fidelity, truthfulness, and justice
    b. Discusses how ethical decisions affect women
    c. Proposes that the value of something is based on its usefulness

13. For the following areas, provide a specific example of how ethical concerns may be involved:
    a. Cost containment
    b. Cultural sensitivity

14. In applying the QSEN competency of informatics, explain how the digital transmission of patient information can be an ethical concern.

Select the best answer for each of the following questions:

15. A professional code of ethics includes:
    1. legal standards for practice.
    2. extensive details on moral principles.
    3. guidelines for approaching common ethical dilemmas.
    4. a collective statement of group expectations for behavior.

16. By administering medication to a patient on a unit in an extended care facility, a nurse is applying the ethical principle of:
    1. justice.
    2. fidelity.
    3. autonomy.
    4. beneficence.

17. A nurse has been working with a patient who had abdominal surgery. The patient is experiencing discomfort and has been calling for assistance often. The ethical principle of fidelity is demonstrated when the nurse:
    1. changes the dressing.
    2. provides a warm lotion back rub.
    3. informs the patient of the actions of the medications administered.
    4. returns to assist the patient with breathing exercises at the agreed-upon times.

18. A student nurse is assigned to work with parents who refuse to have essential medical treatment provided to their child. The medical center is pursuing a court order to force the family to accept the treatment plan that will assist the child. The nurse has strong feelings for the family's position, as well as the importance of the medical treatment. The first step for the nurse to take in attempting to resolve this ethical dilemma is to:
    1. examine personal values.
    2. evaluate the outcomes.
    3. gather all of the facts.
    4. verbalize the problem.

19. An example of advocacy in nursing practice is:
    1. documenting care provided to a patient.
    2. giving medication to a patient.
    3. assessing the patient's comfort level after surgery.
    4. contacting the physician to discuss the patient's response to the plan of care.

20. The last phase in the processing of an ethical dilemma is to:
    1. evaluate the action taken.
    2. consider treatment options.
    3. negotiate the options and outcomes.
    4. identify the problem.

21. Which one of the following situations represents an ethical rather than a legal consideration?
    1. Administering medications
    2. Providing care to someone without health insurance
    3. Sharing patient information with another health care worker
    4. Reporting a communicable disease to the public health officer

STUDY GROUP QUESTIONS

- What are ethics and what is the purpose of a code of ethics in a profession?
- What principles are promoted in a profession?
- How can a nurse be a patient advocate?
- What are the basic standards of ethics?
- What are values and how are they developed?
- How do values relate to ethics?
- How does a professional determine that an ethical dilemma exists?
- What are the steps for processing an ethical dilemma?
- What ethical dilemmas may arise in health care and nursing practice?

STUDY CHART

Create a study chart to identify and compare *Responsibility, Accountability, Confidentiality, Competence, Judgment, and Advocacy,* and provide examples of nursing behaviors for each.

7 Evidence-Based Practice

CASE STUDIES

1. You are working in a home care agency. One of your assigned patients is having difficulty with managing his daily insulin intake. You discover that he is having difficulty in getting an accurate blood glucose reading with his monitor. Because of the problem, the patient is self-administering too much or too little insulin. You remember that some of the other home care patients are also having some trouble with this particular glucose monitor.
   a. Use the PICO format to develop a possible question.
   b. What type of trigger is present in this scenario?

2. As a nurse for a surgical unit in a local medical center, you will be involved in identifying some quality improvement (QI) projects for your unit.
   a. What possible areas may be important for you, your fellow staff members, and the patients on your unit?

CHAPTER REVIEW

Match the description/definition in Column A with the correct term in Column B.

	Column A	**Column B**
C	1. Characteristics, or traits, that vary among subjects	a. Pilot
d	2. Prediction made about the relationship between study variables	b. Abstract
a	3. To trial a new practice	c. Variable
b	4. Brief summary of an article that quickly tells you if the article is research or clinically based	d. Hypothesis

Complete the following:

5. Evidence-based practice is:

6. Identify three valuable sources of non–research-based evidence.

7. A peer-reviewed article is:

8. A qualitative research study focuses on:

9. Provide an example of how a nurse integrates evidence into practice.

10. In the Quality Improvement model, what does PDSA stand for?
   P -
   D -
   S -
   A -

11. Provide an example of a patient outcome and measurement.

12. A randomized control trial (RCT) includes which of the following? Select all that apply.
   a. Subjects _____
   b. Experimental therapies _____
   c. A control group _____
   d. Subjective input from the researcher _____
   e. Analysis of the results _____

13. An evidence-based article includes which of the following? Select all that apply.
    a. An abstract _____
    b. The author's biography _____
    c. A literature review _____
    d. The study's design and methods _____
    e. The author's opinions about the subjects _____
    f. A conclusion relevant to the findings _____

14. Identify three of the competencies for evidence-based practice.

15. Sources for new scientific information are:

16. In a research study, the statistical analysis indicated a "p value" of 0.02. This is understood as being a good result.
    True _____ False _____

17. Two examples of comprehensive databases are:

18. Identify how evidence-based practice change can be communicated to others.

19. Root cause analysis is:

20. For the following study, identify each of the PICOT components:
    Over a 4-month period, the nursing staff on the unit is going to observe whether wound healing of pressure ulcers is improved if they are left open to air for 2 hours each day, rather than covered for 24 hours.
    P -
    I -
    C -
    O -
    T -

Select the best answer for each of the following questions:

21. A nurse recognizes which of the following as a sentinel event?
    1. An error is made and a medication dose is skipped.
    2. A wound infection is noted on a patient who has transferred from a nursing home.
    3. A patient dies within 48 hours of admission to the medical center.
    4. A hip replacement is performed on the wrong leg.

22. Which of the following is the best description of a case control study?
    1. A comparison of one group of subjects to another
    2. A focus on a subgroup with a known condition
    3. A prediction or explanation of phenomena
    4. A description of the responses to an independent variable

STUDY GROUP QUESTIONS

- What is evidence-based practice?
- How does a nurse become involved in the research process?
- What is PICO(T)?
- Where can reliable research-based data be found?
- What databases represent the scientific knowledge of health care?
- What types of evidence or studies are available for reference?
- How are evidence-based findings used in nursing practice?
- How are evidence-based changes communicated and evaluated?
- What is the relationship between evidence-based practice and quality improvement?

8 Critical Thinking

CASE STUDIES

1. You receive reports on your patient assignment for the day. You have six patients who require assessment and have orders for treatments and medications.
   a. How can you use critical thinking to approach this multiple patient assignment?

2. As a home care nurse, you have been assigned to visit a patient who requires dressing changes for a foot ulceration. When you arrive in the home, you see that the patient does not have any commercially packaged dressings or saline solution. You have used the last of your supplies and the drive to the office will take more than 1 hour. The dressing that the patient has on her foot is saturated with purulent drainage.
   a. What options are available to you in this situation?
   b. What further investigation about the patient and her living situation may be necessary?

3. A patient who has just been diagnosed with heart disease is being discharged to his home. He will be on a low-sodium and low-cholesterol diet.
   a. Using critical thinking skills, what areas will you focus on for this patient and his new diet?

CHAPTER REVIEW

Match the description/definition in Column A with the correct term in Column B.

	Column A	**Column B**
_____	1. Process of recalling an event to determine its meaning and purpose	a. Scientific method
_____	2. Series of clinical judgments that result in informal or formal diagnoses	b. Decision making
_____	3. End point of critical thinking that leads to problem resolution	c. Intuition
_____	4. Inner sensing that something is so	d. Diagnostic reasoning
_____	5. Process that moves from observable facts from an experience to a reasonable explanation of those facts	e. Reflection

Complete the following:

6. Identify one example of how critical thinking is used in each of the following steps of the nursing process:
   a. Assessment
   b. Nursing diagnosis
   c. Planning
   d. Implementation
   e. Evaluation

7. Identify the level of critical thinking demonstrated by each of the following:
   a. Trusting experts to have the right answers for every problem
   b. Analyzing and examining problems more independently
   c. Making choices without assistance and accepting accountability

8. Identify the elements of the critical thinking model.

9. Identify the attitude of critical thinking demonstrated for each of the following:
   a. Performing a skill safely and effectively
   b. Questioning an order that appears incorrect
   c. Performing a systematic and thorough pain assessment
   d. Developing a unique way to teach the patient how to change a dressing
   e. Admitting to the nurse manager that a medication was given in error

10. Provide an example of how the nurse can use each of the following critical thinking skills:
    a. Reflection
    b. Language
    c. Learning

11. What are two useful tools for developing critical thinking skills?

12. Which of the following statements are accurate regarding critical thinking attitudes? Select all that apply.
    a. Risk-taking is not desirable in patient care. _____
    b. Using disciplined thinking reduces creativity. _____
    c. Perseverance can indicate that one is always looking for available resources. _____
    d. Personal feelings should not be allowed to influence delivery of care. _____
    e. All sides of each situation should be considered. _____
    f. Intuition should be used as a primary tool in determining patient care. _____

Select the best answer for each of the following questions:

13. In employing critical thinking, the first step that the nurse should use is:
    1. evaluation.
    2. decision making.
    3. self-regulation.
    4. interpretation.

14. Having worked for a number of years in the acute care environment, a nurse achieved the ability to use a complex level of critical thinking. The nurse:
    1. acts solely on his or her own opinions.
    2. trusts the experts to have the answers to problems.
    3. implements creative and innovative options.
    4. applies rules and principles the same way in every situation.

15. Clinical care experiences have recently begun for a student nurse. When beginning to work with patients, the student nurse implements critical thinking in practice by:
    1. asking for assistance if uncertain.
    2. sharing personal ideas with peers.
    3. acting on independent judgments.
    4. relying on standardized, textbook approaches.

16. A nurse has an extremely large patient assignment this evening and begins to feel overwhelmed. Of the following, what is the nurse's priority activity?
    1. Sharing his or her feelings with colleagues
    2. Calling the supervisor and asking for assistance
    3. Reviewing the overall assignment to get his or her bearings
    4. Moving immediately to provide patient care, starting with the room closest to the nurse's station

17. Orientation for new nurses begins. The instructor assembled information on critical thinking and nursing approaches. The instructor recognizes that critical thinkers in nursing:
    1. make quick, single-solution decisions.
    2. act on intuition instead of experience.
    3. review data in a disciplined manner.
    4. alter interventions for every circumstance.

18. A nurse is caring for a patient who is experiencing a respiratory disorder. Intuition is a part of the critical thinking process for the nurse. While caring for the patient, the nurse demonstrates intuition by:
    1. reviewing care with the patient in advance.
    2. observing communication patterns.
    3. establishing a nursing diagnosis.
    4. sensing that the patient is not doing as well this morning as before.

19. Entering a room at 2:00 AM, a nurse notes that the patient is not in bed; the patient is sitting in the chair and states that she is having difficulty sleeping. Employing critical thinking, the nurse responds by:
    1. assisting the patient back into bed.
    2. asking more about the patient's sleep problem.
    3. positioning the patient and providing a warm blanket.
    4. obtaining an order for a hypnotic medication.

20. A nurse has a diverse patient assignment this evening. When reviewing the patients' conditions, the nurse determines that the first individual who should be seen is:
    1. the patient who is hypotensive.
    2. the patient receiving a visit from a family member.
    3. the patient being treated by the respiratory therapist.
    4. the patient waiting for the effects of an analgesic that was given 5 minutes ago.

21. In using the critical thinking skill of self-regulation, a nurse will:
    1. be orderly in data collection.
    2. look at all situations objectively.
    3. use scientific and experiential knowledge.
    4. reflect on his or her own experiences and improve performance.

22. During the process of reflection, what is the most appropriate question for a nurse to ask himself or herself?
    1. "What could I have done differently?"
    2. "What's going on right now?"
    3. "How can the patient's status change?"
    4. "What should I do to communicate this information?"

23. A nurse believes that substance abuse is a serious problem with negative consequences for patients and families. The nurse, however, provides excellent care to a patient who is admitted with this problem. The nurse is displaying the critical thinking attitude of:
    1. integrity.
    2. fairness.
    3. discipline.
    4. perseverance.

STUDY GROUP QUESTIONS

- How is critical thinking integrated into nursing practice?
- What attitudes are needed by a nurse to be a critical thinker?
- How are the competencies of critical thinking applied in clinical practice?
- Why is critical thinking important throughout the nursing process?

9 Nursing Process

CASE STUDIES

1. Mr. B., a 47-year-old male patient, goes to the annual community health fair. During a routine blood pressure screening, it is determined that his blood pressure is significantly above normally expected levels.
   a. What additional assessment data should be obtained from the patient and family?
   b. What limitations exist in this situation for completing an assessment?

2. Mr. B. returns for a follow-up visit at the medical center's adult health clinic. Mr. B. is diagnosed with hypertension and an antihypertensive medication is prescribed, but he appears unsure about how and when he should take the prescription. Mr. B. also identifies that his father died from a heart attack at 54 years old.
   a. Identify the relevant assessment data for this patient.
   b. Based upon this information, identify two nursing diagnoses.

3. During Mr. B.'s appointment at the adult health clinic, he was found to have high blood pressure, and antihypertensive medication was prescribed. Mr. B. did not have any previous knowledge of or experience with either hypertension or hypertensive medication. Mr. B. mentions again that his father died at age 54 years of a heart attack.
   a. Based on the nursing diagnoses that were developed, identify one long-term or short-term goal for each diagnosis and at least one expected outcome for each goal.

Nursing Diagnoses	Long-Term or Short-Term Goals	Expected Outcomes
1.		
2.		

   b. Identify two nursing interventions that may be appropriate in assisting the patient to achieve the expected outcomes and goals.

4. At his next visit to the adult health clinic, Mr. B. tells the nurse that he is taking the antihypertensive medication that was ordered by the physician "when he remembers." He says that he is trying to use the relaxation techniques that he was taught during his last visit, but he does not use them regularly.
   a. What nursing implementation methods should take priority at this time?
   b. What, if any, alterations must be made in the original plan of care?

5. Mr. B. returns to the adult health clinic for evaluation of his status. His blood pressure is lower than before but remains slightly above normal limits. He exercises once or twice a week and states that this is making him feel better. Mr. B. shows the nurse a calendar on which he has written down the times for taking his medication. Mr. B. relates that he has been trying very hard to use the relaxation techniques when he starts to feel anxious or overwhelmed. He identifies that he cannot control all of his "destiny," but he is trying to do things that may help him avoid what happened to his father.
   a. In accordance with previously identified outcomes, what nursing evaluation may be made on this patient's status?
   b. What areas, if any, may require reassessment?

6. A 4-year-old girl is newly diagnosed with diabetes mellitus. You are going to be working with the family to help them adjust to the treatment regimen.
   a. What assessment data is important to collect from the child and family?
   b. Identify a possible nursing diagnosis for the child or the family related to the new diagnosis.

CHAPTER REVIEW

Match the description/definition in Column A with the correct term in Column B.

Column A

_____ 1. Unintended effect of a medication, diagnostic test, or intervention

_____ 2. Observations or measurements made by the nurse during assessment

_____ 3. Comparing data with another source to determine accuracy and relevancy

_____ 4. Multidisciplinary, outcome-based care plan

_____ 5. Clinical judgment about patient responses to health problems or life processes

_____ 6. Information obtained through the senses

_____ 7. Activities performed in the course of a normal day

_____ 8. Support for why a specific nursing action is chosen

_____ 9. Interpretation of cues

_____ 10. Information verbally provided by the patient

Column B

a. Subjective data

b. ADLs

c. Adverse reaction

d. Critical pathway

e. Nursing diagnosis

f. Cue

g. Objective data

h. Scientific rationale

i. Inference

j. Validation

Complete the following:

11. The three phases of an interview are:

12. Based on the following data clusters, identify possible nursing diagnoses for each of the following:
    a. Abdominal pain, three loose liquid stools per day, hyperactive bowel sounds

    b. Fatigue, weakness, tachycardia upon activity, exertional dyspnea

13. Identify at least one goal or expected outcome and one nursing intervention for the following nursing diagnoses:
    a. *Deficient Knowledge related to the need for postoperative care at home*
       Goal:

       Expected outcome:

       Nursing intervention:

    b. *Constipation related to lack of physical activity*
       Goal:

       Expected outcome:

       Nursing intervention:

c. *Risk for injury*
   Goal:

   Expected outcome:

   Nursing intervention:

14. Identify whether the following are examples of cognitive, interpersonal, or psychomotor skills in patient care:
    a. Preparing and administering an injection
    b. Completing a health history
    c. Providing emotional support to a family member
    d. Changing a surgical dressing
    e. Recognizing the patient's need for nutritional instruction

15. Before implementing standing orders, the nurse should check:

16. The steps of the implementation phase of the nursing process are:

17. During interactions with a patient, a nurse gathers more data and identifies a new patient need. The nurse should:

18. A patient with diabetes mellitus goes to the outpatient center for care. There is a written plan for diet counseling, medication, and follow-up care. These specific procedures are termed a(n) _____ for care.

19. An example of an indirect nursing intervention is:

20. Identify all of the following that typically may be delegated to unlicensed assistive personnel:
    a. Skin care _____
    b. Tracheostomy care _____
    c. Hygienic care _____
    d. Personal grooming _____
    e. Urinary catheterization _____
    f. Administration of IV medications _____
    g. Assistance with ambulation _____

21. Specify how the wording of the following patient outcome statements may be improved:
    a. Erythema will be less noticeable
    b. Pulse rate will be normal
    c. Patient's calorie intake will increase

22. Identify at least three (3) ways to create a good environment for an interview with a patient.

23. Indicate whether the following data are subjective or objective:
    a. "I feel tired."
    b. BP 124/64
    c. Pain level of 5 on a scale of 10
    d. Diaphoresis
    e. Wound edges dry and intact

24. What information can be found in a patient's medical record?

25. How would the following data be validated by the nurse?
    a. Patient states that he is fatigued.
    b. The pressure ulcer appears larger.

26. Provide examples of how the nurse can implement each of the following in the plan of care:
    a. Direct care
    b. Counseling
    c. Teaching
    d. Controlling adverse reactions

27. What are the steps in the evaluation process?

28. Provide an example of how the nurse can determine the patient's cultural needs or preferences.

29. For the nursing diagnosis *Feeding Self-care Deficit,* indicate two interventions that the nurse can implement to assist the patient.

Select the best answer for each of the following questions:

30. A new graduate is preparing to work with patients on a medical unit. The nursing process is applied as a:
    1. method for processing the care of many patients.
    2. tool for diagnosing and treating patients' health problems.
    3. guideline for determining the nurse's accountability in patient care.
    4. logical, problem-solving approach to providing patient care.

31. Upon admission, the nurse begins to assess the patient. The patient appears uncomfortable, stating that she has severe abdominal pain. The nurse should:
    1. inquire specifically about the discomfort.
    2. let the patient rest, returning later to complete the assessment.
    3. perform a complete physical examination immediately.
    4. ask the family about the patient's health history.

32. The following nursing diagnoses are proposed for patients on the medical unit. The diagnostic statement that contains all of the necessary components is:
    1. impaired gas exchange related to accumulation of lung secretions.
    2. imbalanced nutrition related to chemotherapy treatment.
    3. complicated grieving.
    4. pain related to abdominal surgery.

33. A nurse is working with patients who go to the community center for health screenings and educational sessions. An example of a wellness nursing diagnosis label that is appropriate for this group is:
    1. *Risk for Impaired Skin Integrity.*
    2. *Readiness for Enhanced Family Coping.*
    3. *Altered Parent-Infant Attachment.*
    4. *Fluid Volume Deficit.*

34. In reviewing the nursing diagnoses written by a new staff member, a supervisor identifies which of the following as a correctly written nursing diagnosis?
    1. *Altered Respiratory Function related to abnormal blood gases*
    2. *Urinary Infection related to long-term catheterization*
    3. *Deficient Knowledge related to need for cardiac monitoring*
    4. *Pain related to severe arthritis in finger joints*

35. A nurse is working with a patient who has the following symptoms: dyspnea, ankle edema, weight gain, abdominal distention, hypertension. The nursing diagnosis that is most appropriate for these signs and symptoms is:
    1. *Ineffective Tissue Perfusion.*
    2. *Disturbed Body Image.*
    3. *Impaired Gas Exchange.*
    4. *Excess Fluid Volume.*

36. A patient is to have abdominal surgery tomorrow. The nurse determines that an outcome for this patient that meets the necessary criteria is:
    1. patient will be repositioned every 2 hours.
    2. patient will express fears about surgery.
    3. patient will achieve normal elimination pattern before discharge.
    4. patient will perform active range-of-motion exercises every 2 hours while in bed.

37. There are a number of activities that are to be performed by a nurse during a clinical shift. In deciding to perform a nurse-initiated intervention, the nurse:
    1. administers oral medications.
    2. orders laboratory tests.
    3. changes a sterile dressing.
    4. teaches newborn hygienic care.

38. A nurse implements a preventive nursing action when:
    1. immunizing patients.
    2. assisting with hygienic care.
    3. inserting a urinary catheter.
    4. providing crisis intervention counseling.

39. A nurse has been working with a patient in the rehabilitative facility for 2 weeks. The nurse is in the process of evaluating the patient's progress. During the evaluation phase, the nurse recognizes that:
    1. nursing diagnoses always remain the same.
    2. time frames for patient outcomes may be adjusted.
    3. evaluative skills differ greatly from those for patient assessment.
    4. the number of nursing diagnoses and outcomes is most important.

40. An expected outcome for a patient is the following: "Pulse will remain below 120 beats per minute during exercise." If the patient's pulse rate exceeds 120 beats per minute one of every three exercise periods, the nurse appropriately evaluates the patient's goal attainment as:
    1. patient has achieved desired behavior.
    2. patient requires further evaluation of progress.
    3. patient's response indicates need for elimination of exercise.
    4. patient does not comply with therapeutic regimen.

41. The nurse is caring for a patient who has been medically stable. During the change-of-shift report, the nurse is informed that the patient is experiencing a slight arrhythmia. To avoid complications during the implementation of care, the nurse plans to first:
    1. evaluate the patient's vital signs.
    2. ask about the patient's previous diagnoses.
    3. contact the physician immediately.
    4. tell the nursing assistant to perform the usual care for the patient.

42. For a patient in the acute care facility, a nurse identifies several interventions. The statement that best communicates the specific nursing intervention to be performed is:
    1. assist with exercises.
    2. take the patient's vital signs.
    3. refer the patient to a therapist.
    4. provide 30 ml of water with the nasogastric tube feedings every 4 hours.

43. The nurse is working with a patient who has diabetes mellitus. The nursing diagnosis is "Deficient fluid volume related to osmotic diuresis." An appropriate patient outcome, based on this nursing diagnosis, is:
    1. patient will have an increased urinary output.
    2. patient will decrease the amount of fluid intake during a 24-hour period.
    3. patient will demonstrate a decrease in edema in the lower extremities.
    4. patient will have palpable peripheral pulses and good capillary refill.

44. A nurse is working with a patient who is experiencing abnormal breath sounds and thick secretions. The nurse identifies a nursing diagnosis of:
    1. *Deficient Fluid Volume.*
    2. *Ineffective Airway Clearance.*
    3. *Risk for Altered Mucous Membranes.*
    4. *Dysfunctional Ventilatory Weaning Response.*

45. In completing a health history, a nurse obtains from the patient psychosocial information that includes:
    1. the reason for seeking health care.
    2. past health problems.
    3. the primary language spoken.
    4. physical safety status.

46. A patient tells the nurse that she feels she may not be using the crutches correctly when ambulating. The best way for the nurse to validate this information is to:
    1. ask the family about the patient's ambulation.
    2. ask the physician how the patient was taught.
    3. discuss the problem with the other staff members.
    4. observe the patient using the crutches.

47. An example of the most appropriately written nursing diagnosis is:
    1. *Acute Pain related to surgery.*
    2. *Shortness of Breath related to immobility.*
    3. *Anxiety related to lack of knowledge about cardiac monitoring.*
    4. *Recurrent Infection related to improper catheterization procedure.*

48. In determining which of the following patients on the medical unit to visit first, a nurse selects the patient with which of the following diagnoses?
    1. *Imbalanced Nutrition: less than body requirements*
    2. *Ineffective Tissue Perfusion*
    3. *Deficient Knowledge regarding home care resources*
    4. *Impaired Physical Mobility*

49. An example of a physician-initiated intervention is:
    1. teaching a patient about the therapeutic diet.
    2. assessing a patient's skin.
    3. providing emotional support.
    4. preparing a patient for a diagnostic test.

STUDY GROUP QUESTIONS

- What is involved in patient assessment, and what priorities does a nurse have in completing an assessment?
- How does the patient assessment fit into the nursing process?
- Why does an error in the assessment phase influence the remaining implementation of the process, and how can a nurse avoid errors?
- What methods may be used to obtain patient data and what type of data is obtained with each method?
- What is involved in a patient interview?
- How can a nurse optimize the environment for a patient interview?
- How can a nurse use different communication strategies to obtain data during patient assessment?
- What is a nursing diagnosis?
- What are the components of a nursing diagnosis?
- How are actual and potential nursing diagnoses different?
- How are medical and nursing diagnoses different?

- What errors are possible in formulating nursing diagnoses, and how can they be avoided?
- Which nursing diagnoses become priorities in planning patient care?
- How are long-term and short-term goals different from each other?
- How are goals and expected outcomes different from each other?
- What are the guidelines for formulating goals and outcomes?
- In selecting nursing interventions, what are three essential nurse competencies?
- How are the three types of nursing interventions different from one another?
- What factors should be considered when selecting nursing interventions?
- What is the purpose of the care plan, and what types are available for use?
- How does a critical pathway differ from a "traditional" care plan?
- How does the consultation process begin, and who and what may be involved in the process?
- What is the focus of the implementation phase of the nursing process?
- What are standing orders and protocols, and how are they used in patient care situations?
- What are the five preparatory nursing activities that are completed before implementing the care plan?
- What are the nursing implementation methods?
- How is nursing implementation communicated to other members of the health care team?
- How is evaluation incorporated into the nursing process?
- How is evaluation used in patient situations and in nursing practice and health care delivery settings?
- What circumstances would lead to a modification of a care plan?

STUDY CHART

Create a study chart to compare the *Steps of the Nursing Process* that identifies the different activities involved in each step.

Create a *Concept Map* for one of the case studies in this chapter.

Informatics and Documentation

CASE STUDIES

1. Mrs. Q. has just been transferred to her room from the postanesthesia care unit (PACU) after right hip replacement surgery. She was accompanied by a nurse from the PACU. Vital signs were taken upon transfer and found to be within expected limits. A dressing is in place on the patient's right hip. Mrs. Q. does not appear to be having any difficulty at the moment.
   a. What information should be provided by the PACU nurse to the primary nurse on the surgical unit when Mrs. Q. is transferred to her room?
   b. What additional information may Mrs. Q.'s primary nurse want to obtain from the PACU nurse?

2. The primary nurse begins to plan and provide care for Mrs. Q. Upon entering the patient's room, Mrs. Q. is found to be grimacing and moaning in pain. She says that she is having intense pain in her right hip area. The dressing to her hip is dry and intact. Mrs. Q. says that she does not want to move because it really hurts. The primary nurse helps Mrs. Q. to get into a more comfortable position and begins to prepare the pain medication ordered by the physician. The primary nurse administers the pain medication, and, after approximately one-half hour, Mrs. Q. states that the pain has been reduced. Using SOAP or DAR methods, document the nursing interaction with Mrs. Q.

3. Mr. W. has just been diagnosed with type 1 diabetes mellitus and needs to learn how to self-administer his insulin injections.
   a. What information should be included in the patient record regarding the teaching provided to Mr. W. on the self-injection of insulin?

CHAPTER REVIEW

Match the description/definition in Column A with the correct term in Column B.

	Column A	Column B
_d_	1. An oral or written exchange of information between health care providers	a. Record
_e_	2. Information about patients provided only to appropriate personnel	b. POMR
_a_	3. Permanent communication with the patient's health care management	c. Acuity recording
_b_	4. Structured method of documentation with emphasis on the patient's problems	d. Report
_c_	5. Documentation that requires staff to identify interventions and allows patients to be compared with one another	e. Confidentiality

Complete the following:

6. The following are guidelines for written documentation. Indicate the correct action to be taken by the nurse for each guideline.
   a. Never erase entries or use correction fluid, and never use pencil.
   b. Do not write retaliatory or critical comments about patients.
   c. Avoid using generalized, empty phrases.
   d. Do not cross out errors.
   e. Do not leave blank spaces.
   f. Do not speculate or guess.
   g. Do not record: "Physician made error."
   h. Never chart for someone else.
   i. Do not wait until the end of shift to record important information.

7. a. HIPAA (Health Insurance Portability and Accountability Act of 1996) has new regulations that require written consent for disclosure of all patient information.
      True _____ False _____
   b. Incident or occurrence reports should be documented in the patient's medical record in the nurse's notes section.
      True _____ False _____
   c. Poor written and verbal communication has been a top ten reason for sentinel events.
      True _____ False _____

8. Standards for health care agencies and documentation are set by the:

27

9. For each of the following, identify an example of how the patient record is used.
   a. Communication:
   b. Finance:
   c. Education:
   d. Research:
   e. Auditing/monitoring:

10. Provide an example of a malpractice issue related to charting:

11. Identify the five characteristics of quality documentation:

12. Subjective statements made by the patient are best documented by:

13. Demonstrate how a student nurse should sign a written patient record:

14. Identify what is wrong with the following notations and how they can be corrected:
   a. "Ate some breakfast."
   b. "Voided an adequate amount."
   c. "Provided wound care qd."

15. For telephone reports, identify what the SBAR acronym represents and give an example of each area:
   S:
   B:
   A:
   R:

16. Provide two items that should be included in a discharge summary:

17. Home care documentation is completed for quality control and as the basis for:

18. Completion of narrative notes only when there are abnormal patient findings is part of the concept of:

19. What are the purposes and advantages of nursing informatics?

20. Identify at least two ways in which electronic records are safeguarded for privacy and security:

21. Identify the four concepts included in informatics:

22. Which of the following are the correct nursing actions for a telephone order? Select all that apply.
   a. Identifying that Mr. J. is in Room 212 _____
   b. Asking the physician to repeat the medication order for Mr. J. three times _____
   c. Checking that 40 mg of the drug is what should be given _____
   d. Writing "TO" (telephone order) in the nurse's notes _____
   e. Asking another nurse to call the physician back to verify the order _____
   f. Having Mr. J.'s doctor cosign the order within 24 hours _____

23. What information is usually available to nurses on a clinical information system (CIS)?

24. A problem-oriented medical record includes: Select all that apply.
   a. Progress notes _____
   b. Narrative notes _____
   c. Initial care plan _____
   d. Problem list _____
   e. Incident reports _____
   f. Discharge summary _____

25. What information should student nurses leave off of written materials that are prepared for class?

26. Identify the errors in the following charting example:
   Patient says she feels ok. 140/82, 88, 14. Gained a little weight. Complained about her doctor. Says she didn't eat much breakfast today.

Select the best answer for each of the following questions:

27. A nurse is working in a facility that uses computerized documentation of patient information. To maintain patient confidentiality with the use of computerized documentation, the nurse should:
   1. delete any and all errors made in the record.
   2. give his or her password only to other nurses working with the patient.
   3. log off the file or computer when not using the terminal.
   4. remove sensitive patient information, such as communicable diseases, from the record.

28. The nurses on a medical unit in an acute care facility are meeting to select a documentation format to use. They recognize that less fragmentation of patient data will occur if they implement:
    1. source records.
    2. focus charting.
    3. charting by exception.
    4. critical pathways.

29. While caring for a patient on the surgical unit, a nurse notes that the patient's blood pressure has dropped significantly since the last measurement. The nurse shares this information immediately with the health care provider in a(n):
    1. flow sheet record.
    2. incident report.
    3. telephone report.
    4. change-of-shift report.

30. Documentation of patient care is reviewed during the orientation to the facility. The new graduate nurse understands that the method for written documentation that is acceptable is:
    1. using red ink to make entries on patients' charts.
    2. charting all of the patient care at the end of the shift.
    3. beginning each entry with the time of the treatment or observation.
    4. leaving space at the end of the notations to allow for additional documentation.

31. A nurse is caring for a patient who has had abdominal surgery. Accurate and complete documentation of the care provided by the nurse is evident by the following notation:
    1. "Vital signs taken."
    2. "Tylenol with codeine given for pain."
    3. "Provided adequate amount of fluid."
    4. "IV fluids increased to 100 mL per hour according to protocol."

32. A nurse is involved in patient care in an agency that uses military time for documentation. Which of the following represents 4:00 PM?
    1. 0400
    2. 0800
    3. 1400
    4. 1600

33. An example of the use of a clinical decision support system (CDSS) is:
    1. access to patient's lab reports.
    2. direct input to the medical orders by the health care provider.
    3. problem-oriented recording.
    4. an alert for incorrect drug dosages.

34. An appropriate action by a student nurse is demonstrated by:
    1. accessing records of other students' patients.
    2. writing the patient's name and room number on assignments.
    3. copying patient records for review and preparation of care plans.
    4. reading the patient's record in preparation for clinical care.

35. A nurse enters a patient's room and discovers a yellow pill on the bed under the patient's pillow. The patient receives Lasix 40 mg daily. Which of the following notations is appropriate to include on an incident or occurrence report?
    1. "Patient refused to take Lasix at 10 AM."
    2. "Yellow pill found on bed under pillow."
    3. "Lasix not administered by primary nurse."
    4. "Patient did not receive 10 AM diuretic."

36. The nursing information system (NIS) that follows a more traditional format is the:
    1. protocol design.
    2. critical pathway design.
    3. nursing process design.
    4. medical diagnosis design.

37. Which of the following statements made by a new staff nurse during a change-of-shift report requires correction?
    1. "The patient is uncooperative about doing his stoma care."
    2. "Oxygen is needed after ambulation. This is a change in priorities."
    3. "Ms. Q. is a 62-year-old with diabetes mellitus."
    4. "The abdominal surgical wound is healing slowly, with no drainage noted."

STUDY GROUP QUESTIONS

- What is the purpose of documentation and reporting?
- What are the legal guidelines for documentation?
- How do the guidelines influence nursing documentation and reporting?
- What methods are available for documentation of patient data?
- How do the different types of documentation (e.g., SOAP, DAR, and narrative) compare with one another?
- How does written documentation compare with computerized systems, and what are the advantages and disadvantages of each method?
- What types of forms are used for patient documentation?
- How does patient documentation change in different health care settings?
- What information is necessary when doing change-of-shift, telephone, transfer, and incident reports?
- What role do informatics play in heath care?
- How do nurses use information systems?
- What safety measures need to be taken by nurses when accessing electronic records?
- What type of patient information is accessible on electronic systems?

Communication

CASE STUDIES

1. For the following patient situations, identify the communication techniques that may be most effective in establishing a nurse-patient relationship:
   a. An older adult patient who has a moderate hearing impairment
   b. The Russian-speaking parents of a young child who has been taken into the emergency department after a bicycle accident
   c. A young adult patient who is blind and requires daily insulin injections
   d. A 60-year-old Hispanic woman who will be having her first internal pelvic examination
   e. A 45-year-old patient on a ventilator

2. You are working with a patient who appears to have literacy issues. There is a need to instruct the patient about the medical diagnosis.
   a. What strategies should you use to assist the patient to understand the diagnosis and treatment plan?

CHAPTER REVIEW

Match the description/definition in Column A with the correct term in Column B.

	Column A	Column B
c	1. Person who initiates interpersonal communication	a. Therapeutic communication
g	2. Information sent or expressed by the sender	b. Metacommunication
f	3. Means of conveying messages	c. Sender
h	4. Person to whom the message is sent	d. Intonation
e	5. Indicates whether the meaning of the sender's message was received	e. Feedback
d	6. Tone of the speaker's voice that may affect a message's meaning	f. Channels
b	7. A message within a message that conveys a sender's attitude toward the self and toward the listener	g. Message
		h. Receiver
a	8. Development of a working, functional relationship by the nurse with the patient, fulfilling the purposes of the nursing process	

Complete the following:

9. Determine what level of communication the following examples illustrate:
   a. Talking to oneself
   b. "He looks uncomfortable, and I want to show him that I'm concerned about his discomfort."
   c. The ability to speak to consumers on health-related topics

10. Provide an example of how compassion fatigue may develop.

11. Individuals maintain distances between themselves during interactions. Identify the zone (Intimate, Personal, Social, or Public) being used in each of the following examples:
    a. Speaking to a group of students in a classroom
    b. Conducting a small group therapy session
    c. Performing a physical examination
    d. Making patient rounds with a physician
    e. Changing a wound dressing
    f. Testifying at a hearing
    g. Completing a change-of-shift report

12. For an older adult with impaired communication, identify the appropriate communication techniques. Select all that apply.
    a. Maintaining a quiet environment that is free of background noise _____
    b. Shifting from subject to subject during the conversation _____
    c. Letting the person know if you are having difficulty understanding him or her _____
    d. Using explorative questions to facilitate conversation _____
    e. Using long sentences to explain subject matter _____

13. The following are examples of inappropriate communication by a nurse. Specify an effective strategy that should be used to correct the situation.
    a. Calling the patient "honey"

    b. Reporting to a nursing colleague about the "gallbladder in room 214"

    c. Talking about a patient to other nurses in the elevator

    d. Running into a patient's room to administer medications and then leaving immediately

    e. Informing a patient that the physician will be performing an abdominal hysterectomy and that she should expect a midline incision of approximately 10 cm

14. For the following examples, identify a question that the nurse could ask that would be more appropriate and obtain better information from the patient:
    a. "You're feeling okay today, right?"

    b. "You don't take any medication at home, do you?"

    c. "Are you having any lymphedema?"

    d. "The physician will be doing a paracentesis today. He said he explained it to you."

15. Identify the communication strategy that is being used for each of the following examples:
    a. Sitting with a patient who is crying

    b. Showing interest in the patient who is discussing concerns or sharing family information

    c. Saying "Go on" or "Tell me more"

    d. Asking the patient to verify the meaning of statements made

    e. Directing the attention of the patient to a particular idea in the discussion

16. For the nursing diagnosis *impaired verbal communication related to aphasia,* identify at least two nursing interventions to promote communication with the patient.

17. Nurses on a medical unit are discussing issues related to their work schedules. Identify the examples of positive responses:
    a. "There's nothing we can do about the staffing situation." _____
    b. "Don't talk to me like that!" _____
    c. "What do you think we can do to improve this situation?" _____
    d. "I want to hear what your concerns are." _____

18. A nurse takes into account cultural considerations when communicating with patients. Identify the appropriate action(s):
    a. Stroking the head of a Southeast Asian patient _____
    b. Assigning a female staff member to care for a female Amish patient _____
    c. Maintaining direct eye contact with a Native American patient _____
    d. Introducing oneself and using the patient's last name _____

19. For the acronym SOLER, identify the skills for attentive listening:
    S:
    O:
    L:
    E:
    R:

20. Identify the nursing actions/responses that occur during the Orientation Phase of the Helping Relationship. Select all that apply.
    a. Achieving a smooth transition for the patient to other caregivers as needed _____
    b. Providing information needed to understand and change behavior _____
    c. Reviewing available data, including the medical and nursing history _____
    d. Expecting the patient to test your competence and commitment _____
    e. Setting the tone for the relationship by adopting a warm, empathetic, caring manner _____
    f. Prioritizing patient problems and identifying patient goals _____

21. Rose is a new nurse on the cardiac unit. Her new colleagues, who have worked there for many years, do not help her and say things like, "Didn't you learn that in school?" This is an example of:

    lateral violence

22. Identify three physiological alterations that could influence communication for the patient.

23. What is going on in the photo below that may interfere with communication between the nurse and the patient?

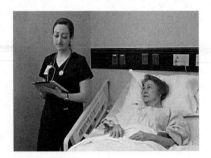

Select the best answer for each of the following questions:

24. A patient tells a nurse that he feels anxious and afraid. The nurse responds by saying, "I will stay here with you." The nurse is using the principle of effective communication known as:
    1. empathy.
    2. courtesy.
    3. availability.
    4. encouragement.

25. A patient states that he believes he may have cancer. The nurse tells him, "I wouldn't be concerned. I'm sure that the tests will be negative." The response by the nurse demonstrates the use of:
    1. assertiveness.
    2. false reassurance.
    3. professional opinion.
    4. hope and encouragement.

26. A nurse is assigned to a young adult male patient. Gender sensitivity is demonstrated when the nurse:
    1. uses sexual innuendo.
    2. engages in gender-oriented joking.
    3. stereotypes male and female roles.
    4. uses direct and indirect communication according to gender.

27. A patient regularly visits a medical clinic. A nurse establishes a helping relationship with the patient. During the working phase of a helping relationship, the nurse:
    1. encourages and helps the patient to set goals.
    2. reminisces about the relationship with the patient.
    3. anticipates health concerns or issues.
    4. identifies a location for the interaction.

28. A nurse is interviewing a patient who is in the outpatient area. The nurse uses paraphrasing communication with the statement:
    1. "This is your blood pressure medication. It will help to lower your blood pressure to the level where it should be."
    2. "Do you mean that the pain comes and goes when you walk?"
    3. "I would like to return to our discussion about your family."
    4. "If I understand you correctly, you are primarily concerned about your dizzy spells."

29. A patient tells a nurse that there are other people in the room who are watching her from under the bed. The nurse employs therapeutic communication when he or she:
    1. identifies that there are no people under the bed.
    2. tells the patient that he or she will help look for the other people.
    3. asks the patient why other people are watching her.
    4. reassures the patient that he or she will tell the people to go away.

30. While speaking with a female patient, a nurse notes that she is frowning. The nurse wants to find out about possible concerns by:
    1. asking why the patient is unhappy.
    2. telling the patient that everything is fine.
    3. identifying that the patient is frowning.
    4. asking if the patient is angry about the health care problem.

31. A patient's condition has deteriorated, and he has been transferred to the intensive care unit. The roommate asks the nurse what is wrong with the patient. The nurse should respond to the roommate by stating:
    1. "The patient's condition is no concern of yours."
    2. "Everything is fine. Don't worry. He'll be okay."
    3. "I recognize your interest in the patient, but I cannot share personal information with you without his permission."
    4. "Your roommate's condition worsened overnight, and he had to be moved to the intensive care unit for observation."

32. A patient is experiencing aphasia as a result of a CVA (cerebrovascular accident, or stroke). To promote communication, a nurse plans to:
    1. speak louder.
    2. use more questions.
    3. use visual clues, such as pictures and gestures.
    4. refer to a speech therapist to communicate with the patient.

33. A patient is talking endlessly about problems in the past with arthritic pain, but the nurse must get specific information for the admission assessment. The nurse's best response is:
    1. "You seem to have had difficulty managing the arthritis. What are you doing now for the pain?"
    2. "You can tell me more at another time. We need to move on to other information now."
    3. "You've given me a lot of information, but I have to ask you something else."
    4. "Are you taking medication for the arthritis?"

34. A nurse enters a room and finds the patient crying. The best action by the nurse is to:
    1. ask the patient why he or she is crying.
    2. tell the patient that things will get better.
    3. let the patient know that you will come back later.
    4. sit quietly with the patient.

35. A patient has a visual impairment. In communicating with this patient, a nurse should:
    1. use flash cards.
    2. use simple sentences.
    3. caution the patient before any physical contact.
    4. speak very loud and slow.

36. A nurse tells the patient's family that recovery may be "difficult." This may lead to an issue with:
    1. pacing.
    2. clarity.
    3. relevance.
    4. connotation.

37. A cultural group that may perceive continuous eye contact as intrusive or threatening is:
    1. Asian.
    2. Hispanic.
    3. African American.
    4. Northern European.

38. A nurse is working with a preschool-age child. An appropriate communication technique to use with an individual in this age-group is to:
    1. speak loudly and forcibly.
    2. communicate directly with the parents to determine the child's needs.
    3. sit or kneel down to be on the same level as the child.
    4. use medical terms when speaking with the parents so the child will not understand.

39. A patient's blood sample was dropped on its way to the lab. The patient asks the nurse why blood needs to be drawn again for the same test. The nurse's best response is:
    1. "One of the vials was dropped and broken by mistake. We will make sure that this sample gets to the lab safely."
    2. "We just have to do the test again."
    3. "Someone didn't do their job right the first time."
    4. "This kind of thing happens. It won't take long."

40. Which one of the following medications has the greatest potential to influence patient communication?
    1. Diuretics
    2. Antipsychotics
    3. Anticholinergics
    4. Antipyretics

41. A nurse is evaluating communication skills used during an interaction with a newly admitted patient. Of the statements made, the nurse responded therapeutically with:
    1. "Why aren't you able to keep taking the prescribed medications?"
    2. "We need to move quickly through the rest of the interview because it will be time for your therapy."
    3. "I can understand why you don't like that physician. I think you need to find another one."
    4. "I noticed that you didn't eat any of the lunch. Is there something that is bothering you?"

STUDY GROUP QUESTIONS

- What is therapeutic communication?
- What are the basic elements of communication?
- How do nurses and patients communicate verbally and nonverbally?
- What factors may influence communication?
- How may a patient's physical, psychosocial, and developmental status influence communication with the nurse?
- How is a helping relationship established with a patient?
- What are the principles/techniques of effective communication?
- How are the principles/techniques used by a nurse in a caring relationship?
- How is communication used within the steps of the nursing process?
- What are some of the barriers to effective communication, and how can they be overcome by the nurse?

STUDY CHART

Create a study chart to compare the *Components of Verbal and Nonverbal Communication* that identifies how each may influence the nurse-patient interaction (e.g., intonation).

12 Patient Education

CASE STUDIES

1. Your patient is a 47-year-old married woman who has gone to the medical clinic for evaluation. She has been diagnosed with hypertension and placed on an antihypertensive medication. She has no previous knowledge or experience with the diagnosis or the medication. There is a family history of coronary disease; her father died of a heart attack at 54 years old.
   a. What information about the patient may affect her motivation to learn?
   b. Formulate a teaching plan for the patient that includes goals and teaching strategies.

2. You are a nurse in a pediatrician's office. An 8-year-old boy has just been diagnosed with diabetes mellitus. His parents are very concerned about what this means for their son.
   a. What general information will the family need?
   b. How will you adapt your teaching for your 8-year-old patient?

3. There is a presentation tomorrow that you will give to a small group of patients.
   a. What do you need to take into consideration when preparing the setting for the teaching session?

CHAPTER REVIEW

Match the description/definition in Column A with the correct term in Column B.

Column A	Column B
_____ 1. Expression of feelings, attitudes, opinions, and values	a. Cognitive learning
_____ 2. Mental state that allows for focus and comprehension of material	b. Motivation
_____ 3. Acquiring skills	c. Attentional set
_____ 4. Intellectual behaviors, including knowledge and understanding	d. Affective learning
_____ 5. Desire to learn	e. Return demonstration
_____ 6. Completion of a procedure to show competence	f. Psychomotor learning

Complete the following:

7. What are the six aspects of the ACCESS model and when would it be used?

8. A mild level of anxiety may motivate learning.
   True _____ False _____

9. From the following, select the appropriate topics for health education related to health maintenance and promotion and illness prevention. Select all that apply.
   a. First aid _____
   b. Occupational therapy _____
   c. Awareness of potential complications after a heart attack _____
   d. Hygiene _____
   e. Origin of symptoms _____
   f. Awareness of signs and symptoms of hypoglycemia _____
   g. Self-help devices _____
   h. Surgical intervention _____

10. Identify teaching activities for a(n):
    a. Infant
    b. Toddler
    c. Preschooler
    d. School-age child
    e. Older adult

11. A learner may find it difficult to concentrate in the presence of:

12. What characteristics does the patient need in order to learn psychomotor skills?

13. When selecting an environment for teaching, a nurse needs to consider:

14. Written materials used for teaching a patient with limited health literacy are usually presented at the _____ grade level.

15. Teaching sessions that are usually tolerated best last for _____ minutes. In planning the teaching session, essential information should be taught _____.

16. The patient becomes fatigued during the teaching session. You should:

17. For the nursing diagnosis *noncompliance with medication regimen related to insufficient knowledge of purpose and actions*, identify possible learning goals and outcomes and nursing interventions.

18. What is the preferred teaching style for the following types of learners?
    a. Visual
    b. Tactile
    c. Auditory

19. For the following, identify the domain of learning.
    a. Self-injection of insulin
    b. Coping with care of a family member
    c. Aware of potential complications after a heart attack
    d. Response of the family to a member's substance abuse
    e. Sterile dressing technique
    f. Aware of signs and symptoms of hypoglycemia

20. Identify an instructional technique that may be used in each of the following situations:
    a. A small group of patients in a cardiac rehabilitation group who need dietary information

    b. A patient with a leg cast who will be using crutches

    c. Students learning therapeutic communication skills to be used on a mental health unit

21. Explaining how a test will feel before the procedure is performed is an example of:

22. a. According to national reports, a total of _____% of adults in the United States have difficulty reading and understanding health information, including pamphlets and charts.
    b. What tools are available to assess your patients' literacy?

23. The nurse tells the patient that the injection will cause pain. What is a more effective way to communicate with the patient about the injection?

24. Identify what "teach-back" is and its purpose.

25. A focused assessment for patient education includes:

26. What should be included in the documentation of patient teaching?

Select the best answer for each of the following questions:

27. A nurse is preparing to teach a group of new parents about infant care. The nurse recognizes that learning can be enhanced with:
    1. previous unfamiliarity with the topic area.
    2. fear of health outcomes.
    3. moderate discomfort.
    4. mild anxiety level.

28. The patient who most likely has the greatest motivation to learn is the individual who is:
    1. waiting for the results of diagnostic tests.
    2. hypertensive, but has no symptoms.
    3. dealing with a family conflict.
    4. recovering from reconstructive surgery.

29. While preparing a teaching plan for a group of patients with diabetes, a nurse integrates the basic principle of education that:
    1. material should progress from complex to simpler ideas.
    2. prolonged teaching sessions improve concentration and attentiveness.
    3. learning is improved when more than one body sense is stimulated.
    4. previous knowledge of a topic area interferes with the acquisition of new information.

30. During a teaching session for a patient with heart disease, the nurse uses reinforcement to stimulate learning. An example of reinforcement for this patient is:
    1. allowing the patient to manage self-care needs.
    2. teaching about the disease process while delivering nursing care.
    3. outlining the exercise plan and providing explicit instructions.
    4. complimenting the patient on his or her ability to identify the action of prescribed medications.

31. After approximately 20 minutes have passed in the educational session, the nurse notices that the patient is slightly slumped in the chair and is no longer maintaining eye contact. The nurse should:
    1. reposition the patient in the chair.
    2. move the patient to a cooler, brighter room.
    3. reschedule the remainder of the teaching for another time.
    4. continue with the teaching session in order to cover the necessary content.

32. When preparing to teach the self-injection technique to a patient, the nurse begins with:
    1. having the patient demonstrate the procedure.
    2. discussing the procedure and the equipment used.
    3. providing written materials and having the patient practice the technique.
    4. demonstrating to the patient how to perform the procedure correctly.

33. After teaching a patient about a cerebrovascular accident (CVA/stroke), the nurse prepares to evaluate the patient's psychomotor domain of learning. This is accomplished by:
    1. observing the patient use a cane to ambulate.
    2. asking the patient about the basic etiology of a stroke.
    3. determining the patient's attitudes about the treatment regimen.
    4. having the patient complete a written schedule for daily activities at home.

34. When the teaching session has been completed, a nurse evaluates the patient's cognitive domain of learning to see if there are areas that require additional instruction. The nurse evaluates the patient's ability to:
    1. perform the range-of-motion exercises independently.
    2. identify the equipment necessary for surgical wound care.
    3. demonstrate the proper use of crutches to ambulate up and down stairs.
    4. discuss concerns about the difficulty in maintaining accurate records of the treatments.

35. Which patient appears to be demonstrating the greatest readiness to learn? The patient who says:
    1. "There's nothing wrong with me."
    2. "I think the doctor made a mistake."
    3. "I can manage on my own."
    4. "What do I need to know about this?"

36. A type of reinforcement that works well with children is:
    1. material.
    2. social.
    3. activity.
    4. negative.

37. A nurse recognizes that the most effective teaching strategy for a patient in the acceptance stage is to:
    1. share small bits of information.
    2. introduce only reality.
    3. provide simple explanations while doing care.
    4. focus on future skills and knowledge.

38. A patient is having difficulty communicating with other family members. Which one of the following would be the most effective teaching strategy for this patient?
    1. Demonstration
    2. Role-playing
    3. Telling
    4. Analogy

STUDY GROUP QUESTIONS

- What are the standards (e.g., The Joint Commission) for patient education?
- How does patient education promote, maintain, and restore health?
- What are the principles of teaching and learning?
- What factors may influence a patient's ability to learn?
- How does an individual's developmental status influence the selection of teaching methodologies?
- How does the teaching process compare with the communication and nursing processes?
- How does the nurse develop a teaching plan for a patient?
- What teaching approaches and instructional methods may be used by a nurse?
- How is patient education documented?

13 Managing Patient Care

CASE STUDY

1. As a nurse working on a busy surgical unit, this evening you have eight postoperative patients assigned to you.
   a. What types of activities could be delegated to an unlicensed nursing assistant?
   b. What determination do you need to make before safely delegating activities to the nursing assistant?
   c. What opportunities are available for doing more than one intervention at a time with the patient?

CHAPTER REVIEW

Complete the following:

1. Identify three responsibilities of a nurse manager.

2. A person who is reasonably independent and self-governing in decision making and practice is demonstrating:

3. The five rights of delegation are:

4. Provide the correct term for the following definitions:
   a. Duties and activities an individual is employed to perform:
   b. Official power to act:
   c. Being answerable for one's actions:

5. Case management is:

6. Provide at least one example of how staff members can be actively involved when decentralized decision making exists on a nursing unit:

7. For the QSEN competency of Teamwork and Collaboration, identify ways that team communication can be promoted.

8. A patient on the unit, who was admitted 2 days ago with ketoacidosis, has a blood glucose level of 425, which is far above the expected range. The patient was receiving a longer-acting insulin. There are concerns about the type of insulin and dietary management. Identify the way this information should be reported with the SBAR:
   S -
   B -
   A -
   R -

Select the best answer for each of the following questions:

9. A student nurse is working with a patient who has begun to have respiratory difficulty. It is the student nurse's initial responsibility to:
   1. call the pharmacy.
   2. alert the primary nurse.
   3. contact the attending physician.
   4. administer the prescribed medication.

10. The nurses on a medical unit are discussing plans to change the focus of the unit to the primary nursing care model. With this model, the assignment for nurse A is:
    1. Mrs. J., Mrs. R., and Mrs. T. for the length of their stays.
    2. to receive reports from the nursing assistant on the care of Mrs. J., Mrs. R., and Mrs. T.
    3. side 1 of the unit in cooperation with nurse B and the nursing assistant.
    4. medication administration for all of the patients on the unit while nurse B does the physical care with the nursing assistant.

11. A nurse in the long-term care facility is delegating care to the nursing assistant. It is appropriate for the nurse to delegate the care of the patient who requires:
    1. catheter care.
    2. an admission history.
    3. administration of oral medications.
    4. vital sign measurements after episodes of arrhythmias.

12. A student nurse is assigned to care for a patient in the hospital. While taking the patient's vital signs, the student cannot obtain the blood pressure reading after two attempts. The student should:
    1. keep trying to get the blood pressure measurement.
    2. use the closest measurement to the last reading.
    3. ask another nurse to obtain the blood pressure measurement.
    4. inform the instructor about the difficulty and request assistance.

13. A nurse is working with a patient who has just returned from surgery. The nurse has no experience working with the patient's postoperative surgical dressing. During an assessment, the nurse notices that the dressing has come loose and has fallen away from the surgical wound. The patient tells the nurse, "Oh, you can fix it." The nurse:
    1. asks the patient to help replace the dressing.
    2. replaces the loosened dressing as best as possible.
    3. asks the surgeon to replace the dressing.
    4. covers the wound with a sterile dry dressing until assistance is obtained.

14. A nurse has been assigned to work on a very busy medical unit in the hospital. It is important for the nurse to employ time management skills. The nurse implements a plan to:
    1. have all the patients' major needs met in the morning hours.
    2. anticipate possible interruptions by therapists and visitors.
    3. complete assessments and treatments for each patient at different times each day.
    4. leave each day unstructured to allow for changes in treatments and patient assignments.

15. The staff on a medical unit in an acute care facility is moving to a system where the nurse manager will lead a group of other RNs, LPNs, and aides. This is an example of:
    1. functional nursing.
    2. primary nursing.
    3. total patient care.
    4. team nursing.

16. A student nurse has a multiple patient assignment. In reviewing the report obtained from the primary nurse, the student should decide to see which patient first? The patient who is:
    1. experiencing nausea
    2. using a bedpan
    3. having a severe anxiety attack
    4. thirsty and wants another drink with breakfast

STUDY GROUP QUESTIONS

- To whom may a nurse delegate care responsibilities? What types of responsibilities may be delegated legally and safely?
- What is involved in decentralized decision making?
- How does the nurse manager function within the health care team?
- How do the different types of nursing care delivery models differ from one another?
- What is quality improvement (QI), and what does it mean to nurses?
- What is necessary for effective coordination and prioritization of care?

STUDY CHART

Create a study chart to compare and contrast the different *Nursing Care Delivery Models.*

Infection Prevention and Control

CASE STUDIES

1. An 86-year-old woman in an extended care facility has a urinary catheter attached to a drainage system.
   a. What precautions should be taken for this patient to prevent a urinary tract infection?

2. Yesterday a 45-year-old man had abdominal surgery. He has a large midline abdominal incision covered by a sterile dressing. He will require dressing changes twice daily.
   a. What precautions should be taken for this patient to prevent wound infection?

3. An 85-year-old man with MRSA requires isolation precautions. He is oriented to his surroundings and is concerned about whether his family will be able to visit him.
   a. What specific nursing care should be implemented for this patient?

CHAPTER REVIEW

Match the description/definition in Column A with the correct term in Column B.

	Column A	**Column B**
k	1. Arises from microorganisms outside the patient	a. Exudate
f	2. Cellular response to injury or infection	b. Aseptic technique
j	3. Microorganisms that cause another infection because they are resistant to antibiotics	c. Health care–acquired infection
c	4. Infection that developed that was not present at the time of patient admission	d. Sterilization
b	5. Methods to reduce or eliminate disease-producing microorganisms	e. Colonization
g	6. Microorganisms that do not cause disease but help to maintain health	f. Inflammation
d	7. Process that eliminates all forms of microbial life	g. Flora
h	8. Disease-producing microorganism	h. Pathogen
a	9. Substance formed through the inflammatory process that may ooze from openings in the skin or mucous membranes	i. Endogenous infection
e	10. Microorganism that grows but does not cause disease	j. Suprainfection
L	11. Ability of microorganisms to produce disease	k. Exogenous infection
m	12. Being more than normally vulnerable to a disease	l. Virulence
i	13. Alteration of a patient's flora with a resulting overgrowth	m. Susceptibility

Complete the following:

14. Identify whether the following are performed using sterile technique in an acute care environment:
    a. Hand hygiene _____
    b. Postoperative dressing change _____
    c. Urinary catheter insertion _____
    d. Barrier precautions _____
    e. Intramuscular injection _____

15. An outcome for a patient with a 3-cm–diameter wound is:

16. Immunizations are available for which of the following? Select all that apply.
    a. Hepatitis A _____
    b. Diphtheria _____
    c. Rubella _____
    d. Tuberculosis _____
    e. AIDS _____
    f. Varicella _____

17. For the following, select all actions that require that equipment be discarded and/or the sterile field be redone.
    a. A mask is worn when opening the sterile tray. _____
    b. The sterile dressing package is torn. _____
    c. The tip of the sterile syringe touches the surface of a clean, disposable glove. _____
    d. A sterile basin is held out over the sterile field. _____
    e. A cup on the sterile field is touched with a sterile gloved hand. _____
    f. Sterile dressings are placed within the 1-inch edge of the sterile field. _____

18. Identify specific actions that a nurse can implement to interrupt the chain of infection.
    a. Control or eliminate the infectious agent:

    b. Control or eliminate the reservoir:

    c. Control the portals of exit:

    d. Control transmission:

    e. Control susceptibility of host:

19. What results would be expected for the following laboratory studies in the presence of an infection?
    a. WBC count
    b. Erythrocyte sedimentation rate
    c. Iron level
    d. Neutrophils
    e. Basophils

20. In relation to health care–acquired infections (HAI):
    a. How can they be reduced?

    b. Which patients are more susceptible to HAI?

21. A patient's gastrointestinal defenses against infection are altered by:

22. Select all the appropriate techniques for isolation precautions.
    a. Wash hands in the clean utility room after patient care. _____
    b. Provide for the patient's sensory needs during care. _____
    c. Prevent visitors from entering the patient's room. _____
    d. Keep face mask below the level of eyeglasses or goggles. _____
    e. Place disposable items in paper bags. _____
    f. Maintain each patient's personal protective equipment (PPE) within the patient's room. _____
    g. Keep PPE at the door to the room or in an anteroom area. _____

23. Handling of biohazardous waste includes:

24. Specify the order in which the following PPE should be applied before entering an isolation room:

    a. Mask _____
    b. Gloves _____
    c. Gown _____

25. If a mask, gown, and gloves are worn into an isolation room, the first item(s) of PPE to be removed when exiting the room is/are the:

26. Select all of the following in which appropriate asepsis has occurred:
    a. Handling a sterile dressing with clean gloves _____
    b. Holding a sterile bowl above waist level using sterile gloves _____
    c. Keeping the hands above the elbows after a surgical scrub _____
    d. Turning away from and placing one's back to the sterile field _____
    e. Talking or coughing over the sterile field _____
    f. Discarding sterile packages that are wet _____
    g. Placing objects to the edge of the sterile field _____
    h. Discarding a small amount of solution before pouring the remainder into a sterile container on the field _____

27. For the nursing diagnosis *Impaired Skin Integrity related to 2-inch-diameter pressure ulcer on sacrum*, identify a patient outcome and nursing interventions.

28. Number the flaps on the sterile package in the figure according to which should be opened first, second, and last.

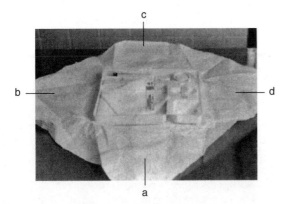

29. Proper disposal of contaminated sharps includes:

30. Provide an example of how the nurse needs to be aware of his or her own breaks in aseptic technique.

31. What equipment is needed to collect a urine specimen from the patient with an indwelling urinary catheter?

32. Select all of the following actions that are appropriate for hand hygiene.
    a. Cleaning under artifical nails _____
    b. Removing rings during washing _____
    c. Leaning against the sink _____
    d. Keeping the water temperature hot _____
    e. Washing the hands for at least 15 seconds _____
    f. Turning off the faucet with the elbows _____
    g. Keeping hands and forearms lower than the elbows during washing _____
    h. Drying from the forearms to the fingers _____

33. The patient sees the nurse using the hand sanitizer frequently and remarks, "I must be full of germs, since you're always cleaning your hands." How should the nurse respond?

34. Information on the current immunizations schedule can be found at the:

35. What are the three most common infections in long-term care?

36. Which of the following infectious organisms are transmitted through blood? Select all that apply.
    a. *Candida albicans* (fungi) _____
    b. HIV _____
    c. *Staphylococcus aureus* _____
    d. *Plasmodium falciparum* (protozoa) _____
    e. Streptococcus _____
    f. Hepatitis B _____

37. Place the following steps for specimen collection in an isolation room in the correct order. After changing the bed linens and changing the gloves, the nurse should:
    a. Perform hand hygiene _____
    b. Check the container label and send the specimen to the lab _____
    c. Place the specimen container on a clean paper towel in the bathroom _____
    d. Transfer the specimen to the containers _____
    e. Collect the specimen _____

38. When splashing or spraying of bodily fluids is anticipated, the nurse should use a:

39. Identify the breaks in isolation technique in each photo below:

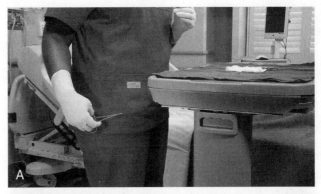

A

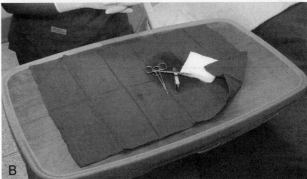

B

Select the best answer for each of the following questions:

40. At the community health fair, a nurse is asked by one of the residents about the influenza vaccine. The nurse responds to the resident that the influenza vaccine is recommended for individuals who are:
    1. Health care workers
    2. Traveling to other countries
    3. Younger than 6 years of age
    4. Between 40 and 65 years of age

41. A nurse is preparing a room for a patient with tuberculosis. The specific aspect for this tier of Standard Precautions that is different than tier 1 is that the care should include:
    1. a private room with negative air flow.
    2. hand hygiene after gloves are removed.
    3. eye protection if splashing is possible.
    4. disposal of sharps in a puncture-resistant container.

42. A nurse is preparing a teaching plan for patients about the hepatitis B virus. The nurse informs them that this virus may be transmitted by:
    1. mosquitoes.
    2. droplet nuclei.
    3. blood products.
    4. improperly handled food.

43. A nurse is working on a unit with a number of patients who have infectious diseases. One of the most important methods for reducing the spread of microorgaisms is:
    1. sterilization of equipment.
    2. the use of gloves and gowns.
    3. maintenance of isolation precautions.
    4. hand hygiene before and after patient care.

44. The assignment today for a nurse includes a patient with tuberculosis. In caring for a patient on droplet precautions, the nurse should routinely use:
    1. regular masks and eyewear.
    2. regular masks, gowns, and gloves.
    3. surgical hand hygiene and gloves.
    4. particulate filtration masks and gowns.

45. A nurse is caring for a patient who has a large abdominal wound that requires a sterile saline soak and dressing. While performing the care, the nurse drops the saline-soaked 4 × 4 gauze near the wound on the patient's abdomen. The nurse:
    1. discontinues the procedure.
    2. throws the gauze away and prepares a new 4 × 4 gauze.
    3. picks up the 4 × 4 with sterile forceps and places it on the wound.
    4. rinses the 4 × 4 with saline and places it on the wound using sterile gloves.

46. A nurse is checking the laboratory results of a male patient admitted to the medical unit. The nurse is alerted to the presence of an infectious process based on the finding of:
    1. iron: 80 g/100 mL.
    2. neutrophils: 65%.
    3. erythrocyte sedimentation rate (ESR): 13 mm per hour.
    4. white blood cells (WBC): 16,000/mm^3.

47. The individual most at risk for a latex allergy is the patient with a history of:
    1. hypertension.
    2. congenital heart disease.
    3. diabetes mellitus.
    4. cholecystitis.

48. A nurse is working with a patient who has a deep laceration to the right lower extremity. To reduce a possible reservoir of infection, the nurse:
    1. wears gloves and a mask at all times.
    2. isolates the patient's personal articles.
    3. has the patient cover the mouth and nose when coughing.
    4. changes the dressing to the extremity when it becomes soiled.

49. A nurse implements droplet precautions for the patient with:
    1. pulmonary tuberculosis.
    2. varicella.
    3. rubella.
    4. herpes.

50. A patient who has had a transplant will require what type of isolation?
    1. Contact
    2. Airborne
    3. Droplet
    4. Protective

51. For a patient with hepatitis A, the nurse is aware that the disease is transmitted through:
    1. feces.
    2. blood.
    3. skin.
    4. droplet nuclei.

52. A sign that is indicative of a systemic infection resulting from a wound is:
    1. redness.
    2. drainage.
    3. edema.
    4. fever.

53. There are small open wounds on the hands of the nurse. The nurse's most appropriate action is:
    1. asking to work at the nurse's station for the day.
    2. using clean, disposable gloves for patient care.
    3. applying antibacterial ointment before patient contact.
    4. providing patient care as usual and washing the hands more frequently.

54. A nurse is aware that older adults are more susceptible to infection as a result of:
    1. thickening of the dermal and epidermal skin layers.
    2. increased production of T lymphocytes.
    3. increased production of digestive juices.
    4. drying of the oral mucosa.

STUDY GROUP QUESTIONS

- What is the nature of the infectious process?
- What are the components of the chain of infection?
- What are the body's normal defenses against infection?
- What is a health care–associated infection, who are the patients at risk, and how can a nurse prevent this infection?
- How is the nursing process applied to infection control in the acute, extended care, and home care environments?
- What nursing measures may be implemented to prevent or control the spread of infection?
- What is included in Standard Precautions?
- What information may be taught to the patient and the patient's family for prevention or control of infectious processes?
- How does the nurse perform the procedures that are important for infection control?

15 Vital Signs

CASE STUDIES

1. You are volunteering at a community health fair. You have been asked to take blood pressure (BP) readings for the residents participating in the event.
   a. What blood pressure readings indicate that follow-up care should be recommended?
   b. What other information may be obtained from a patient while taking the blood pressure reading?

2. You are assigned to an orthopedic unit in the medical center. A patient was involved in an automobile accident and has bilateral casts on the upper arms.
   a. How will you obtain the patient's pulse rate and blood pressure?

3. You have just started your shift at the extended care facility. The nurse reporting off identifies that one of your assigned patients is febrile.
   a. What signs and symptoms do you expect to find with a patient who is febrile?
   b. What interventions are indicated for febrile patients?

4. The patient has been brought to the emergency room with signs of heat stroke.
   a. What interventions are anticipated for this patient?
   b. What teaching should be done to prevent the occurrence in the future?

5. A postoperative patient is being monitored with pulse oximetry. You are checking the reading, but the device does not appear to be working.
   a. What are the expected readings for oxygen saturation?
   b. What "troubleshooting" can you perform to determine if the pulse oximeter is working properly?
   c. How can you help postoperative patients to improve their saturation level?

CHAPTER REVIEW

Match the description/definition in Column A with the correct term in Column B.

	Column A	Column B
_____	1. Decrease of systolic and diastolic pressures below normal	a. Tachypnea
_____	2. Another word for fever	b. Bradypnea
_____	3. Rate and depth of respirations increase	c. Hypothermia
_____	4. Widening of blood vessels	d. Apnea
_____	5. Pulse rate less than 60 beats per minute for an adult	e. Bradycardia
_____	6. 140/90 mm Hg for two or more readings	f. Hypotension
_____	7. Rate of breathing abnormally rapid	g. Hyperventilation
_____	8. Decreased body temperature	h. Hypertension
_____	9. No respirations for several seconds	i. Vasodilation
_____	10. Rate of breathing abnormally slow	j. Febrile
_____	11. Normal breathing	k. Auscultatory gap
_____	12. Temporary disappearance of sounds between Korotkoff sounds	l. Eupnea

Complete the following:

13. Convert the following temperature readings:
    a. 97° F = _____ ° C
    b. 38.4° C = _____ ° F
    c. 102° F = _____ ° C
    d. 39.4° C = _____ ° F

14. What are the Fahrenheit and centigrade temperature readings that should alert the nurse to an alteration in the patient's temperature regulation?

15. Indicate on the model where the following pulses should be palpated:

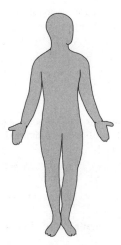

    a. Carotid
    b. Brachial
    c. Radial
    d. Apical
    e. Dorsalis pedis

16. Indicate on the aneroid scale where the following blood pressure reading would be noted:
    a. Korotkoff sounds first heard at 164 mm Hg and inaudible at 92 mm Hg

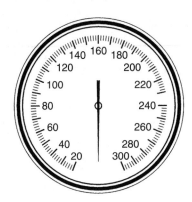

17. Vital sign measurements may not be delegated to unlicensed assistive personnel.
    True _____ False _____

18. Identify actions that will reduce body temperature in the following ways:
    a. Conduction:
    b. Convection:
    c. Evaporation:

19. A patient is on isolation precautions and temperature measurements are being used to monitor the status of the fever. The thermometer of choice in this situation is a(n):

20. A nurse identifies a pulse deficit. How was this assessed?

21. For a patient who has had a right mastectomy, the nurse should take the blood pressure:

22. Vital signs are usually recorded on the:

23. Decreasing hemoglobin levels will _____ the respiratory rate.

24. To obtain arterial oxygen saturation for an adult patient, the pulse oximeter may be applied to:

25. The pulse pressure for a patient with a BP of 150/90 is:

26. Which of the following are correct for blood pressure measurement? Select all that apply.
    a. The cuff is 40% of the circumference of the limb being used. _____
    b. The bladder encircles 50% of the arm of an adult. _____
    c. The cuff is deflated at a rate of 2 to 3 mm Hg per second. _____
    d. The arm is kept below the level of the heart. _____
    e. The cuff is inflated to 30 mm Hg above the point where the pulse disappears. _____
    f. The systolic blood pressure is identified as the first onset of Korotkoff sounds. _____
    g. A difference of 30 mm Hg is expected between the left and right arm measurements. _____

27. A nurse is preparing to take the patient's oral temperature but discovers that he has just had a cup of coffee. The appropriate action is to:

28. Identify a situation when a patient's blood pressure may have to be palpated.

29. How are the following vital signs measured differently in children?
    a. Temperature:
    b. Blood pressure:

30. Which of the following are correct techniques for a tympanic temperature measurement? Select all that apply.
    a. Using the right ear if the patient has been lying on his/her left side in bed _____
    b. Pointing the probe midpoint between the eyebrows and sideburns for children younger than 3 years of age _____
    c. Pulling the ear pinna backward and down for an adult _____
    d. Moving the thermometer back and forth a little during the assessment _____
    e. Fitting the speculum tip loosely into the ear canal _____
    f. Waiting 2 to 3 minutes before repeating the measurement in the same ear _____

31. A patient's pulse is expected to be increased in the presence of which of the following factors? Select all that apply.
    a. Anxiety _____
    b. Hypothermia _____
    c. Unrelieved severe pain _____
    d. Asthma _____
    e. Hemorrhage _____
    f. Administration of beta blockers _____

32. What are the contraindications for the following temperature assessments?
    a. Axillary temperature
    b. Rectal temperature

33. End-tidal carbon dioxide ($ETCO_2$) values are used commonly for patients with:

34. For a blood pressure taken in the lower extremity:
    a. How should the patient be positioned?
    b. What artery is used for palpation?
    c. Is the reading expected to be higher or lower than the upper extremity?

35. Place the following steps for apical pulse measurement in the correct order:
    a. Count the rate for 1 minute. _____
    b. Replace the gown and position the patient for comfort. _____
    c. Locate anatomical landmarks. _____
    d. Place the diaphragm over the fifth intercostal space at the left midclavicular line. _____

e. Warm the diaphragm in the hand for 5 to 10 seconds. _____
f. Position the patient supine or sitting. _____

36. The danger of an increased temperature in young children is the potential for:

37. Provide three examples of antipyretic medications that may be ordered for a febrile patient.

38. How is orthostatic hypotension assessed?

39. Indicate the following for core temperature readings:
    a. Readings are invasive or noninvasive?
    b. Sites for core readings include:

40. What are the uses for the diaphragm and the bell of the stethoscope?

41. Indicate whether the body temperature is increased or decreased for the following individuals:
    a. Ovulating female
    b. Older adult

42. Indicate the correct techniques for pulse oximetry. Select all that apply.
    a. Recording the first reading after application of the probe _____
    b. Using the earlobe for a patient with tremors _____
    c. Applying the probe to the bridge of a toddler's nose _____
    d. Using fingers with acrylic nails, but no nail polish _____
    e. Expecting readings between 80% and 90% _____

43. How do the following influence respiration?
    a. Anxiety:
    b. Analgesic medications:
    c. Body position:

44. Which of the following can lead to hypotension? Select all that apply.
    a. Hemorrhage _____
    b. Stress _____
    c. Obesity _____
    d. Fluid deficit _____
    e. Cigarette smoking _____

Select the best answer for each of the following questions:

45. A nurse is working on a pediatric unit and assessing the vital signs of an infant admitted for gastroenteritis. The nurse expects that the vital signs are normally the following (BP is blood pressure in units of mm Hg, P is pulse rate in units of beats per minute, and R is respirations in units of breaths per minute):
    1. BP = 90/50, P = 122, R = 46
    2. BP = 90/60, P = 80, R = 20
    3. BP = 100/60, P = 140, R = 32
    4. BP = 110/50, P = 98, R = 40

46. While working in an extended care facility, a nurse expects the vital signs of an older adult patient to be:
    1. BP = 98/70, P = 60, R = 12
    2. BP = 120/60, P = 110, R = 30
    3. BP = 140/90, P = 74, R = 14
    4. BP = 150/100, P = 90, R = 25

47. A student nurse is taking vital signs for her assigned patients on the surgical unit. The student is aware that a patient's body temperature may be reduced after:
    1. exercise.
    2. emotional stress.
    3. periods of sleep.
    4. cigarette smoking.

48. While working in an emergency department, a nurse is carefully monitoring the vital signs of the patients who have been admitted. The nurse is alert to the potential for a decrease in a patient's pulse rate as a result of:
    1. hemorrhage.
    2. hypothyroidism.
    3. respiratory difficulty.
    4. epinephrine (adrenaline) administration.

49. A patient is being treated for hyperthermia. The nurse anticipates that the patient's response to this condition will be:
    1. generalized pallor.
    2. bradycardia.
    3. reduced thirst.
    4. diaphoresis.

50. Several friends have gone on a ski trip and have been exposed to very cold temperatures. One of the individuals appears to be slightly hypothermic. The best initial response by the nurse in the ski lodge is to give this individual:
    1. soup.
    2. coffee.
    3. brandy.
    4. warm cola.

51. When checking the temperature of a patient, a nurse notes that he is febrile. A nonsteroidal antipyretic medication is ordered. The nurse prepares to administer:
    1. digoxin.
    2. prednisone.
    3. theophylline.
    4. acetaminophen

52. A nurse has been assigned a number of different patients in the long-term care unit. When taking vital signs, the nurse is alert to the greater possibility of tachycardia for the patient with:
    1. anemia.
    2. hypothyroidism.
    3. a temperature of 95° F.
    4. a patient-controlled analgesic (PCA) pump with morphine drip.

53. While reviewing the vital signs taken by the aide this morning, a nurse notes that one of the patients is hypotensive. The nurse will be checking to see if the patient is experiencing:
    1. lightheadedness.
    2. a decreased heart rate.
    3. an increased urinary output.
    4. increased warmth to the skin.

54. Vital sign measurements have been completed on all assigned patients. The nurse will need to immediately report a finding of:
    1. pulse pressure of 40 mm Hg.
    2. apical pulses of 78, 80, 76 beats per minute.
    3. apical pulse of 82 beats per minute; radial pulse of 70 beats per minute.
    4. BP of 140/80 mm Hg left arm, 136/74 mm Hg right arm.

55. A nurse is preparing to take vital signs for the patients on the acute care unit. A tympanic temperature assessment is indicated for the patient:
    1. after rectal surgery.
    2. wearing a hearing aid.
    3. experiencing otitis media.
    4. after an exercise session.

56. Blood pressure monitoring is being conducted on a cardiac care unit. The nurse is determining whether an automatic blood pressure device is indicated for use. This device is selected for the patient with:
    1. an irregular heartbeat.
    2. Parkinson's disease.
    3. peripheral vascular disease.
    4. a systolic blood pressure greater than 140 mm/Hg.

57. A 34-year-old patient has gone to a physician's office for an annual physical examination. The nurse is completing the vital signs before the patient is seen by the physician. The nurse alerts the physician to a finding of:
    1. T: 37.6° C
    2. P: 120 beats per minute
    3. R: 18 breaths per minute
    4. BP: 116/78 mm Hg

58. A nurse is assigned to the well-child center that is affiliated with the acute care facility. A mother takes her 1½-year-old son to the center for his immunizations. The nurse assesses the child's pulse rate by checking the:
    1. radial artery.
    2. apical artery.
    3. popliteal artery.
    4. femoral artery.

59. A nurse determines that a patient's pulse rate is significantly lower than it has been during the past week. The nurse reassesses and finds that the pulse rate is still 46 beats per minute. The nurse should first:
   1. document the measurement.
   2. administer a stimulant medication.
   3. inform the charge nurse or physician.
   4. apply 100% oxygen at maximum flow rate.

60. The most important sign of heat stroke is:
   1. hot, dry skin.
   2. nausea.
   3. excessive thirst.
   4. muscle cramping.

61. The most accurate temperature measurement for an adult patient experiencing tachypnea and dyspnea is:
   1. oral.
   2. rectal.
   3. axillary.
   4. tympanic.

62. A nurse should insert a rectal thermometer into the adult patient:
   1. ¼ to ½ inch
   2. 1 to 1½ inches
   3. 1½ to 2 inches
   4. 2 to 2½ inches

63. A patient is determined to have an intermittent fever. This is supported by which of the following observations?
   1. A constant body temperature greater than 38° C (100.4° F)
   2. A fever that spikes and falls but does not return to normal
   3. Long periods of normal temperatures with febrile episodes
   4. Spikes in readings mixed with normal temperatures

64. Which of the following values indicates the correct pulse pressure for a patient with a blood pressure of 170/90?
   1. 80
   2. 170
   3. 260
   4. Value not known based on the information given

65. For a patient who is experiencing a febrile state, the nurse should:
   1. ambulate the patient frequently.
   2. restrict fluid intake.
   3. keep the patient warm.
   4. provide oxygen as ordered.

66. A nurse anticipates that bradycardia will be evident if a patient is:
   1. exercising.
   2. hypothermic.
   3. asthmatic.
   4. extremely anxious.

67. A nurse anticipates that a patient with hypertension will be receiving:
   1. diuretics.
   2. antipyretics.
   3. narcotic analgesics.
   4. anticholinergics.

68. To determine the arterial blood flow to a patient's feet, the nurse should assess the:
   1. radial artery.
   2. brachial artery.
   3. popliteal artery.
   4. dorsalis pedis artery.

69. A nurse anticipates an increase in blood pressure for the patient who is:
   1. sleeping.
   2. overweight.
   3. taking narcotics.
   4. hemorrhaging.

70. Prehypertension is classified as an average of repeated readings of:
   1. Systolic: 120 to 139 mm Hg; diastolic: 80 to 89 mm Hg
   2. Systolic: 140 to 159 mm Hg; diastolic: 90 to 99 mm Hg
   3. Systolic: 160 to 179 mm Hg; diastolic: 90 to 99 mm Hg
   4. Systolic: greater than 180 mm Hg; diastolic: greater than 100 mm Hg

STUDY GROUP QUESTIONS

- What are the guidelines for measurement of vital signs?
- When should vital signs be taken?
- How does the nurse determine what sites and equipment to use for measurement of vital signs?
- What body processes regulate temperature?
- What factors influence body temperature?
- How is the temperature measurement converted from centigrade to Fahrenheit and vice versa?
- What sites and equipment are used for temperature measurement?
- What nursing interventions are appropriate for increases and decreases in a patient's body temperature?
- What factors influence pulse rate?
- What sites may be used for pulse rate assessment?
- How should the stethoscope be used in pulse rate assessment?
- What changes may occur in the pulse rate and rhythm?
- What nursing interventions are appropriate for alterations in pulse rate?
- What is blood pressure?
- What factors may increase or decrease blood pressure?
- What are abnormal alterations in blood pressure?
- What equipment is used for blood pressure measurement?
- What nursing interventions are appropriate for increases and decreases in blood pressure?
- What body processes are involved in respiration?

- How are respirations assessed?
- What alterations may be noted in a patient's respirations?
- How does pulse oximetry function and what is its purpose?
- What are the procedures for assessment of temperature, pulse rate, respirations, blood pressure, and pulse oxygen saturation?
- What should be included in patient and family teaching for measurement and evaluation of vital signs?

STUDY CHART

Create a study chart to compare the *Vital Signs Across the Life Span* that identifies expected temperature, pulse rate, respiration, and blood pressure for each age group.

16 Health Assessment and Physical Examination

CASE STUDIES

1. You are assigned to assist with physical examinations in the outpatient clinic. On the schedule for today are three patients. One of the patients is a 72-year-old Hispanic woman, another is a 16-year-old girl, and the last is a 4-year-old boy.
   a. How can you assist each of these patients to feel more at ease before and during the physical examination?

2. A patient in the physician's office informs you that he is having trouble hearing when other people are speaking to him.
   a. What specific assessments will you perform on this patient?

3. You observe a lesion on the patient's abdomen that is draining fluid.
   a. What specific assessments should be made?
   b. How should you prepare to assess the lesion?

CHAPTER REVIEW

Match the description/definition in Column A with the correct term in Column B.

	Column A	Column B
_____	1. Black, tarry stools	a. Ptosis
_____	2. Fluid accumulation, swelling	b. Alopecia
_____	3. Loss of hair	c. Edema
_____	4. Drooping of eyelid over the pupil	d. Jaundice
_____	5. Tiny, pinpoint red spots on the skin	e. Bruit
_____	6. Curvature of the thoracic spine	f. Melena
_____	7. Yellow-orange discoloration	g. Kyphosis
_____	8. A hardened area	h. Petechiae
_____	9. Blowing, swishing sound in blood vessel	i. Erythema
_____	10. A red discoloration	j. Induration

Complete the following:

11. Identify the five skills used in physical assessment and briefly describe each.

12. Identify the following positions for physical examination.

a.

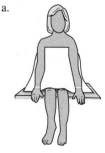

b.

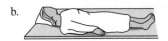

c.

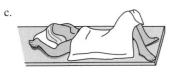

d.

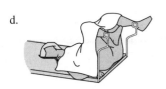

e.

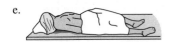

f.

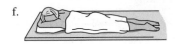

g.

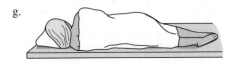

h.

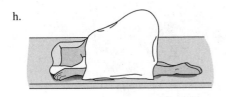

13. Identify which of the pulses is being palpated in each illustration.

a.

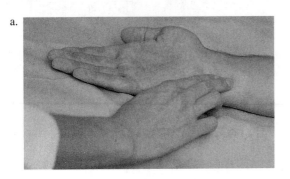

b.

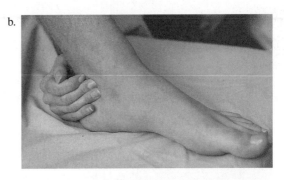

c.

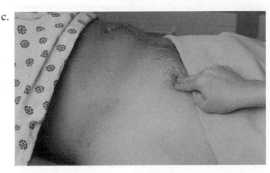

d.

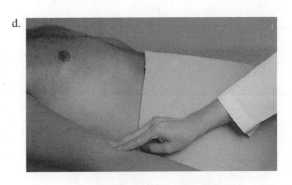

e.

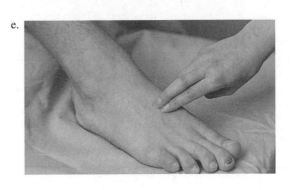

14. Correctly identify the primary skin lesion in each illustration.

a.

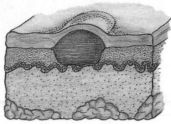

b.

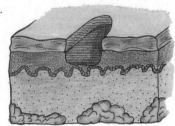

c.

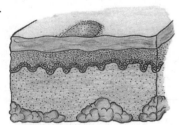

d.

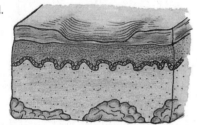

e.

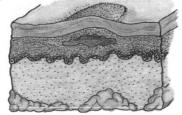

15. Identify on the illustration where the PMI is located.

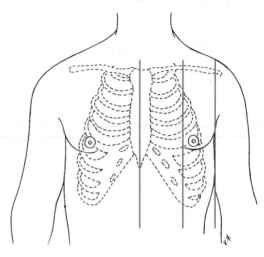

16. Identify a physical and a behavioral finding that may indicate abuse for the following:

	Physical	Behavioral
a. Child sexual abuse	_____	_____
b. Domestic abuse	_____	_____
c. Older adult abuse	_____	_____

17. Identify the abdominal structures that are assessed.

a.

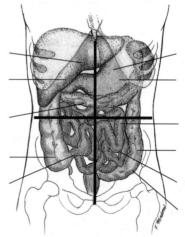

b.

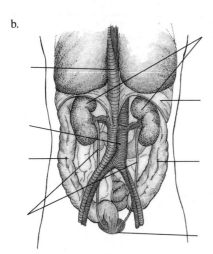

18. Mark each of the following physical assessment findings as either expected or unexpected. For unexpected findings, investigate what may be the possible etiology.

	Expected	*Unexpected*
a. Skin lifts easily and snaps back	_____	_____
b. Erythema noted over bony prominences	_____	_____
c. Hair evenly distributed over scalp and pubic area	_____	_____
d. Brown pigmentation of nails in longitudinal streaks (dark-skinned patient)	_____	_____
e. Pallor in face and nail beds	_____	_____
f. Clubbing of nails	_____	_____
g. PEERLA	_____	_____
h. Pupils cloudy	_____	_____
i. Yellow discoloration of sclera	_____	_____
j. Eardrum translucent, shiny, and pearly gray	_____	_____
k. Light brown or gray cerumen	_____	_____
l. Nasal septum midline	_____	_____
m. Nasal mucosa pale with clear, watery discharge	_____	_____
n. Sinuses tender to touch	_____	_____
o. Teeth chalky white, with black discoloration	_____	_____
p. Tongue medium red, moist, and slightly rough on top	_____	_____
q. Soft palate rises when patient says "ah"	_____	_____
r. Uvula reddened and edematous, tonsils with yellow exudate	_____	_____
s. Thyroid gland small, smooth, and free of nodules	_____	_____
t. Lungs resonant to percussion	_____	_____
u. Costal angle greater than 90 degrees between costal margins	_____	_____
v. Bulging of intercostal spaces	_____	_____
w. No carotid bruit present	_____	_____
x. Extra heart sound noted	_____	_____
y. Jugular vein distention at 45-degree angle	_____	_____
z. Dependent edema in ankles	_____	_____
aa. Female breasts smooth, symmetrical, without retraction	_____	_____
bb. Soft, well-differentiated, moveable lumps in the breasts noted	_____	_____
cc. Bowel sounds active and audible in all four quadrants	_____	_____
dd. Bulging flanks	_____	_____
ee. Flat or concave umbilicus	_____	_____
ff. Rebound tenderness found	_____	_____
gg. Perineal skin smooth and slightly darker than surrounding skin	_____	_____
hh. Bartholin glands palpable with discharge evident	_____	_____
ii. Glans penis smooth and pink on all surfaces	_____	_____
jj. Testes smooth and ovoid	_____	_____
kk. No crepitus found on range of motion	_____	_____
ll. Hips and shoulders aligned parallel	_____	_____
mm. Lordosis of spine noted	_____	_____
nn. Reflexes symmetrical	_____	_____
oo. Able to recall past events, unable to repeat series of five numbers	_____	_____
pp. Able to perform rapidly alternating movements	_____	_____

19. A patient has an area of discomfort. The nurse will examine this area:
    1. first.
    2. last.

20. When using the stethoscope, high-pitched sounds are heard best with a:
    1. diaphragm.
    2. bell.

21. To inspect an adult patient's ear canal, the nurse pulls the auricle:
    1. up and back.
    2. down and back.

22. The position to place the patient in for a genital examination is:

23. The position to place the patient in for an abdominal examination is:

24. Identify what a nurse is able to assess in a general survey of a patient:

25. A weight gain of 5 lb or 2.2 kg/day indicates:

26. What techniques are appropriate when assessing patients of different ages? Select all that apply.
    a. Speaking privately with adolescents about their concerns _____
    b. Using closed-ended questions to increase the speed of the examination _____
    c. Calling children and their parents by their first names _____
    d. Providing time for children to play _____
    e. Performing the examination for an older adult near bathroom facilities _____
    f. Proceeding rapidly through the examination of an older adult to finish it as quickly as possible _____

27. Patients older than 65 years should be instructed to have yearly eye examinations.
    True _____ False _____

28. A nurse is preparing to perform a skin assessment for an average adult patient. Select all of the following techniques that are correct:
    a. Using fluorescent lighting _____
    b. Keeping the room very warm _____
    c. Using disposable gloves to inspect lesions _____
    d. Looking for coloration changes by checking the tongue and nail beds _____

29. During a physical examination, a nurse notes that the patient appears to be very anxious. The nurse should:

30. One example of a test for colorectal cancer is:

31. Select the three best positions that a patient may be placed in for a cardiac assessment:
    a. Prone _____
    b. Supine _____
    c. Lithotomy _____
    d. Sitting _____
    e. Left lateral recumbent _____
    f. Dorsal recumbent _____
    g. Sims _____

32. Identify signs and symptoms that a patient may have if he or she has cardiopulmonary disease.

33. What are the risk factors associated with osteoporosis? Select all that apply.
    a. An active lifestyle _____
    b. Smoking _____
    c. African American background _____
    d. A history of falls _____
    e. A history of Cushing disease _____
    f. Exposure to sunlight _____
    g. A thin, light body frame _____

34. Identify at least two techniques that are used in assessment of the lymph nodes:

35. Continuous dilation of the pupils is found with the patient experiencing:

36. An expected response when testing the pupils for accommodation is:

37. What is used to weigh the following patients?
    a. Newborn infant
    b. Mobile adult

38. The primary nurse tells the student that the patient is experiencing tinnitus. The student expects that the patient will describe:

39. Three possible causes of hearing loss are:

40. To assess for a pulse deficit, the nurse should:

41. An irregular pulse is counted for _____ seconds.

42. Identify all of the risk factors for breast cancer. Select all that apply.
    a. Under 40 years old _____
    b. Recent use of oral contraceptives _____
    c. Late onset menarche _____
    d. Family history _____
    e. Childless _____

43. The nurse is preparing to do an assessment of the abdomen.
    a. The correct sequence for the abdominal exam is:
    b. Bowel sounds usually occur _____/minute.
    c. What finding is expected for the patient with ascites?
    d. Absent bowel sounds can result from:

44. When teaching the patient about the signs and symptoms of prostate cancer, the nurse should include what information?

45. How can the nurse test recent and past memory?

46. A patient is suspected of substance abuse. What physical findings would be found on the skin? Select all that apply.
    a. Loss of pigment _____
    b. Spider angiomas _____
    c. Hematomas _____
    d. Red, dry areas _____
    e. Burns on the fingers _____
    f. Irregularly shaped moles _____

Select the best answer for each of the following questions:

47. A nurse is assessing a patient's nail beds. An expected finding is indicated by:
    1. softening of the nail bed.
    2. a concave curve to the nail.
    3. brown, linear streaks in the nail bed.
    4. a 160-degree angle between the nail plate and nail.

48. A young adult woman arrives at the family planning center for a physical examination. For this patient with mature breasts, the nurse expects to find that the:
    1. breast tissue is softer.
    2. nipples project and areolae have receded.
    3. areolae are dark and have increased diameter.
    4. breasts are elongated and nipples are smaller and flatter.

49. A nurse has checked the medical record and found that a patient has anemia. The presence of anemia is accompanied by the nurse's finding of:
    1. pallor.
    2. erythema.
    3. jaundice.
    4. cyanosis.

50. A patient with asthma has gone to an urgent care center for treatment. On auscultation of the lungs, a nurse hears rhonchi. These sounds are described as:
    1. dry and grating.
    2. loud, low-pitched, and coarse.
    3. high-pitched, fine, and short.
    4. high-pitched and musical.

51. A patient is admitted to a medical center with a peripheral vascular problem. A nurse is performing the initial assessment of the patient. While assessing the lower extremities, the nurse is alert to venous insufficiency as indicated by:
    1. marked edema.
    2. thin, shiny skin.
    3. coolness to touch.
    4. dusky red coloration.

52. A nurse is performing a complete neurological assessment on a patient after a cerebrovascular accident (CVA/stroke). To assess cranial nerve III, the nurse:
    1. uses the Snellen chart.
    2. lightly touches the cornea with a wisp of cotton.
    3. whispers into one ear at a time.
    4. measures pupil reaction to light and accommodation.

53. Student nurses are practicing neurological assessment and determination of cranial nerve functioning. To assess cranial nerve X, the student nurse should ask the patient to:
    1. say "ah."
    2. shrug the shoulders.
    3. smile and frown.
    4. stick out the tongue.

54. While completing a physical examination, a nurse assesses and reports that a patient has petechiae. The nurse has found:
    1. light perspiration on the skin.
    2. moles with regular edges.
    3. thickness on the soles of the feet.
    4. pinpoint-size, flat, red spots.

55. A nurse reviews a chart and sees that a patient who has been admitted to the unit this morning has a hyperthyroid disorder. The nurse anticipates that an examination of the eyes will reveal:
    1. diplopia.
    2. strabismus.
    3. exophthalmos.
    4. nystagmus.

56. In preparation for an examination of the internal ear, a nurse anticipates that the color of the eardrum should appear:
    1. white.
    2. yellow.
    3. slightly red.
    4. pearly gray.

57. A patient with a history of smoking and alcohol abuse has gone to a clinic for a physical examination. Based on this history, the nurse is particularly alert during an examination of the oral cavity to the presence of:
   1. spongy gums.
   2. pink tissue.
   3. thick, white patches.
   4. loose teeth.

58. A patient in a physician's office has an increased antero-posterior diameter of the chest. The nurse should inquire specifically about the patient's history of:
   1. smoking.
   2. thoracic trauma.
   3. spinal surgery.
   4. exposure to tuberculosis.

59. When auscultating a patient's chest, a nurse hears what appears to be an S3 sound. This is an expected finding if the patient is:
   1. 10 years old.
   2. 35 years old.
   3. 56 years old.
   4. 82 years old.

60. A patient in a medical center has been prescribed bed rest for a prolonged period of time. There is a possibility that the patient may have developed phlebitis. The nurse assesses for the presence of this condition by:
   1. palpating the ankles for pitting edema.
   2. checking the popliteal pulses bilaterally.
   3. inspecting the thighs for clusters of ecchymosis.
   4. checking the appearance and circumference of the lower legs.

61. When teaching a 45-year-old patient in the gynecologist's office about breast cancer, a nurse includes information on recommendations for screening. The patient is informed that a woman her age should have:
   1. annual mammograms.
   2. biannual CT scans.
   3. physical examinations every 3 years.
   4. breast self-examinations every 3 months.

62. A patient has been experiencing some lightheadedness and loss of balance over the past few weeks. A nurse wants to check the patient's balance while waiting for the patient to have other laboratory tests. The nurse administers the:
   1. Allen test.
   2. Rinne test.
   3. Weber test.
   4. Romberg test.

63. Screenings are being conducted at the junior high school for scoliosis. A nurse is observing the students for the presence of:
   1. an S-shaped curvature of the spine.
   2. an exaggerated curvature of the thoracic spine.
   3. an exaggerated curvature of the lumbar spine.
   4. a bulging of the cervical vertebrae and disks.

64. While reviewing a medical record, a nurse notes that a patient has suspected pancreatitis. The nurse assesses the patient for:
   1. positive rebound tenderness.
   2. midline abdominal pulsations.
   3. hyperactive bowel sounds in all quadrants.
   4. bulging of the flanks with dependent distention.

65. An 80-year-old woman is being assessed by a nurse in an extended care facility. The nurse is assessing the genitalia of this patient and suspects that there may be a malignancy present. The nurse's suspicion is due to the finding of:
   1. scaly, nodular lesions.
   2. yellow exudates and redness.
   3. small ulcers with serous drainage.
   4. extreme pallor and edema.

66. A screening for osteoporosis is being conducted at an annual health fair. To determine the risk factors for osteoporosis, a nurse is assessing individuals for:
   1. multiparity.
   2. a heavier than recommended body frame.
   3. an African American background.
   4. a history of dieting and/or alcohol abuse.

67. A patient in a rehabilitation facility has experienced a cerebrovascular accident (CVA/stroke) that has left the patient with an expressive aphasia. The nurse anticipates that this patient will:
   1. be unable to speak or write.
   2. be unable to follow directions.
   3. respond inappropriately to questions.
   4. have difficulty interpreting words and phrases.

68. To assess a patient's visual fields, a nurse should:
   1. ask the patient to read text.
   2. turn the room light on and off.
   3. move a finger at arm's length toward the patient from an angle.
   4. shine a penlight into the patient's eye at an oblique angle.

69. A nurse exerts downward pressure on the thigh. This assessment is determining the muscle strength of the:
   1. triceps.
   2. trapezius.
   3. quadriceps.
   4. gastrocnemius.

70. Light palpation involves depressing the part being examined:
   1. ½ inch.
   2. 1 inch.
   3. 1½ inches.
   4. 2 inches.

71. A nurse teaches the male patient that he should notify a health care provider if he finds the following during a testicular self-examination:
    1. loose, deeper color scrotal skin with a coarse surface.
    2. cordlike structures on the top of the testicles.
    3. small, pea-sized lumps on the front of the testicle.
    4. smegma under the foreskin.

72. A nurse manager observes a new nurse on the unit performing a patient assessment. The new nurse's assessment should be interrupted if the manager observes the nurse:
    1. using the pads of the first three fingers to palpate the breast tissue.
    2. auscultating the abdomen continuously for 5 minutes.
    3. palpating both carotid arteries simultaneously.
    4. testing sensory function on random locations with the patient's eyes closed.

73. A nurse assesses a patient's skin and documents that vesicles are present. This observation is based on the nurse finding:
    1. flat, nonpalpable changes in skin color.
    2. palpable, solid elevations smaller than 1 cm.
    3. irregularly shaped, elevated areas that vary in size.
    4. circumscribed elevations of skin filled with serous fluid.

74. A nurse is assessing a patient's level of consciousness using the Glasgow Coma Scale. The following findings are documented: Eyes open to speech, responses are oriented, localized pain is noted. The score for this patient is:
    1. 15.
    2. 13.
    3. 11.
    4. 9.

75. To assess the temperature of the patient's skin, the nurse should use the:
    1. thumbs.
    2. fingertips.
    3. palm of the hand.
    4. dorsal surface of the hand.

76. The patient needs to sit upright to breathe easier. This is recorded by the nurse as:
    1. apnea.
    2. dyspnea.
    3. orthopnea.
    4. tachypnea.

STUDY GROUP QUESTIONS

- What are the purposes of the physical examination?
- How is physical assessment integrated into patient care?
- How does a nurse incorporate cultural sensitivity and awareness of ethnic physiological differences into the physical examination?
- What are the physical assessment skills, and what information is obtained through their use?
- How does a nurse prepare a patient and environment for a physical examination?
- What similarities and differences exist in the preparation and procedure for a physical examination of a child, adult, and older adult?
- What information is obtained through a general survey?
- What positions and equipment are used for completion of the physical examination?
- What is the usual sequence for performing the physical examination?
- What are the expected and unexpected findings of a complete physical examination?
- What self-screening procedures may be taught to patients?
- How does a nurse report and record the findings of a physical examination?

STUDY CHART

Create a study chart to compare the *Expected vs. Unexpected Findings in a Physical Examination,* working in sequential order of the exam from the integumentary system through the neurological system.

17 Administering Medications

CASE STUDIES

1. You are visiting a patient at home who has poor eyesight and occasional forgetfulness. The patient has four oral medications to take at different times of the day. He tells you that he doesn't think that he can remember to take them all and that he can't remember what information he was given by the prescriber.
   a. What strategies may be implemented to assist this patient in maintaining the medication regimen?

2. You are preparing to give medications to the patient in the long-term care facility, but the prescriber's handwriting is difficult to read.
   a. What should you do to prevent medication errors?

3. A patient in a long-term care facility is about to receive her medications, but you notice that she does not have an identification band.
   a. What is the appropriate next action?

4. You are going to administer an injection to a 6-year-old child on a pediatric acute care unit.
   a. What safety measures should you implement?

5. The patient has just received an immunization and appears to be having an anaphylactic reaction.
   a. What treatments are anticipated?

6. You are about to prepare a narcotic medication for administration to a patient. The record shows that 24 tablets should remain in the box but there are only 23 tablets left.
   a. What should you do?

7. You are caring for a patient who requires an antipyretic medication that is ordered for oral administration, but the patient has been experiencing severe nausea.
   a. What are your actions?

CHAPTER REVIEW

Match the description/definition in Column A with the correct term in Column B.

Column A

_____ 1. Placing medication under the tongue

_____ 2. The effect of two medications combined is greater than each given separately

_____ 3. Secondary effects of medication, such as nausea

_____ 4. Unpredictable effect of medications

_____ 5. Fluid administered and retained in a body cavity

_____ 6. Injection into tissues below the dermis of the skin

_____ 7. Severe allergic response characterized by bronchospasm and laryngeal edema

_____ 8. Inserting medication into the eye

_____ 9. Administering medications through the oral, nasal, or pulmonary passages

_____ 10. Patient taking many medications

_____ 11. Placing solid medication against the mucous membranes of the cheek

_____ 12. Injecting medication into body tissues

Column B

a. Parenteral administration

b. Inhalation

c. Instillation

d. Buccal

e. Subcutaneous

f. Intraocular

g. Idiosyncratic reaction

h. Polypharmacy

i. Sublingual

j. Synergistic effect

k. Side effects

l. Anaphylactic reaction

Complete the following:

13. Provide an example of how a nurse's professional responsibility in administering medications is controlled or regulated.

14. a. Identify a strategy for a nurse to implement to avoid errors with medications that appear the same.

    b. Specify two acceptable patient identifiers.

15. Provide an example of how each of the following factors can influence the actions of medications.
    a. Dietary factors
    b. Physiological variables
    c. Environmental conditions

16. Identify the four routes for parenteral administration of medications.

17. For the following medication orders, identify the essential component that is missing. (Note: All have been correctly signed by the prescriber.)
    a. Apresoline IM stat
    b. Morphine sulfate 10 mg q3-4h
    c. Vancomycin 1 g IV
    d. Lasix 40 mg bid

18. Identify the six guidelines or "rights" that a nurse uses for administering medications.

    1. _____

    2. _____

    3. _____

    4. _____

    5. _____

    6. _____

19. Place the following steps in the correct sequence for removing medication from a vial for an IM injection.
    a. Select the correct needle and syringe. _____
    b. Dislodge air bubbles. _____
    c. Insert the needle through the rubber seal of the vial. _____
    d. Remove the syringe from the vial. _____
    e. Perform hand hygiene. _____
    f. Inject the air in the syringe into the air space in the vial. _____
    g. Remove the needle cap. _____
    h. Pull back on the plunger of the syringe and withdraw air equal to the volume of medication to be administered. _____
    i. Invert the vial and fill the syringe to the correct volume of medication. _____
    j. Remove the cap from the vial. _____

20. Identify the form of medication for the following.
    a. Solid dose form for oral use; medication in a powder, liquid, or oil form and encased by a gelatin shell:
    b. Solid dose form mixed with gelatin and shaped in form of pellet for insertion into body cavity:
    c. Clear liquid containing water and/or alcohol; designed for oral use; usually has a sweetener added:
    d. Finely divided drug particles dispersed in a liquid medium; when the liquid is left standing, particles settle to the bottom of the container:
    e. Semiliquid suspension used to cool, protect, or clean the skin:

21. An example of a commonly abused over-the-counter medication is:

22. Adherence to medication therapy:
    a. Noncompliance with or nonadherence to medication therapy may be related to:
    b. Identify at least one strategy to promote medication adherence.

23. MedWatch is a _____.

24. For each of the following pairs, identify which of the two has the faster absorption or action in the body:
    a. IV _____   or   Oral _____
    b. IM _____   or   Subcutaneous _____
    c. Acidic oral   or   Alkaline oral
       medication _____   medication _____
    d. Tablets _____   or   Solutions _____
    e. Large surface   or   Smaller surface area _____
       area _____
    f. Less lipid   or   Highly lipid soluble _____
       soluble _____
    g. Albumin   or   Nonalbumin binding _____
       binding _____

25. The time that it takes for a medication to reach its highest effective concentration is its:

26. Oral medication is contraindicated for a patient with:

27. What is a potential problem with this medication order?
    Lasix 40.0 mg

28. Identify the appropriate equivalents for the following:
    a. 1 mL = _____ gtt
    b. 60 mL = _____ ounces
    c. _____ L = 1 quart
    d. 3 g = _____ mg
    e. 0.25 L = _____ mL
    f. _____ mL = 1 teaspoon

29. Identify the five different types of medication orders and provide an example of each:
    1.
    2.
    3.
    4.
    5.

30. Verbal orders are usually required to be signed by the prescriber within what time frame?

31. A nurse calculates the medication order and determines that six tablets should be given to the patient for each dose. What should the nurse do first?

32. Describe the difference between an adverse and a side effect.

33. After a patient is given medications, the patient tells the nurse that the medicine looks different from the previous administrations of the medication. The nurse should:

34. Identify the correct techniques for medication administration. Select all that apply.
    a. Discard the patient's unopened unit-dose medication that was refused. _____
    b. Crush medication and mix it in a large amount of food to mask the taste. _____
    c. Note in the record if a patient refuses a medication. _____
    d. Record medications before administration. _____
    e. Give another nurse's medications to the patient. _____
    f. Administer non-time-critical medications within 1 to 2 hours of the scheduled time. _____
    g. Aspirate when giving immunizations. _____
    h. Document the patient's response in the record. _____

35. Identify the generic names for the following drugs:
    a. Levaquin
    b. Lasix
    c. Advil
    d. Haldol

36. A triple check to compare the medication label to the order should be done:
    1.
    2.
    3.

37. Identify a technique that may be used to facilitate administration of medications to children.
    a. Oral medications:
    b. Injections:

38. Identify a way that a nurse may minimize the discomfort of an injection.

39. How should a medication that is irritating to the tissues be injected?

40. Identify the correct angle for each of the following illustrations and the type of injection that is being administered.
    a. _____ b. _____ c. _____

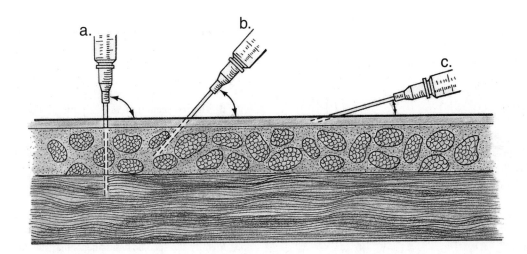

41. Identify three ways in which medication may be administered intravenously.
    a.
    b.
    c.

42. A wireless barcode scanner is usually used to identify:
    a.
    b.
    c.

43. Identify the meaning of the following abbreviations.
    a. ac: _____
    b. bid: _____
    c. prn: _____
    d. q4h: _____
    e. stat: _____

44. Check the orders and calculate the correct dosages for the following medication orders.
    a. Prescriber's order: Synthroid 0.15 mg PO daily
       In stock: Split tablets in a container labeled 75 mcg
       How many tablets should be given?
    b. Prescriber's order: Prilosec 40 mg PO bid
       In stock: Prilosec 20 mg tablets
       How much of the medication should be given?
    c. Prescriber's order: Lasix 20 mg IM stat
       In stock: Lasix 10 mg/mL
       How much medication should be given?

d. Prescriber's order: hydrocortisone succinate 200 mg/day in two equal doses
   In stock: hydrocortisone succinate 50 mg/mL
   How much medication should be given for each dose?
   Mark the amount to be administered on the syringe.

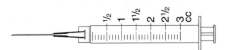

e. Prescriber's order: regular insulin 24 units
   In stock: regular insulin U-100
   How much medication should be administered?
   Mark the amount to be administered on the syringe.

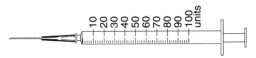

f. Prescriber's order: cefazolin 500 mg q8h
   In stock: Keflex 250 mg tablets
   How many tablets should be given?
g. The medication is mixed in 50 mL of fluid in a volume-controlled set and will be infused with a minidrip over 1 hour.
   The nurse sets the rate to infuse at: _____ drops/minute

45. Identify an area of patient assessment before administration of a parenteral injection.

46. Identify on the figure the sites recommended for subcutaneous injections.

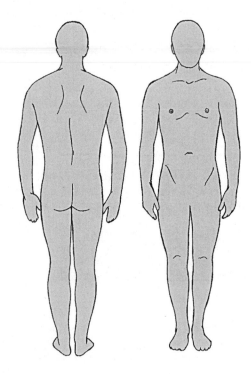

47. Select all of the following actions that are correct for the administration of medications to a patient with dysphagia.
    a. Do not allow the patient to self-administer, even if able. _____
    b. Position the patient upright. _____
    c. Turn the patient's head toward the weaker side to help the patient swallow. _____
    d. Use thinner liquids for the patient to take with the medications. _____
    e. Use a straw for liquids. _____
    f. Crush medication and mix with pureed food, if indicated. _____

48. For medication administration through an enteral/nasogastric tube:
    a. A priority assessment specifically for the patient receiving medication through a nasogastric tube is for the nurse to:
    b. The tube should be flushed with _____ mL of _____ in between each medication, and flushed after all medications are given with _____ mL.

49. Before administration of a topical, the nurse needs to:

50. Identify the following for the administration of ear drops:
    a. Position the patient:
    b. Pull ear pinna _____ for an adult patient.
    c. Irrigate with _____ mL of _____ temperature fluid.

51. For the use of a pressured metered-dose inhaler (pMDI):
    a. When the patient has difficulty coordinating the inhaler, a(n) _____ should be used.
    b. The patient should inhale for _____ seconds while pressing down on the canister and hold the breath for _____ seconds.
    c. How much time should be given in between administration of the same medication?
    d. The medication order is 2 puffs of the inhaler qid. The canister contains 160 puffs total.
       How many days will the canister last? _____
    e. After the administration of a corticosteroid inhalation, the patient should:

52. The patient should be placed in _____ position for the administration of a rectal suppository.

53. Identify the specific assessments that should be completed before administration of the following types of medications:
    a. Anticoagulant
    b. Antihypertensive
    c. Analgesic
    d. Cardiotonic

54. Eye drops should be administered directly onto the cornea.
    True _____ False _____

55. From the following, identify the guidelines that are appropriate for pediatric medication administration. Select all that apply.
    a. Identify the dosage based on the child's weight in pounds. _____
    b. Pediatric doses are usually given in micrograms and small syringes. _____
    c. IM doses are very small and usually do not exceed 1 mL in small children. _____
    d. Most medications are rounded to the nearest tenth. _____
    e. Mentally estimate a patient's dose before beginning the calculation, comparing the answer with the estimate before preparing the medication. _____
    f. Dosage ranges for 24-hour periods are similar to adult dosages. _____

56. Identify the correct sequence of actions for a saline flush.
    a. Pulling back gently on syringe plunger and checking for blood return _____
    b. Cleaning the lock's injection port with antiseptic swab _____
    c. Flushing the IV site with normal saline by pushing slowly on plunger _____
    d. Removing the saline-filled syringe _____
    e. Preparing two syringes filled with 2 to 3 mL of normal saline (0.9%) _____
    f. Inserting the syringe with normal saline 0.9% through injection port of IV lock _____

57. A nurse is responsible for administering an incorrect medication or dosage.
    True _____ False _____

58. For IV push or bolus medication administration:
    a. The medication should be infused at a rate of 2 mL over 2 minutes; this is how many milliliters (mL) every 30 seconds? _____.
    b. If the medication is incompatible with the IV fluid that is infusing, the nurse should:

59. Identify the site that may be used for an intradermal injection.

60. A tuberculin test has been administered.
    a. Results should be read in _____ hours.
    b. A positive test for an individual with no known risk factors is: _____.

61. The patient is to receive a vaginal cream medication.
    a. The preferred position is: _____.
    b. The applicator is inserted: _____ cm or _____ in.

62. Provide examples of positive and negative synergistic effects.

63. An advantage of computerized physician order entry to medications is:

64. When do medication orders have to be rewritten by the prescriber?

65. What safety measures are used when withdrawing medication from an ampule?

66. The patient needs to have multiple subcutaneous injections. The basic rule for site rotation is to:

67. Place the steps for administration of an oral medication in the correct order.
    a. Label the medication. _____
    b. Compare the medication with the MAR. _____
    c. Identify the patient. _____
    d. Pour the liquid from the bottle into the cup. _____
    e. Perform hand hygiene. _____
    f. Compare the prepared medication with the MAR. _____
    g. Obtain the medication from the patient's drawer. _____

68. Identify the four (4) pharmacokinetic processes and an example of how each may be influenced.
    a.
    b.
    c.
    d.

Select the best answer for each of the following questions:

69. A nurse determines the location for an injection by identifying the greater trochanter of the femur, anterosuperior iliac spine, and iliac crest. The injection site being used by the nurse is the:
    1. rectus femoris muscle.
    2. ventrogluteal area.
    3. dorsogluteal area.
    4. vastus lateralis muscle.

70. Upon receiving the assignment for the evening, a nurse notices that two of the patients have the same name. The best way to identify two patients on a medical unit who have the same name is to:
    1. ask the patients their names.
    2. verify their names with the family members.
    3. check the patients' ID bands.
    4. ask another nurse about their identities.

71. A nurse is to administer a subcutaneous injection to an average-size adult. The nurse selects a:
    1. 27-gauge, ½-inch needle and 0.5-mL syringe.
    2. 25-gauge, ⅝-inch needle and 1-mL syringe.
    3. 22-gauge, 1-inch needle and 3-mL syringe.
    4. 20-gauge, 1-inch needle and 3-mL syringe.

72. A nurse has administered medications to all assigned patients on the medical unit. Upon assessing the response of the medications given, the nurse is alert to the possibility of a toxic reaction. This is indicated by the patient experiencing:
    1. itching.
    2. nausea.
    3. dizziness.
    4. respiratory depression.

73. The nursing staff is completing a review of the procedures used for the storage and administration of narcotics. A nurse implements the required procedure when:
    1. narcotics are kept together with the patient's other medications.
    2. small amounts of medication may be discarded without notation.
    3. the narcotic count is checked daily by the medication nurse.
    4. a separate administration record is kept in addition to the patient's medication administration record (MAR).

74. An order is written for a patient to receive potassium chloride (KCl) and vitamins intravenously. The nurse expects that this medication will be given via a(n):
    1. IV bolus administration.
    2. tandem administration.
    3. piggyback administration.
    4. large-volume administration.

75. While completing an admission assessment, a nurse discovers that a patient is allergic to shellfish. Later that morning when the nurse is preparing medications for this patient, the nurse will withhold medication that contains:
    1. iodine.
    2. alcohol.
    3. glucose.
    4. calcium carbonate.

76. A patient in a nurse practitioner's office is receiving penicillin for the first time. The nurse asks the patient to wait in the office after the administration of the medication. The nurse is observing for a possible anaphylactic response that would be demonstrated by:
    1. drowsiness.
    2. pharyngeal edema.
    3. an increased blood pressure reading.
    4. a decreased respiratory rate.

77. A drug that is to be given on a q4h schedule may be administered at:
    1. 10 AM and 10 PM.
    2. 10 AM, 2 PM, and 10 PM.
    3. 10 AM, 2 PM, 6 PM, and 10 PM.
    4. 10 AM, 2 PM, 6 PM, 10 PM, and 2 AM.

78. A specific assessment that a nurse should make before the administration of an anticoagulant is to check for:
    1. an allergy history.
    2. evidence of bruising.
    3. the patient's level of discomfort.
    4. increased blood pressure.

79. In the event of a mistake in the administration of medications, the first action that a nurse should take is to:
    1. complete an occurrence report.
    2. inform the patient of the problem.
    3. report the error to the nurse in charge or the physician.
    4. provide an appropriate antidote for the medication given.

80. The subcutaneous site that is most commonly used for low-molecular-weight heparin injections is the:
    1. abdomen.
    2. anterior thigh.
    3. scapular region.
    4. outer aspect of the upper arm.

81. A prescriber indicates to a nurse that a patient will be receiving an intermediate-acting insulin. The nurse anticipates that the patient will receive:
    1. insulin glargine (Lantus).
    2. insulin lispro (Humalog).
    3. isophane insulin suspension (NPH).
    4. protamine zinc insulin suspension (PZI).

82. A charge nurse is evaluating the injection technique of a new staff member. The correct technique for a Z-track injection is noted when the new staff member:
    1. uses the deltoid site.
    2. pulls the skin 1 to 1½ inches laterally.
    3. removes the needle immediately after the injection.
    4. releases the skin before the needle is removed.

83. For a subcutaneous injection to an average-size adult, which of the following techniques requires correction? The student nurse:
    1. selects a 25-gauge, ⅝-inch needle.
    2. injects the needle at a 45-degree angle.
    3. recaps the needle after injecting the medication.
    4. does not massage the injection site after administration.

84. A nurse is aware that a parenteral administration of a concentrated dose of medication in a small amount of fluid is a:
    1. bolus injection.
    2. piggyback infusion.
    3. volume control infusion.
    4. mini-infuser administration.

85. The patient who will most likely have a difficulty with the excretion of medication from the body is the individual who has:
    1. diabetes mellitus.
    2. renal failure.
    3. circulatory insufficiency.
    4. Parkinson's disease.

86. Which prescriber's order takes priority when preparing medications?
    1. PRN
    2. Now
    3. Stat
    4. Standing

87. The nurse anticipates that the medication that will be prescribed as an intraocular disk for the patient with glaucoma is:
    1. pilocarpine.
    2. azithromycin.
    3. iodoxamide.
    4. silver nitrate.

64

88. The medication that the patient is taking is ototoxic. Based on this information, the nurse knows to specifically assess the patient's:
    1. respiratory rate.
    2. urinary output.
    3. blood pressure.
    4. hearing.

89. The recommended maximum amount of IM medication that can be given safely at one time to an average-size older adult is:
    1. 0.5 mL.
    2. 1 mL.
    3. 2 mL.
    4. 3 mL.

STUDY GROUP QUESTIONS

- How are medications named and classified, and what forms of medications are available?
- What legislation and standards guide medication administration?
- How are medications absorbed, distributed, metabolized, and excreted from the body?
- What are the different types of medication actions?
- What are the different routes for medication administration, and what are the advantages, disadvantages, and contraindications for each route?
- What are the systems used for drug measurement, and how are amounts converted within and between the systems?
- How are dosages calculated for oral, parenteral, and pediatric medications?
- What are the roles of the health team members in the administration of medications?
- What are the six "rights" of medication administration?
- What patient assessment data are critical to obtain before administering medications?
- What equipment is used for the administration of medications via different routes?
- What are the sites or body landmarks for parenteral administration?
- What are the procedures for administration of medications?
- How can IV medication be administered?
- How is administration of medications adapted to patients of different ages and levels of health?
- What information is included in patient/family teaching for medication administration?
- How has technology influenced the administration of medications?

STUDY CHART

Create a study chart to compare *Parenteral Medication and Preparation* that identifies the equipment, needle gauge, amount of medication, site to be used, and angle of injection for subcutaneous, intramuscular, and intradermal injections.

18 Fluid, Electrolyte, and Acid-Base Balances

CASE STUDIES

1. The patient is diagnosed with heart failure and will be taking Digoxin and Lasix on a daily basis.
   a. What patient teaching is indicated in relation to possible fluid and electrolyte imbalances?

2. You are working with two patients today. One of the patients is unconscious and is experiencing a period of prolonged immobility. The other patient has a long history of alcoholism. You are alert to possible alterations in fluid and electrolyte imbalance.
   a. What specific signs and symptoms may these patients exhibit as a result of their present conditions?

3. An adult male patient has come to the outpatient clinic for an examination. During the initial interview, the patient tells you that he has smoked 2½ packs of cigarettes each day for the last 25 years.
   a. What physical signs do you anticipate finding because of the patient's history?
   b. What acid-base imbalance is this patient most likely to experience?

4. Following a motor vehicle accident, the patient had traumatic injuries and a significant hemorrhage. He will be receiving blood transfusions.
   a. What are the priority assessments that should be completed before administration of the blood?
   b. What safety measures should be implemented to reduce the possibility of complications?

CHAPTER REVIEW

Match the description/definition in Column A with the correct term in Column B.

	Column A	Column B
_____	1. Positively charged electrolytes	a. Anions
_____	2. Having the same osmotic pressure	b. Diffusion
_____	3. Movement of water across a semipermeable membrane	c. Filtration
_____	4. Movement of molecules from an area of higher concentration to an area of lower concentration	d. Active transport
_____	5. Negatively charged electrolytes	e. Cations
_____	6. Movement of solutes out of a solution with greater hydrostatic pressure	f. Isotonic
_____	7. Overall particle concentration	g. Hypotonic
_____	8. Having a lower osmotic pressure	h. Osmosis
_____	9. Movement of molecules to an area of higher concentration	i. Osmolality

Complete the following:

10. Identify the following terms:
    a. All fluids outside of the cell:
    b. Fluid between the cells and outside the blood vessels:
    c. All fluids within the cell:

11. Identify if the following electrolytes are cations or anions and whether they are primarily extracellular or intracellular:
    a. Sodium
    b. Potassium
    c. Calcium
    d. Magnesium
    e. Chloride
    f. Bicarbonate

12. Acid-base balance in the body is regulated by:

13. What age groups are most susceptible to fluid and acid-base imbalances?

14. Identify whether the following solutions are isotonic, hypertonic, or hypotonic:
    a. Dextrose 5% in water (D_5W)
    b. 0.45% sodium chloride (0.45% NS)
    c. 0.9% sodium chloride (0.9% NS)
    d. Lactated Ringer's (LR)
    e. Dextrose 5% in 0.45% sodium chloride ($D_5\frac{1}{2}NS$)

15. Identify three types of medications that may cause fluid, electrolyte, or acid-base imbalances.

16. Specify two possible nursing diagnoses for patients experiencing fluid, electrolyte, or acid-base imbalances.

17. Identify the sites for an IV infusion.

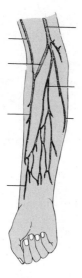

18. A patient who is NPO, with normal renal function, needs to have _____ added to the solution.

19. Identify the signs and symptoms that are associated with phlebitis at an IV site.

20. A patient with a peripherally inserted central catheter (PICC) line develops a fever and increased white blood cell (WBC) count. The nurse anticipates that the health care provider will order:

21. The patient had a rapid infusion of IV fluids and has developed crackles in the lungs, shortness of breath, and tachycardia. The nurse should:

22. Transfusion of a patient's own blood is termed:

23. Identify the electrolyte imbalance that is associated with each of the following test results:
    a. Serum sodium level—125 mEq/L
    b. Serum potassium level—5.8 mEq/L
    c. Serum ionized calcium level—3.7 mEq/L
    d. Serum magnesium level—1.2 mEq/L

24. Calculate the following IV infusion rates:
    a. IV 500 mL of D_5W to infuse in 5 hours; drop factor = 15 gtt/mL. How many gtt/min should infuse?
    b. IV 1000 mL of NS to infuse in 8 hours; drop factor = 10 gtt/mL. How many gtt/min should infuse?
    c. IV 200 mL of NS to infuse in 4 hours; drop factor = 60 gtt/mL. How many gtt/min should infuse?
    d. IV 2 L of D_5W to infuse in 18 hours. How many mL/hour should be set on the infusion pump?

25. Identify the following hormones that control fluid balance:
    a. Pituitary
    b. Adrenal

26. If a hypotonic solution is given intravenously to a patient, the fluid will move into the cells.
    True _____ False _____

27. Arterial pH is an indirect measurement of:

28. Oxygen moves into the lungs via the process of:

29. An average adult's daily intake of fluid is approximately _____ mL.

30. The nurse is going to perform a venipuncture to initiate IV therapy. Place the following steps in the correct order.
    a. Prepare the IV infusion tubing and solution. _____
    b. Re-apply the tourniquet. _____
    c. Perform hand hygiene. _____
    d. Cleanse the site. _____
    e. Select a large-enough vein. _____

31. The nurse is calculating the patient's intake and output for the last 8 hours. During this time, the patient consumed 1 cup of gelatin, ½ cup of juice, 1 cup of water, and 1 cup of tea. The IV infusion started with 750 mL in the bag, with 125 mL remaining at the end of the shift. The urinary output was 340 mL and there was 30 mL of drainage from the nasogastric tube.

    Cup = 8 oz

    What is the patient's intake and output?

    I = _____   O = _____

32. Which of the following is/are most likely to lead to a fluid volume deficit? Select all that apply.
    a. Vomiting _____
    b. Heart failure _____
    c. Corticosteroid administration _____
    d. Fever _____
    e. Increased sodium intake _____
    f. Diuretic administration _____

33. A patient has a nursing diagnosis of *Deficient Fluid Volume related to excessive diaphoresis* from fever. Identify a related outcome and two nursing interventions for this patient.

34. When selecting a site to start an IV, the nurse should begin with the site that is: _____

35. The IV site is located in the right antecubital space. The nurse notes that the rate fluctuates when the patient flexes his right arm. The nurse should:

36. Identify the correct order of the following steps for the removal of an IV.
    a. Turn off the roller clamp _____
    b. Remove the IV catheter _____
    c. Remove the dressing _____
    d. Record the fluid infusion _____
    e. Inspect the tip of the IV catheter _____
    f. Perform hand hygiene and apply clean gloves _____
    g. Place gauze over the site and apply light pressure _____

37. The nurse is preparing the IV fluid infusion. What should be checked when looking at the IV fluid?

38. In preparing to administer a blood transfusion, what are the critical assessments that need to be made?

39. It is suspected that the patient is experiencing hypokalemia. Identify all of the signs that support this assessment. Select all that apply.
    a. Bilateral muscle weakness _____
    b. Positive Chvostek's sign _____
    c. Bradycardia _____
    d. Diminished bowel sounds _____
    e. Tetany _____
    f. ECG abnormalities _____

40. Identify which of the following are correct when performing an IV site dressing. Select all that apply.
    a. Apply tape over the IV insertion site. _____
    b. Cleanse the site horizontally, vertically, and then in a outward circular pattern. _____
    c. Use skin protectant where the tape will be. _____
    d. Anchor the IV tubing. _____
    e. Use clean technique for the procedure. _____
    f. Use a catheter stabilization device. _____

Select the best answer for each of the following questions:

41. The IV site is swollen, pale, and cool to the touch. The nurse identifies this as:
    1. phlebitis.
    2. infiltration.
    3. local infection.
    4. allergic response.

42. A hypotonic IV solution is expected to be administered to a patient who is experiencing:
    1. hypernatremia.
    2. hypocalcemia.
    3. hypervolemia.
    4. hypokalemia.

43. The patient has hypernatremia with a fluid deficit. The nurse anticipates finding:
    1. dry, sticky mucous membranes.
    2. orthostatic hypotension.
    3. abdominal cramping.
    4. diarrhea.

44. The patient who is experiencing a gastrointestinal problem has had periods of prolonged vomiting. The nurse is observing the patient for signs of:
    1. metabolic acidosis.
    2. metabolic alkalosis.
    3. respiratory acidosis.
    4. respiratory alkalosis.

45. The nurse is working with a patient who has had emphysema for many years. The nurse believes that the patient has uncompensated respiratory acidosis. This belief is a result of an analysis of the patient's blood gas values that reveals:
    1. pH = 7.35, $PaCO_2$ = 40 mm Hg, HCO_3^- concentration = 22 mEq/L
    2. pH = 7.40, $PaCO_2$ = 45 mm Hg, HCO_3^- concentration = 28 mEq/L
    3. pH = 7.30, $PaCO_2$ = 50 mm Hg, HCO_3^- concentration = 24 mEq/L
    4. pH = 7.45, $PaCO_2$ = 55 mm Hg, HCO_3^- concentration = 18 mEq/L

46. The patient has been admitted to the medical center for stabilization of congestive heart failure. The physician has prescribed Lasix (a diuretic) for the patient. This patient should be observed for:
    1. diarrhea.
    2. edema.
    3. dysrhythmia.
    4. hyperactive reflexes.

47. The patient has a potassium level above the normal value. The nurse anticipates that treatment for this patient with hyperkalemia will include:
    1. fluid restrictions.
    2. foods high in potassium.
    3. administration of diuretics.
    4. IV infusion of calcium.

48. The patient has lost a large amount of body fluid. In assessment of this patient with hypovolemia (fluid volume deficit, FVD), the nurse expects to find:
    1. oliguria.
    2. hypertension.
    3. periorbital edema.
    4. neck vein distention.

49. The nurse is determining the care that is to be provided to the patients on the medical unit. There are a number of patients who have the potential for a fluid and electrolyte imbalance. A nurse-initiated (independent) intervention for these patients is:
    1. administration of IV fluids.
    2. monitoring of intake and output.
    3. performance of diagnostic tests.
    4. dietary replacement of necessary fluids/electrolytes.

50. For a patient who is experiencing a fluid volume excess, the nurse plans to determine the fluid status. The best way to determine the fluid balance for the patient is to:
    1. obtain diagnostic test results.
    2. monitor IV fluid intake.
    3. weigh the patient daily.
    4. assess vital signs.

51. The patient is admitted to the trauma unit after an accident while using power tools at home. The patient experienced significant blood loss and required a large infusion of citrated blood. The nurse assesses this patient for the development of:
    1. urinary retention.
    2. poor skin turgor.
    3. increased blood pressure reading.
    4. positive Chvostek's sign.

52. The patient is experiencing a severe anxiety reaction and the respiratory rate has increased significantly. Nursing intervention for this patient who may develop respiratory alkalosis is:
    1. placing the patient in a sitting position.
    2. providing the patient with nasal oxygen.
    3. having the patient breathe into a paper bag.
    4. having the patient cough and deep breathe.

53. A patient with normal renal function is to be maintained NPO. An IV of 1000 mL of D_5W is ordered to infuse over 8 hours. The nurse should:
    1. infuse the IV at a faster rate.
    2. add multivitamins to the solution.
    3. provide oral fluids as a supplement.
    4. question the prescriber about adding potassium to the IV.

54. A patient with an IV infusion may develop phlebitis. The nurse recognizes this condition by the presence at the IV infusion site of:
    1. pallor.
    2. swelling.
    3. redness.
    4. cyanosis.

55. The patient has had an IV line inserted. Upon observation of the IV site, the nurse notes that there is evidence of an infiltration. The nurse should first:
    1. slow the infusion.
    2. discontinue the infusion.
    3. change the IV bag and tubing.
    4. contact the prescriber immediately.

56. The nurse is reviewing the hospital policy for maintenance of IV infusions. The current guidelines for changing continuous IV tubing (non–blood administration sets) are every:
    1. 36 hours.
    2. 48 hours.
    3. 72 hours.
    4. 96 hours.

57. The patient has just started to receive the blood transfusion. The nurse is performing the patient assessment and notes the patient has chills and flank pain. The nurse stops the infusion and then:
    1. calls the physician.
    2. administers epinephrine.
    3. collects a urine specimen.
    4. sets up new tubing with an IV infusion of 0.9% saline.

58. A patient who has been admitted with a renal dysfunction is demonstrating signs and symptoms of a fluid volume excess (hypervolemia). Upon completing the patient assessment, the nurse anticipates finding:
    1. poor skin turgor.
    2. decreased blood pressure.
    3. neck vein distention.
    4. increased urine specific gravity.

59. The nurse is assisting the patient with a fluid volume deficit to select an optimum replacement fluid. The nurse suggests that the patient drink:
    1. tea.
    2. milk.
    3. coffee.
    4. fruit juice.

60. A patient with congestive heart failure and fluid retention is placed on a fluid restriction of 1000 mL/24 hours. On the basis of guidelines for patients with restrictions, for the time period from 7:00 AM to 3:30 PM the nurse plans to provide the patient:
    1. 250 mL.
    2. 400 mL.
    3. 500 mL.
    4. 750 mL.

61. The patient has come to the orthopedist's office for treatment of osteoporosis. The nurse is explaining to the patient some of the possible complications from this disorder that may affect fluid and electrolyte balance. The nurse informs the patient to report:
    1. low back pain.
    2. tingling in the fingers.
    3. muscle twitching.
    4. positive Trousseau's sign.

62. The patient has a history of alcoholism and is admitted to the medical center in a malnourished state. The nurse specifically checks the lab values for:
    1. hypercalcemia.
    2. hyponatremia.
    3. hyperkalemia.
    4. hypomagnesemia.

63. The patient who is most prone to respiratory acidosis is the individual who is experiencing:
    1. hyperthyroidism.
    2. an acute asthma episode.
    3. renal failure.
    4. an anxiety reaction.

64. Older adults have a greater risk of fluid imbalance as a result of:
    1. increased thirst response.
    2. decreased glomerular filtration.
    3. increased body fluid percentage.
    4. increased basal metabolic rate.

65. An example of a type of medication that can lead to metabolic acidosis is:
    1. aspirin.
    2. Lasix.
    3. potassium.
    4. Benadryl.

66. An appropriate technique when initiating an intravenous infusion is to:
    1. use hard, stiff veins.
    2. shave the arm hair with a razor.
    3. use the proximal site in the dominant arm.
    4. apply the tourniquet 4 to 6 inches above the selected site.

67. A unit of packed cells or whole blood usually transfuses over:
    1. ½ hour.
    2. 1 hour.
    3. 2 hours.
    4. 5 hours.

68. An individual with type O blood is able to receive:
    1. type A or type B.
    2. type AB.
    3. type O.
    4. all types.

69. A specific technique for initiating intravenous therapy for an older adult is to:
    1. select sites in the hands.
    2. use the largest possible IV cannula gauge.
    3. set the IV flow rate at 150 to 200 mL/hr.
    4. insert at a decreased angle of 10 to 15 degrees.

70. The patient lost 4 pounds since last week as a result of taking Lasix. This is approximately:
    1. ½ L of fluid.
    2. 1 L of fluid.
    3. 2 L of fluid.
    4. 4 L of fluid.

STUDY GROUP QUESTIONS

- How are body fluids distributed in the body?
- What is the composition of body fluids?
- How do fluids move throughout the body?
- How is the intake of body fluids regulated?
- What are the major electrolytes, and what is their function in the body?
- How is acid-base balance maintained?
- What are the major fluid, electrolyte, and acid-base imbalances and their causes?
- What signs and symptoms will the patient exhibit in the presence of a fluid, electrolyte, or acid-base imbalance?
- What diagnostic tests are used to determine the presence of imbalances?
- What information is critical to obtain in a patient assessment to determine the presence of a fluid, electrolyte, or acid-base imbalance?
- What health deviations increase a patient's susceptibility to an imbalance?
- What nursing interventions should be implemented for patients with various fluid, electrolyte, and acid-base imbalances?
- What information should be included in patient/family teaching for prevention of imbalances, or restoration of fluid, electrolyte, or acid-base balance?
- What are the nursing responsibilities associated with the initiation and maintenance of IV therapy?
- What are the responsibilities of the nurse with regard to blood transfusions?

STUDY CHARTS

Create study charts to compare

a. *Electrolyte Imbalances and Patient Responses,* including etiology, diagnostic test results, patient assessment, and nursing interventions for sodium, potassium, calcium, and magnesium imbalances

b. *Acid-Base Imbalances and Patient Responses,* including etiology, diagnostic test results, patient assessment, and nursing interventions for metabolic acidosis and alkalosis and for respiratory acidosis and alkalosis

19 Caring in Nursing Practice

CASE STUDIES

1. The daughter of a patient in an extended care facility has traveled from another state to visit. When she arrives with her husband and teenage son, she finds that her mother has deteriorated dramatically from the last time she spoke with her. The patient, in the terminal stages of liver disease, is now only minimally responsive with episodes of agitation and disorientation. The family, especially the daughter, is emotionally distraught.
   a. What can be done by the nurse to demonstrate caring for this patient's family?
   b. What can be done for the patient to demonstrate caring?

2. The nurse observes the student giving a bath to a bedridden patient. The door to the room is open and the patient is exposed. In addition, the student is not being very gentle with the patient.
   a. What caring behaviors are missing?
   b. How can the nurse help the student to recognize and incorporate caring behaviors?

CHAPTER REVIEW

Complete the following:

1. Match the theorists with the theoretical concepts:
   Patricia Benner and Judith Wrubel
   Jean Watson
   Madeleine Leininger
   Kristen Swanson
   a. Five processes and subdimensions _____
   b. Transpersonal caring _____
   c. Caring is primary _____
   d. Transcultural caring _____

2. For the following nursing behaviors, identify an example of a clinical intervention.
   a. Providing presence
   b. Touch
   c. Listening
   d. Knowing the patient

3. A patient is to have an IV line inserted. The nurse demonstrates caring behaviors by:

4. Describe how caring and spirituality are connected.

5. How can nurses care for each other?

Select the best answer for each of the following questions:

6. A nurse is discussing with her peers how much a patient matters to her. She states that she does not want the patient to suffer. The nurse is implementing the theory described by:
   1. Patricia Benner.
   2. Jean Watson.
   3. Kristen Swanson.
   4. Madeleine Leininger.

7. A patient was admitted to the hospital to have diagnostic tests to rule out a cancerous lesion in the lungs. The nurse is sitting with the patient in the room awaiting the results of the tests. The nurse is demonstrating the caring behavior of:
   1. knowing.
   2. comforting.
   3. providing presence.
   4. maintaining belief.

8. A nurse manager would like to promote more opportunities for the staff on the busy unit to demonstrate caring behaviors. The manager elects to implement:
   1. more time off for the staff.
   2. a strict schedule for patient treatments.
   3. staff selection of patient assignments.
   4. staff appointment to hospital committees.

9. A new graduate is looking at theories of caring. He selects Leininger's theory because it is most agreeable with his belief system. Leininger defines caring as a(n):
   1. new consciousness and moral idea.
   2. nurturing way of relating to a valued other.
   3. central, unifying domain necessary for health and survival.
   4. improvement in the human condition using a transcultural perspective.

10. A nurse is working with a patient who has been admitted to the oncology unit for treatment of a cancerous growth. This nurse is applying Swanson's theory of caring and demonstrating the concept of maintaining belief when:
    1. performing the patient's dressing changes.
    2. providing explanations about the medications.
    3. keeping the patient draped during the physical exam.
    4. discussing how the radiation therapy will assist in decreasing the tumor's size.

11. A new graduate is assigned to a surgical unit in which there are a large number of procedures to be performed during each shift. This nurse demonstrates a caring behavior in this situation by:
    1. avoiding situations that may be uncomfortable or difficult.
    2. attempting to do all the treatments independently and quickly.
    3. seeking assistance before performing new or difficult skills.
    4. telling patients that he or she is a new graduate and unfamiliar with all the procedures.

12. An example of the caring process of "enabling" is:
    1. performing a catheter insertion quickly and well.
    2. reassuring the patient that the lab results should be fine.
    3. providing pain medication before a procedure.
    4. assisting a patient during the birth of a child.

13. A subdimension of Swanson's process of caring—"doing for others as he/she would do for self"—involves:
    1. being there.
    2. performing skillfully.
    3. generating alternatives.
    4. offering realistic optimism.

14. In the Caring Assessment Tool (CAT), an example of mutual problem solving with a patient is when a nurse:
    1. discusses health issues with the patient and family.
    2. pays attention to the patient.
    3. provides privacy for the patient.
    4. includes the family members in the patient's care.

15. A nurse attempts to understand the specific cultural concerns of a patient and how they relate to his illness. What caring factor is applied?
    1. Attentive reassurance
    2. Encouragement
    3. Provision of basic human needs
    4. Appreciation of unique meanings

16. Additional teaching is required if a nurse observes that a nursing assistant working with an older adult patient:
    1. has the patient select the clothes to wear.
    2. addresses the patient as "Honey."
    3. carefully organizes the patient's personal items.
    4. combs and styles the patient's hair.

STUDY GROUP QUESTIONS

- What is "caring" in the nursing profession?
- What are the major theories of caring and the key concepts in each one?
- How is caring perceived by patients?
- What are caring behaviors?
- How can a nurse demonstrate caring to patients and families?

20 Cultural Awareness

CASE STUDY

1. For the following situations, identify how a nurse should approach the patient and significant others to recognize cultural concerns and health care needs:
   a. Large numbers of family members surround the patient on the acute care unit.
   b. Dietary practices of the patient prohibit the eating of meat or meat products.
   c. A traditional healer makes calls to the patient's home between the patient's visits to the physician.
   d. The patient and her family speak another language.

CHAPTER REVIEW

Complete the following:

1. Identify two possible nursing diagnoses that may be related to a patient's cultural needs.

2. Provide an example for how the nurse may develop each of the following.
   a. Cultural awareness
   b. Cultural skills

3. Identify an example of a question a nurse could use to elicit specific cultural information from a patient.

4. Identify a specific transcultural communication issue and an appropriate intervention.

5. Explain linguistic competence.

6. Identify four disadvantaged groups and their health care challenges.

7. What should be incorporated into "Teach-Back" to address cultural considerations?

8. Identify four important aspects for working with an interpreter.

9. What are the parts of the LEARN and RESPECT mnemonics?

   L - ~~learn~~ listen   R - rapport
   E - explain   E - empathy
   A - acknowledge   S - support
   R - recommend   P - partnership
   N - negotiate   E - explanations
                            C - cultural competence
                            T - trust

Select the best answer for each of the following questions:

10. A nurse is meeting a patient for the first time for the admission interview. There are eight family members sitting around the patient's bed. After introductions, the most appropriate nursing action is to:
    1. ask the family members to leave immediately.
    2. proceed with the admission interview.
    3. come back at another time.
    4. ask the patient if he or she wants a family member present.

11. The community center where a nurse volunteers has a culturally diverse population. The nurse wants to promote communication with all the patients from different cultures. A beneficial technique for the nurse is to:
    1. explain nursing terms that are used.
    2. use direct and consistent eye contact and touch with all patients.
    3. call patients by their first names to establish rapport.
    4. expect and wait for responses to all questions that are asked.

74

Chapter **20** **Cultural Awareness**

12. A patient expresses to the nurse that traditional Western or American practices are used in the home for health promotion. The nurse expects that the patient will use:
    1. acupuncture.
    2. guided imagery.
    3. aromatic therapy.
    4. over-the-counter medications.

13. When working with an interpreter for a patient who speaks another language, the nurse should:
    1. direct questions to the interpreter.
    2. expect word-for-word translation.
    3. ensure that the interpreter speaks the patient's dialect.
    4. ask the interpreter to evaluate the patient's nonverbal behaviors.

14. The pregnant patient says that she goes to a woman who provides advice and comfort during and after childbirth. The nurse recognizes that the patient is referring to a(n):
    1. *Ayurvedic provider.*
    2. *Sabador.*
    3. *Imam.*
    4. *Doula.*

STUDY GROUP QUESTIONS

- What is culture?
- What are the major ethnocultural groups in the country/community, their health and illness beliefs and practices, and their traditional remedies?
- How can a nurse promote communication with individuals who are from other cultures and/or individuals who speak different languages?
- How can a nurse identify and respond to a patient's cultural needs?
- What information may be obtained from a cultural assessment?
- What nursing approaches may be successful in assisting multicultural patients in health care settings?
- What resources are available to assist a nurse in learning about and working with patients from other cultures?

21 Spiritual Health

CASE STUDY

1. A nurse is working in an acute care facility with a patient who practices Buddhism.
   a. What information should be obtained in relation to the patient's spiritual practices?
   b. What adaptations may have to be made by the nurse, the other members of the health care team, and the acute care facility to meet the patient's spiritual needs?

CHAPTER REVIEW

Match the description/definition in Column A with the correct term in Column B.

Column A

 1. Does not believe in the existence of a supreme spiritual being or god

 2. Cultural or institutional religion

_e_ 3. Awareness of one's inner self and a sense of connection to a higher being

_b_ 4. Multidimensional concept that gives comfort while a person endures hardship and challenges

_f_ 5. Awareness of that which cannot be seen or known in ordinary ways

_g_ 6. Belief that ultimate reality is unknown or unknowable

_c_ 7. Having close spiritual relationships with oneself, others, and a god or other spiritual being

Column B

a. Faith

b. Hope

c. Connectedness

d. Atheist

e. Spirituality

f. Self-transcendence

g. Agnostic

Complete the following:

8. Identify general nursing interventions for promotion of spiritual health.

9. An example of a nursing intervention for a patient who has had a near-death experience is:

10. Identify two possible nursing diagnoses and patient outcomes relating to spirituality or spiritual health.

11. Identify what each letter in the FICA assessment tool acronym designates:
    F:
    I:
    C:
    A:

12. Formulate a question that may be asked to determine a patient's spiritual belief system.

13. There is an order for whole blood replacement for a patient. Before the blood administration, a nurse will check to see if the patient is a member of what religion(s)?

14. Provide at least two examples of rituals or practices associated with spirituality or religion.

15. Religious or spiritual practices may have an impact upon the provision of health care to a patient. For an individual who is of the Islamic faith, which of the following may have to be considered by a nurse and other health care providers? Select all that apply.
    a. Organ donation will be approved. _____
    b. Women prefer female providers/examiners. _____
    c. Euthanasia is practiced. _____
    d. Time will have to be set aside during the day for prayer. _____
    e. Faith healing may be used. _____
    f. Blood products and medicines may be refused. _____

16. Identify the four (4) dimensions of spiritual well-being.

17. Indicate which of the following statements about spirituality is/are correct. Select all that apply.
    a. Patients who identify a religious belief will all practice similar rituals. _____
    b. Promoting spirituality can help a patient cope with illness. _____
    c. Promoting a patient's spirituality may reduce the incidence of depression. _____
    d. The link between spirituality and physical health is well understood. _____
    e. Spirituality exists in all people regardless of their religious beliefs. _____

18. How does the nurse use *presence* to promote spiritual well-being?

19. The nurse wants to assist patients to achieve spiritual health. The nurse should:
    Select all that apply.
    a. Solve their spiritual problems. _____
    b. Employ his/her own personal religious practices with the patient. _____
    c. Explore meditation with the patient to assist in reducing stress. _____
    d. Integrate patient preferences into the plan of care. _____
    e. Provide an environment for expression of beliefs. _____
    f. Recognize that all patients experience spiritual problems. _____

Select the best answer for each of the following questions:

20. A patient is admitted to a medical center for surgery to repair a fractured hip. Upon reviewing the patient's admission history, a nurse finds that the patient attends religious services routinely. The nurse supports the patient's spiritual needs by stating:
    1. "Do you really go to services often?"
    2. "Don't worry. God will take care of you."
    3. "I'll call your minister and have him stop by to see you."
    4. "Is there any way that I may be able to help you with your spiritual needs?"

21. A patient who is of the Jewish faith is admitted to the long-term care facility. A nurse seeks to provide support of the usual health practices that are part of this religion. The nurse learns that one component of usual Jewish tradition states:
    1. No euthanasia should be used.
    2. A faith healer will be involved.
    3. Modern medical treatment should be refused.
    4. Physical exams should be performed only by individuals of the same sex.

22. While caring for a patient in the intensive care unit, the patient has a cardiac arrest. The patient is successfully resuscitated. After this near-death experience, the patient is progressing physically but appears withdrawn and concerned. The nurse assists the patient by stating:
    1. "The experience that you had is easy to explain and understand."
    2. "That was a very close call. It must be very frightening for you."
    3. "Other people have had similar experiences and worked through their feelings."
    4. "If you would like to talk about your experience, I will stay with you."

23. For a patient with a diagnosis of a chronic disease, a nurse wishes to encourage feelings of hope. The nurse recognizes that hope provides:
    1. a meaning and purpose for the patient.
    2. an organized approach to dealing with the disease process.
    3. a connection to the cultural background of the patient.
    4. a binding relationship with the divine being of the patient's religion.

24. A nurse is reviewing the plan of care for a 66-year-old home care patient who is experiencing the beginning stages of Alzheimer's disease. Several nursing diagnoses have been identified from the initial home visit and assessment. The nurse believes that the patient may need to be assessed for spiritual needs based on the diagnosis of:
    1. Impaired Memory.
    2. Altered Health Maintenance.
    3. Ineffective Coping.
    4. Altered Thought Process.

25. According to Erikson's stages of psychosocial development, with regard to spiritual beliefs it is expected that a 6-year-old child will:
    1. begin to ask about a god or supreme being.
    2. have spiritual well-being provided by the parents.
    3. interpret meanings literally.
    4. begin to learn the difference between right and wrong.

26. A nurse recognizes that a group whose members may reject modern medicine based on religious beliefs is:
    1. Hindu.
    2. Islamic.
    3. Catholic.
    4. Navajo.

27. According to Erikson's stages of psychosocial development, with regard to spiritual beliefs it is expected that a middle-age person will begin to:
    1. reflect on inconsistencies in religious stories.
    2. form independent beliefs and attitudes.
    3. review value systems during a crisis.
    4. sort fantasy from fact.

28. A young adult is diagnosed with a very aggressive form of cancer. He yells at the nurse, "Why did this happen to me?" The nurse's best response is:
    1. "Do you think that you did something wrong?"
    2. "You sound upset about your situation. Let's talk about it."
    3. "Tell me why you think this is unfair."
    4. "What makes you say that?"

STUDY GROUP QUESTIONS

- What is spirituality and how does it relate to an individual's health status?
- What are the concepts of spirituality/spiritual health?
- What spiritual or religious problems may arise during patient care?
- How can a nurse assess a patient's spirituality/spiritual health?
- What is the role of a nurse in promoting spiritual health?
- How can a nurse avoid imposing his or her own beliefs on a patient?
- What are the differences and similarities in spiritual practices and health beliefs between the major religious sects?
- How is hope related to spirituality?

22 Growth and Development

CASE STUDIES

1. A student nurse with an inpatient pediatric unit in a medical center has three patients: an infant, a 5-year-old child, and a 16-year-old adolescent.
   a. How should the nurse promote growth and developmental needs for these patients in the acute care environment?
   b. What would be included in a teaching plan for the new parents of the infant?

2. A patient in the extended care facility is an 86-year-old woman who is occasionally disoriented to time, place, and person.
   a. How should a nurse approach this patient to assist her in meeting her developmental needs?

3. A student nurse is working as a summer camp nurse with children 8 to 10 years old. It is the nurse's turn to select diversional activities for a group.
   a. What types of games or activities are appropriate for this age group?

4. A nurse is teaching the parents of adolescents the signs that may indicate a potential suicidal tendency in their children.
   a. What signs/behaviors will the nurse identify for these parents?

CHAPTER REVIEW

Match the description in Column A with the correct theorist in Column B.

	Column A	Column B
d	1. Development of cognition	a. Freud
a	2. Psychosexual focus	b. Erikson
c	3. Based on human needs	c. Maslow
e	4. Moral development	d. Piaget
b	5. Psychosocial development	e. Kohlberg

Complete the following:

6. An example of a teratogen is:

7. The leading cause of death in the toddler and preschool age groups is:

8. Select the age group (infant, toddler, preschool age, school age, adolescent, young adult, middle-aged adult, or older adult) in which each of the following behaviors is evident or usually begins:
   a. Toilet training _____
   b. Tripling of birth weight _____
   c. Use of script handwriting _____
   d. Separation anxiety _____
   e. Moving away from the family _____

f. Parallel play _____
g. Search for personal identity _____
h. Menopause _____
i. Speaking in short sentences _____
j. More graceful running and jumping _____
k. Development of fears _____
l. Presbycusis _____
m. Loss of primary teeth _____
n. Development of primary and secondary sexual characteristics _____
o. Low risk of chronic illness _____
p. Diminished skin turgor and appearance of wrinkles _____
q. Socioeconomic stability _____
r. Recognition of objects by their outward appearance _____

9. To promote awareness of time, place, and person in an extended care environment, a nurse implements:

10. Prescriptive use or administration of more medication than indicated clinically is termed:

11. Identify safety concerns in the home environment for the following age groups:
    a. Toddler
    b. Older adult

12. What are the expected physical assessment findings for a middle-aged adult? Select all that apply.
    a. Abnormal visual fields and ocular movements _____
    b. Palpable lateral thyroid nodes _____
    c. Pulse rate of 60 to 100 beats per minute _____
    d. Decreased strength of abdominal muscles _____
    e. Responsive sensory system _____
    f. Diminished motor responses _____

13. Identify a topic area that is age appropriate for a group of older adults in a senior housing development.

14. Indicate ways that the nurse can reduce stress for a hospitalized child.

15. What is a potential nursing diagnosis for an adolescent individual?

16. What are the characteristics of the adolescent age group? Select all that apply.
    a. Preference for same sex peers _____
    b. Risk-taking _____
    c. Search for personal identify _____
    d. Following the rules of new authority figures _____
    e. Adoption of the parents' moral standards _____
    f. Development of secondary sex characteristics _____

17. How is the "Sandwich Generation" a challenge for nurses?

18. Identify at least one health concern for toddlers and school-age children.

19. Indicate which of the following are true for older adult individuals. Select all that apply.
    a. Cognitive impairment is expected. _____
    b. Strong visual memory is retained. _____
    c. Delirium is potentially reversible. _____
    d. Depression is becoming more common in this population. _____
    e. Short-term memory is unaffected. _____
    f. Sense of touch remains strong. _____

Select the best answer for each of the following questions:

20. A nurse is assigned to prepare a teaching plan for a group of preschool-age children. For this age group, the nurse includes:
    1. appropriate use of medications.
    2. cooking safety including use of the stove.
    3. information on prevention of obesity and hypertension.
    4. guidelines for crossing the street or actions to take during a fire.

21. Children who are admitted to a hospital may be afraid about the hospitalization. To reduce the fear of school-age children in an acute care environment, a nurse:
    1. restrains them for all assessments and procedures.
    2. shows them the equipment that is to be used for procedures.
    3. provides in-depth information on how procedures are done.
    4. tells them that everything will be all right and the procedures will not hurt.

22. During a clinical rotation a student nurse is observing children in a day care center. The student is asked to assist with the activities for the preschool-age children. Children in this age group are usually able to:
    1. make detailed drawings.
    2. skip, throw, and catch balls.
    3. easily hold a pencil and print letters.
    4. use a vocabulary of more than 8000 words.

23. Parents of a toddler ask a nurse what their child should be able to do at the age of 2½ years old. The nurse identifies that the toddler will be able to:
    1. classify objects by size and color.
    2. speak in short sentences.
    3. solve difficult problems.
    4. recognize safety hazards.

24. Parents of a 1-year-old are asking about what can be expected of a child this age. A nurse informs the parents that a major milestone for a 1-year-old child is:
    1. tripling of the birth weight.
    2. sleeping 6 to 7 hours each day.
    3. walking with good balance.
    4. playing well with others.

25. A nurse is working with a group of young adults at the community center. There are many discussions about life and health issues. The nurse is aware that a health-related concern for young adults is that:
    1. attachment needs must be enhanced.
    2. "labeling" may alter their self-perceptions.
    3. adaptation to chronic disease is developing.
    4. fast-paced lifestyles may place them at risk for illnesses or disabilities.

26. A nurse is seeking to evaluate the effectiveness of information provided to the parents of an infant. The nurse determines that teaching has been successful when the parents:
    1. place small pillows in the infant's crib.
    2. position the infant on the stomach for sleeping.
    3. purchase a crib with slats that are less than 2 inches apart.
    4. prop up a bottle for the infant to suck on while falling asleep.

27. When presenting a program for a group of individuals in their middle-aged adult years, a nurse informs the members to expect the following physical change:
    1. A decrease in skin turgor
    2. An increased breast size
    3. Palpable lateral thyroid lobes
    4. A visual acuity that is greater than 20/50

28. Parents of a 3½-year-old boy are concerned when, after hospitalization, the boy begins to suck his thumb again. The boy had not sucked his thumb for over a year. A nurse informs the parents that:
    1. their health care provider must be informed about this behavior.
    2. the child was probably not ready to stop this behavior previously.
    3. the child is feeling neglected by his parents and they should spend more time with him.
    4. the behavior should be ignored as it is common for a child to regress when anxious.

29. An adolescent girl has gone to a family planning center for information about birth control. The patient asks a nurse what she should use to avoid getting pregnant. The nurse responds:
    1. "Are your parents aware of your sexual activity?"
    2. "You've been using some kind of protection before, right?"
    3. "What are your friends doing to protect themselves?"
    4. "What can you tell me about your past sexual experiences?"

30. A patient has gone to an outpatient obstetric clinic for a routine checkup. The patient asks a nurse what is happening with the baby now that she is in her third trimester. The nurse informs the patient that:
    1. the heartbeat can be heard.
    2. the fingers and toes are well developed.
    3. the organ systems are just beginning to develop.
    4. the brain is undergoing a tremendous growth spurt.

31. For a patient in a nursing center, the nurse suspects the potentially reversible cognitive impairment of:
    1. delirium.
    2. dementia.
    3. depression.
    4. disengagement.

STUDY GROUP QUESTIONS

- What are the principles of growth and development?
- How can growth and development be influenced internally and externally?
- What are the differences and similarities of the major developmental theorists?
- How can a nurse apply the different developmental theories to patient situations?
- What are the major physical, psychosocial, and cognitive changes that occur throughout the life span?
- What are the specific health needs for each developmental stage?
- How does the approach of a nurse differ for individuals in each developmental stage to meet their developmental needs?
- What are the different teaching/learning needs of each developmental stage?

STUDY CHART

Create a study chart to compare *Growth and Development Across the Life Span* that identifies the physical abilities, psychosocial/cognitive activities, and health promotion behaviors and strategies for each age group from infancy to older adulthood.

23 Self-Concept and Sexuality

CASE STUDIES

1. A 22-year-old man is admitted to a rehabilitation facility. He was seriously injured in an automobile accident and now is paraplegic. Although he is medically stable, it appears that he is having difficulty dealing with his physical limitations. The patient speaks frequently about his girlfriend and his involvement in athletics and other social activities.
   a. What self-concept and sexuality issues are involved in this situation?
   b. Formulate a plan of care for this patient.

2. A nurse suspects that a patient is the victim of sexual abuse.
   a. What behaviors may the patient be exhibiting that would lead to this assessment?
   b. What questions should the nurse ask to get more information from the patient about the possible abuse?

CHAPTER REVIEW

Match the description/definition in Column A with the correct term in Column B.

Column A	Column B
1. Set of conscious and unconscious feelings and beliefs about oneself	a. Sexuality
2. Set of behaviors that have been approved by family, community, and culture as appropriate in particular situations	b. Self-concept
	c. Transgender
3. Clear, persistent preference for persons of one sex	d. Self-esteem
4. Emotional evaluation of self-worth	
5. Experiences and attitudes related to appearance and physical abilities	e. Sexual orientation
	f. Role
6. Sense of femaleness or maleness	
	g. Identity
7. People whose gender identity or expression is different than their sex at birth	h. Body image
8. Persistent individuality and sameness of a person over time and in various circumstances	

Complete the following:

9. Identify at least two examples of the following.
   a. Positive influences on self-concept

   b. Stressors to self-concept

10. Which of the following behaviors may indicate an altered self-concept? Select all that apply.
    a. Eye contact maintained _____
    b. Straight posture _____
    c. Hesitant speech _____
    d. Overly angry response _____
    e. Independence _____
    f. Passive attitude _____
    g. Able to make decisions _____
    h. Unkempt appearance _____

11. For the following patients, identify the potential concerns related to self-concept and sexuality.
    a. A woman who has had a mastectomy

    b. A woman who is undergoing chemotherapy for cancer and who has a young child at home

    c. A 7-year-old child who has been severely burned

    d. A middle-aged adult man who has had a heart attack

12. A way in which a nurse may promote self-concept in an acute care setting is by:

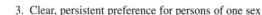

13. An example of an alteration in sexual health is:

14. Specify an area for patient education to promote sexual health.

15. For the nursing diagnosis *Situational Low Self-Esteem related to being unable to successfully pass a required college course*, identify a patient goal/outcome and nursing interventions.

16. The capacity for sexuality diminishes significantly in older adults.
    True _____ False _____

17. Cultural background does not directly influence self-concept.
    True _____ False _____

18. The best method of birth control to reinforce with patients is the least expensive selection.
    True _____ False _____

19. An example of an intervention that a nurse may implement to promote self-concept for an older adult is:

20. For tattoos and body piercings, identify the statements that are correct. Select all that apply.
    a. They are less common practices today _____
    b. There are more complications from piercings than tattoos _____
    c. Federal regulations are in place for these practices _____
    d. Sterile technique should be used for the procedures _____
    e. They are ways of expressing individuality _____

21. Provide an example of a role performance stressor.

22. The vaccine that is recommended for early adolescent males and females to reduce the risk for HPV-related cancers is:

23. What medical diagnoses can interfere with sexual functioning?

Select the best answer for each of the following questions:

24. A nurse recognizes that which of the following age groups is most vulnerable to identity stressors?
    1. Infancy
    2. Preschool
    3. Adolescence
    4. Middle-aged adulthood

25. An adolescent has gone to the nurse's office in a school to discuss some personal issues. The nurse wishes to determine the sexual health of this adolescent. The nurse begins by asking:
    1. "Do you use contraception?"
    2. "Have you already had sexual relations?"
    3. "Are your parents aware of your sexual activity?"
    4. "Do you have any concerns about sex or your body's development?"

26. During an interview and physical assessment of a female patient in the clinic, a nurse finds that the patient has multiple lacerations and bruises and that she has experienced headaches and difficulty sleeping. The nurse suspects:
    1. sexual dysfunction.
    2. emotional conflict.
    3. sexually transmitted infection.
    4. physical and/or sexual abuse.

27. A patient is admitted to a coronary care unit after an acute myocardial infarction. He tells the nurse, "I won't be able to do what I used to at the hardware store." The nurse recognizes that the patient is experiencing a problem with the self-concept component of:
    1. role.
    2. identity.
    3. self-esteem.
    4. body image.

28. An adolescent patient has just been diagnosed with scoliosis and will need to wear a corrective brace. She tells the nurse angrily, "I don't know why I have to have this stupid problem!" The nurse responds most appropriately by saying:
    1. "Tell me what you do when you get angry and upset."
    2. "Don't be angry. You'll be getting the best care available."
    3. "You'll heal quickly and the brace can come off pretty soon."
    4. "It's okay to be angry around your friends, but try not to be upset around your parents."

29. During an initial assessment at an outpatient clinic, a nurse wants to determine a patient's perception of identity. The nurse asks the patient:
    1. "What is your usual day like?"
    2. "How would you describe yourself?"
    3. "What activities do you enjoy doing at home?"
    4. "What changes would you make in your personal appearance?"

30. A patient has been in the rehabilitation facility for several weeks after a cerebral vascular accident (CVA/stroke). During the hospitalization, a nurse has identified that the patient has become progressively more depressed about his physical condition. Although the patient is able, he will not participate in personal grooming and now is refusing any visitors. At this point, the nurse intervenes by:
    1. telling the patient to think more positively about the future.
    2. helping the patient to get washed and dressed every day.
    3. leaving the patient to complete activities of daily living independently.
    4. contacting the physician to discuss a psychological consultation.

31. A nurse is working with a patient who has had a colostomy. The patient asks about resuming a sexual relationship with a partner. The nurse begins by determining:
    1. the patient's knowledge about sexual activity.
    2. how the patient has dealt with other life changes in the past.
    3. the partner's feelings about the colostomy.
    4. how comfortable the patient and the partner are in communicating with each other.

32. A nurse who is using Erikson's theory expects that a 5-year-old boy will begin to:
    1. accept body changes and maturation.
    2. incorporate feedback from peers into his personality.
    3. distinguish himself from the environment around him.
    4. identify with a specific gender group.

33. A patient asks a nurse about a prescription for tadalafil (Cialis). The nurse recognizes, however, that this drug is contraindicated for the patient who is taking:
    1. antibiotics.
    2. beta blockers.
    3. antihistamines.
    4. nonsteroidal antiinflammatory agents.

34. A nurse is aware that which of the following strategies is appropriate for teaching a patient for promotion of a positive sexual experience?
    1. Encouraging the use of only one position for intercourse
    2. Instructing couples to work harder at the beginning of intercourse
    3. Discussing side effects of medications that may alter responsiveness
    4. Emphasizing a shorter period of foreplay

35. Correction is required if a new nurse in the women's clinic is observed:
    1. closing the door during an examination.
    2. determining the patient's cultural beliefs.
    3. identifying physiological changes for the patient.
    4. discussing findings with the patient in the waiting room.

36. Which of the following is anticipated as a sexual change related to the aging process?
    1. Increased vaginal secretions
    2. Decreased time for ejaculation to be achieved
    3. Decreased time for maintenance of an erection
    4. Increased orgasmic contractions

37. During an initial assessment at an outpatient clinic, a nurse wants to determine a patient's level of self-esteem. The nurse asks the patient:
    1. "What is your usual day like?"
    2. "How do you feel about yourself?"
    3. "What hobbies do you enjoy doing at home?"
    4. "What changes would you make in your personal appearance?"

STUDY GROUP QUESTIONS

- What are the components of self-concept?
- What stressors may influence an individual's self-concept?
- How can a nurse promote an individual's self-concept in different health care settings?
- What is sexuality and how does it develop throughout the life span?
- How can sexual health be defined?
- What are some of the current issues related to sexuality and sexual health?
- How may sexual health be altered?
- What health-related factors may influence sexual function?
- How are self-concept and sexuality related?
- How can a nurse determine an individual's self-concept and sexual health?
- What adaptations may be made by a nurse in approaching different age groups for the assessment and promotion of self-concept and sexual health?
- How can a nurse apply critical thinking and nursing processes to the areas of self-concept and sexuality?
- What resources are available to assist individuals to promote optimum self-concept and sexual health?
- How can a nurse make the patient feel more at ease when completing an assessment of sexual health?

STUDY CHART

Create a study chart on *Stressors Affecting Self-Concept* that identifies how the components of self-concept may be influenced and nursing interventions that may be implemented to promote a patient's self-concept.

Family Context in Nursing

CASE STUDIES

1. A 65-year-old man has been admitted to the coronary care unit in a medical center. The patient experienced a myocardial infarction (heart attack) while working late in his store. His wife, who accompanied him to the medical center, not only has been the "home-maker" for the family for more than 25 years but also has assisted in the family business run by her husband. They have two children who live on their own. Their son lives with his male partner, whereas their younger daughter is married and has two children of her own. The patient and his wife speak readily about their daughter but avoid talking about their son.
   a. What factors related to family roles and function are involved in this situation?
   b. What stage of the family life cycle is this family in currently?
   c. What strategies may a nurse use to promote communication in this family?
   d. How may the role of the patient and his wife influence the health education plan?
   e. Identify a family-oriented nursing diagnosis for this situation.

2. The visiting nurse is working with a patient who has just been discharged from a rehabilitation facility after hip surgery.
   a. What should be included in the environmental assessment for this patient?
   b. What information about the patient's family should be assessed?

CHAPTER REVIEW

Match the family stage in Column A with the key principle identified for that stage in Column B.

	Column A (Family Stages)	Column B (Key Principles)
b	1. Unattached young adult	a. Increasing flexibility of family's boundaries to include children's independence
d	2. Newly married couple	b. Accepting parent-offspring separation
a	3. Family with adolescents	c. Accepting shifting of generational roles
e	4. Family with young adults	d. Committing to a new system
c	5. Family in later life	e. Accepting a multitude of exits from and entries into the family system

Complete the following:

6. What is a family?

7. What genetic factors may have an influence upon a family?

8. Identify what is meant by the following:
   a. Family hardiness

   b. Family resiliency

   c. Family diversity

9. Identify the major concerns or challenges that may influence families today.

10. For families providing care for a family member:
    a. Identify possible indicators of caregiver stress.

    b. Identify a nursing diagnosis for a family coping with the difficult care of an older adult parent in the home.

11. Which of the following are correct statements regarding today's society? Select all that apply.
    a. Families are larger. _____
    b. Divorce rates have tripled since the 1950s. _____
    c. Fewer people are living alone. _____
    d. From the 1970s to the 1990s, the number of single-parent families has doubled. _____
    e. Less than one third of gay male couples live together. _____
    f. Father-only families have increased. _____
    g. The fastest growing age group is 65 years and older. _____

12. Identify an effect that inadequate functioning may have on a family.

13. What questions may be asked to determine the influence of culture on a family?

14. Provide examples of health promotion interventions for a family.

15. Identify factors that contribute to domestic violence.

16. How can the nurse care for a family that has experienced death?

17. What is a danger for a family with a rigid structure?

Select the best answer for each of the following questions:

18. A nurse is working with a family in which the parents, both previously divorced, have brought a total of three unrelated children together. This type of family structure is classified as:
    1. nuclear.
    2. extended.
    3. blended.
    4. multi-adult.

19. A community health nurse has been assigned to work with a patient who is being discharged from a psychiatric facility. The nurse recognizes when dealing with the family that:
    1. all family members do not need to understand and agree to the plan of care.
    2. health behaviors of the family do not influence the health of individual family members.
    3. a nurse needs to change the structure of the family to meet the needs of the patient.
    4. health promotion behaviors need to be tied to the developmental stage of the family.

20. Preparation for working with families includes understanding the life cycle stage that the patient is experiencing. A nurse is working with a family that is in the "launching children and moving on" stage. It is expected that a family in this stage may also need to deal with:
    1. a review of life events.
    2. determining career goals.
    3. the death of an older parent.
    4. development of intimate peer relationships.

21. A nurse is working with a family that has been taking care of a parent with Alzheimer's disease for several years in their home. A nursing diagnosis of *Risk for Caregiver Role Strain* is identified. The nurse initially plans for:
    1. respite care.
    2. more medication for the parent.
    3. placement in a long-term care facility.
    4. consultation with a family therapist.

22. After initial assessment of a family, a nurse determines that this is a healthy family. This assessment is based on the finding that:
    1. the family responds passively to stressors.
    2. change is viewed negatively and strongly resisted.
    3. the family structure is flexible enough to adapt to crises.
    4. minimum influence is exerted by the members upon their environment.

23. An older adult patient who had surgery is going to be discharged tomorrow. The patient has a visual deficit and will need dressing changes twice a day. To meet this specific need, the nurse first:
    1. refers the patient to an adult day care center.
    2. arranges for a private duty nurse to take care of the patient 24 hours a day.
    3. informs the patient that the dressing changes will have to be managed independently.
    4. investigates the availability of a family member or neighbor to perform the dressing changes.

24. A nurse is working in the community with an adult woman who is newly diagnosed with diabetes mellitus. The patient is married, has two school-age children, and works part time. The nurse is focused on assisting the patient to learn to manage the diabetes. At this point, the nurse is viewing the family as:
    1. patient.
    2. context.
    3. process.
    4. caregiver.

25. The concept of a family being able to transcend divorce and remarriage is termed:
    1. family resiliency.
    2. family diversity.
    3. family hardiness.
    4. family functioning.

26. To determine family form and membership, a nurse asks the patient:
    1. "How are financial decisions made?"
    2. "Who drives the children to school?"
    3. "Where do you go on vacation?"
    4. "Who do you consider your family?"

27. The nurse is asking the family how the tasks are divided in the household. This question is used to establish the family's:
    1. structure.
    2. function.
    3. status.
    4. form.

STUDY GROUP QUESTIONS

- What are the attributes of a family?
- What are the different family forms?
- What are the current issues/trends influencing families?
- How do the structure and function of a family influence family relationships?
- How does communication affect family relationships?
- How are the nursing approaches to the family as patient and the family as context similar/different?
- How may critical thinking and nursing processes be applied to family nursing?
- What specific assessments should a nurse make in relation to a family?
- How does a nurse plan for the educational needs of a patient within a family?
- What must a nurse consider to meet the health needs of patients within families?
- How are psychosocial/cultural factors involved in family processes and the nursing approach to families?
- What resources are available within the health care setting and community to assist and support family functioning?

STUDY CHART

Create a study chart for your own family and identify the relationships between the members and each person's role and function.

25 Stress and Coping

CASE STUDY

1. A young adult woman is preparing to be married in a few months. She has also received a recent job promotion that requires many additional hours to be spent at work. She is seen in a nurse practitioner's office for vague symptoms.
   a. What possible signs and symptoms may be demonstrated if this patient is experiencing a stress reaction?
   b. Identify a possible nursing diagnosis for this patient.
   c. Indicate an outcome for the nursing diagnosis.
   d. What relaxation techniques may be presented to this patient?

CHAPTER REVIEW

Complete the following:

1. Evaluating an event for its personal meaning is called:

2. Which of the following are correct statements about stress? Select all that apply.
   a. Increased self-confidence results in decreased tension. _____
   b. The emotional concern of others can increase negative effects. _____
   c. Shorter, less intense stressors increase the stress response. _____
   d. The same event can cause different stress levels in different people. _____
   e. The greater the perceived magnitude of the stressor, the greater the stress response. _____
   f. Stress is decreased if a person is unable to anticipate the occurrence of an event. _____

3. A priority nursing intervention for safety for a patient under extreme stress is to determine:

4. Depression in later adulthood is a common problem.
   True _____ False _____

5. An example of a positive benefit of exercise for stress reduction is:

6. For the following, select the type of stress-producing factor that is indicated: *Situational, Maturational, Sociocultural*
   a. Divorce _____
   b. Poverty _____
   c. Immigration status _____
   d. Job change _____
   e. Adolescent identity crisis _____
   f. Hypertension _____
   g. Children moving away from home _____
   h. Homelessness _____

7. Identify an indicator of stress for each of the following areas:
   a. Cognitive
   b. Cardiovascular
   c. Gastrointestinal
   d. Behavioral
   e. Neuroendocrine

8. Identify what stress management techniques can be taught to a patient.

9. The nurse is teaching the patient about reducing the sympathetic nervous system response to stress. A self-regulating approach is to do _____ exercises.

10. Indicate an area that the nurse would discuss with the patient when using Pender's Health Promotion theory.

11. a. Compassion fatigue is most likely to be seen in a nurse who is working in a(n) _____ setting.
    b. What are the signs/symptoms of compassion fatigue?

12. In applying the QSEN competency of safety, what should the nurse assess in relation to stress and coping?

13. When does stress become a crisis?

14. The nurse is assessing a patient and is looking for outward indicators of stress. The following are objective signs associated with stress. Select all that apply.
    a. Twitching _____
    b. Hypotension _____
    c. Tachycardia _____
    d. Maintenance of eye contact _____
    e. Disheveled appearance _____
    f. Picking at the fingernails _____

15. Which of the following are components of cognitive therapy? Select all that apply.
    a. Empowerment _____
    b. Conflict resolution _____
    c. Change perspective _____
    d. Establishing support networks _____
    e. Interaction to express needs and desires _____
    f. Examine whether there is overestimation of the nature of the situation _____

Select the best answer for each of the following questions:

16. An individual who is coping by regressing will demonstrate which behavior?
    1. Becoming numb to the surroundings
    2. Refusing to discuss feelings
    3. Starting to act out in class
    4. Experiencing a loss of appetite

17. A patient has been hospitalized with a serious systemic infection. If the patient is in the resistance stage of the general adaptation syndrome and moving toward recovery, the nurse expects that the patient will demonstrate a:
    1. stabilization of hormone levels.
    2. greater degree of tissue damage.
    3. reduction in cardiac output.
    4. greater involvement of the sympathetic nervous system.

18. While working in a psychiatric emergency department, a nurse is alert to patients who are having severe difficulty in coping. A priority for the nurse is the safety of the patient and others; therefore the nurse asks patients:
    1. "How can we help you?"
    2. "Are you thinking of harming yourself?"
    3. "What physical symptoms are you having?"
    4. "What happened that is different in your life?"

19. As a result of a patient's health problem, the family is experiencing economic difficulty and demonstrating signs of crisis. As part of crisis intervention, a nurse:
    1. refers the patient for financial assistance.
    2. recommends inpatient psychiatric therapy.
    3. plans to teach the family about long-term health needs.
    4. has the patient avoid discussions about personal feelings and emotions.

20. A nurse working for the surgical unit notes that a patient has been exhibiting nervous behavior the evening before a surgical procedure. To assess the degree of stress that the patient is experiencing, the nurse asks:
    1. "Would you like me to call your family for you?"
    2. "How dangerous do you think the surgery will be?"
    3. "You seem anxious. Would you like to talk about the surgery?"
    4. "How would you like to speak with another patient who has had the procedure already?"

21. A nurse identifies that a patient is experiencing a stress reaction. To determine how the patient may cope with the event, the nurse should ask:
    1. "Are you taking any hypnotics?"
    2. "What do you think caused your stress?"
    3. "How long have you felt this way?"
    4. "Have you dealt with this reaction before?"

22. An 80-year-old patient was admitted to the hospital with a diagnosis of pneumonia. The patient is very lethargic and not communicating, and the patient's respirations are extremely labored. The nurse assesses that the patient is experiencing the general adaptation stage of:
    1. alarm.
    2. resistance.
    3. exhaustion.
    4. reflex response.

23. A patient has gone to the employee support center with complaints of fatigue and general uneasiness. The patient believes that the symptoms may be related to the increased amount of work that is expected in the job. The nurse initially recommends that the patient should attempt to reduce or control the stress by:
    1. leaving the job immediately.
    2. enrolling in a self-awareness course.
    3. seeking the assistance of a psychiatrist.
    4. employing relaxation techniques, such as deep breathing.

24. According to general adaptation syndrome (GAS), a nurse expects which of the following signs as part of an alarm reaction?
    1. Pupil dilation
    2. Decreased blood glucose levels
    3. Decreased heart rate
    4. Stabilized hormone levels

25. A nurse identifies that a patient is under stress. To determine the patient's perception of the stress, the nurse should ask:
    1. "Are you sure you are not taking drugs or alcohol?"
    2. "What does the situation mean to you?"
    3. "How did you handle this in the past?"
    4. "Why aren't you seeing a counselor?"

26. Which of the following patient observations does a nurse associate with the ego-defense mechanism of conversion?
    1. Assuming more job responsibilities
    2. Having difficulty sleeping
    3. Acting out inappropriately
    4. Refusing to talk about a problem

27. A patient has been having a hard time at home. He goes outside and begins to yell about the car and starts kicking the tires. This is an example of which of the following ego-defense mechanisms?
    1. Displacement
    2. Compensation
    3. Identification
    4. Denial

28. A nurse wants to assess whether a patient is using maladaptive coping strategies. The patient should be asked specifically about his or her:
    1. dietary intake.
    2. social activities.
    3. cigarette smoking.
    4. exercise plan.

STUDY GROUP QUESTIONS

- What is stress?
- What theories are associated with stress and the stress response?
- How does the general adaptation syndrome (GAS) work?
- How do nursing theorists explain stress and the stress response?
- What factors influence the response to stress?
- What assessment data may indicate the presence of a stress reaction?
- How does stress relate to illness?
- What are coping/defense mechanisms and how may they be used by individuals to deal with stress?
- What is the role of a nurse in reducing or eliminating stress for patients in health promotion, acute care, and restorative care settings?
- What is involved in crisis intervention?
- What are possible relaxation/stress reduction techniques?

26 Loss and Grief

CASE STUDIES

1. A woman's husband committed suicide and she is devastated by the event. In anticipation of potential difficulties, a nurse should be alert to the possibility of a complicated bereavement.
   a. What assessment data may indicate that the woman is experiencing a complicated period of bereavement?
   b. Identify a possible nursing diagnosis, goals/outcomes, and nursing interventions for an individual who is experiencing a complicated bereavement.

2. The family tells the nurse that the patient is interested in hospice care. The siblings have questions about what services are available. As the nurse, what do you tell them about hospice care?

CHAPTER REVIEW

Match the description/definition in Column A with the correct term in Column B.

Column A	Column B
_____ 1. A lifetime of normal developmental processes	a. Actual loss
_____ 2. Loss that is uniquely experienced by a grieving person and often less obvious to others	b. Perceived loss
	c. Situational loss
_____ 3. The result of an unpredictable life event	d. Maturational loss
_____ 4. When a person can no longer touch, hear, see, or have valued people or objects	

Complete the following:

5. Grief resolution may be affected by:

6. Unexpected unemployment may be perceived as a loss. True _____ False _____

7. Provide an intervention that a nurse should implement for a family dealing with a patient's diagnosis of a terminal illness.

8. Which of the following interventions are appropriate for a terminally ill patient with constipation? Select all that apply.
   a. Maintenance of complete bed rest _____
   b. Increased intake of coffee _____
   c. Consumption of fresh vegetables _____
   d. Consumption of whole grain products _____
   e. Reducing fluid intake _____
   f. Obtaining an order for stool softeners _____

9. Identify at least two nursing measures that may be implemented to facilitate the mourning process.

10. Patients in the terminal stage of their lives may experience a sense of abandonment. What actions should a nurse implement to prevent or reduce this occurrence?

11. After a patient's death, there is federal and state legislation regarding policies and procedures for:

12. Formulate a question that a nurse could ask a patient regarding:
   a. The nature of a loss
   b. His/her cultural beliefs about loss
   c. How the family is coping with the loss

13. A patient has been in hospice care at home. A family member is taking care of the patient and is concerned about the patient's impending death, particularly what will happen to the patient. The nurse informs the family member that the signs of impending death include:

14. According to Worden, moving through the four tasks typically takes _____ (time frame).

15. What are the Rs in Rando's R Process Model?

16. In performing postmortem care, which are the correct actions? Select all that apply.
    a. Position the patient upright at 45 to 90 degrees. _____
    b. Ask the family members if they want to help with the care. _____
    c. Discard remaining personal items. _____
    d. Close the patient's eyes. _____
    e. Leave dentures in the patient's mouth. _____
    f. Remove all of the tubes and devices before an autopsy is performed. _____

17. Identify nursing interventions for the following symptoms that may be experienced by a patient who is dying.
    a. Fatigue:

    b. Decreased appetite

18. Provide an example of delayed grief.

19. When would an autopsy be performed?

20. Identify what should be included in the documentation after a patient's death.

21. What physical signs and symptoms can be associated with grief?

Select the best answer for each of the following questions:

22. A nurse is working with a patient who has been diagnosed with a terminal disease. The patient, who is moving into Kübler-Ross's denial stage of grieving, may respond:
    1. "I understand what the diagnosis means, and I know that I may die."
    2. "I would like to be able to make it to my son's wedding in June."
    3. "I think that the diagnostic tests are wrong, and they should be re-done."
    4. "I don't think that I can stand to have any more treatments. I just want to feel better."

23. While working with young children in a day care center, a nurse responds to instances that occur in their lives. Toddlers at the center generally experience loss and grief associated with:
    1. anticipation of loss.
    2. separation from parents.
    3. changes in physical abilities.
    4. development of their identities.

24. In a senior citizen center, a nurse is talking with a group of older adults. The recurrent theme associated with loss for this age group is a:
    1. confusion of fact and fantasy.
    2. perceived threat to their identity.
    3. change in status, role, and lifestyle.
    4. determination to reexamine life goals.

25. A nurse who has recently graduated from nursing school is employed by an oncology unit. There are a number of patients who will not improve and will need assistance with dying. The nurse prepares for this experience by:
    1. completing a detailed course on legal aspects of end of life issues.
    2. controlling his or her emotions about dying patients.
    3. experiencing the death of a close family member.
    4. identifying his or her own feelings about death and dying.

26. A patient has had a long illness and is now approaching the end stages of his life. To assist this patient to meet his need for self-worth and support during this time, the nurse:
    1. arranges for a grief counselor to visit.
    2. leaves the patient alone to deal with his life issues.
    3. asks the patient's family to take over his care.
    4. plans to visit the patient regularly throughout the day.

27. The spouse of a patient who has just died is having more frequent episodes of headaches and generalized joint pain. The initial nursing intervention for this individual is to:
    1. complete a thorough pain assessment.
    2. encourage more frequent use of analgesics.
    3. sit with the patient and encourage discussion of feelings.
    4. refer the patient immediately to a psychologist or grief counselor.

28. A patient is experiencing a very serious illness that may not be curable. The nurse promotes hope for this patient when:
    1. establishing firm goals.
    2. encouraging the development of supportive relationships.
    3. withholding information about the illness and its treatment.
    4. referring the patient for psychological counseling.

29. A patient in the long-term care facility is to receive palliative care measures only during the end stages of a terminal illness. The nurse anticipates that this will include:
    1. pain relief measures.
    2. emergency surgery.
    3. pulmonary resuscitation.
    4. transfer to intensive care if necessary.

30. A patient arrives for outpatient chemotherapy. During this visit the patient tells the nurse that she is experiencing periods of nausea. The nurse promotes patient comfort by providing:
    1. milk.
    2. coffee.
    3. ginger ale.
    4. orange juice.

31. The loss of a known environment is associated with:
    1. being hospitalized for several days.
    2. the death of a pet.
    3. amputation of the right leg.
    4. a recent burglary in the home.

32. Of the following, a situational loss occurs when a:
    1. parent requires physical assistance.
    2. family friend dies.
    3. child goes to college.
    4. job demotion and pay reduction occur.

33. An individual in Bowlby's second phase of mourning, yearning, and searching may be expected to:
    1. be unable to believe the loss.
    2. endlessly examine how the loss occurred.
    3. acquire new skills and build new relationships.
    4. experience emotional outbursts and sobbing.

34. A nurse recognizes exaggerated grief in the person who:
    1. has an active period of mourning that does not decrease and continues over time.
    2. postpones or holds back grieving and responds much later to the event.
    3. cannot function and is overwhelmed, with resulting substance abuse or phobias.
    4. is not aware that behaviors are interfering with daily activities, such as sleeping and eating.

35. The nurse is using Worden's four tasks of mourning to assess the family member's response to the death of a loved one. What is expected when the individual moves into Task III: *Adjust to the environment in which the deceased is missing*?
    1. Realizing that the loved one is gone
    2. Suppressing feelings over the loss
    3. Taking on roles of the loved one
    4. Forgetting the deceased and moving on

STUDY GROUP QUESTIONS

- What are loss and grief?
- What are the different types of loss and possible reactions to these losses?
- What are the differences and similarities between the theories of grief and loss?
- What is anticipatory grief?
- How may the grieving process be influenced by special circumstances?
- How are hope, spirituality, and self-concept related to loss and grieving?
- What behaviors are associated with loss and grieving?
- What resources are available for patient, family, and nurse that assist in the grieving process?
- What principles facilitate mourning?
- How may a nurse apply critical thinking and nursing processes to the patient/family experiencing loss and grieving?
- How are religious and cultural beliefs associated with loss, grief, death, and dying?
- How may a nurse intervene to assist a patient/family with loss and the grieving process?
- What is involved in care of the body after death?

27 Exercise and Activity

CASE STUDY

1. A nurse is assigned to work with an 80-year-old woman residing in a nursing home. There is conflicting information in the chart about her ability to move around independently. The nurse is concerned about meeting her needs for proper body mechanics as well as her safety.
   a. What important assessment information is needed to plan meeting the patient's needs?
   b. If the patient is unable to ambulate independently, what nursing interventions should be planned?

CHAPTER REVIEW

Match the description/definition in Column A with the correct term in Column B.

	Column A	*Column B*
_i_	1. Awareness of the position of the body and its parts	a. Body mechanics
_g_	2. Resistance that a moving body meets from the surface on which it moves	b. Prone
_h._	3. Manner or style of walking	c. Range of motion
_f_	4. Lying face up	d. Posture
_b_	5. Lying face down	e. Dorsiflexion
_e_	6. Movement of the foot where the toes point upward	f. Supine
_a_	7. Maintenance of optimal body position	g. Friction
_d._	8. Body alignment during walking, turning, lifting, or carrying	h. Gait
_c._	9. Mobility of the joint	i. Proprioception

Complete the following:

10. Identify at least three components to assess to determine a patient's mobility.

    range of motion, gait, balance, posture

11. Which of the following are correct principles of body mechanics? Select all that apply.
    a. Maintain a narrow base of support. _____
    b. Face the direction of movement. _____
    c. Maintain a higher center of gravity. _____
    d. Divide balanced activity between the arms and legs. _____
    e. Increase friction between the object and surface. _____
    f. Alternate periods of rest and activity. _____

12. The best way to determine a patient's level of pain is to observe for redness or swelling of the joints.
    True _____ False _X_

13. For a patient who has been on prolonged bed rest:
    a. What should the nurse do to prepare the patient before ambulation? *Sitting position w/ legs dangling*
    b. Transfers and position changes for this patient can lead to the development of:
    orthostatic hypotension

14. Identify at least two pathological influences on alignment, exercise, or activity.

    Congenital defects
    defects of joints, bones + muscles
    CNS damage

15. Range of motion can be determined by observing the patient's gait and ability to perform activities of daily living.
True ✗   False _____

16. An example of a physiological factor that may influence activity tolerance is:

diminished cardiovascular or respiratory function

17. Identify a nursing diagnosis associated with a change in a patient's ability to maintain physical activity.

Activity intolerance, risk for injury, impaired physical mobility, acute or chronic pain

18. For a patient who has severe arthritis and is unable to perform activities of daily living because of discomfort on movement, the priority is to:

pain relief

19. A patient with a respiratory condition should be positioned in:

Fowlers 45-60° or semi-fowlers 30°

20. Complete the following about transferring patients.
    a. The general "rule of thumb" for transfers is: Get help
    b. A nurse's priority during patient transfers is: Safety

21. Identify the following patient positions:

a. _Supine_

b. _prone_

c. _lateral_

22. Which of the following are expected findings for assessment of a patient while standing? Select all that apply.
    (a.) Head is erect and midline. _____
    b. Body parts are asymmetrical. _____
    c. The spine has a lateral curve. _____
    d. The abdomen protrudes. _____
    (e.) The knees are in a straight line between the hips and ankles. _____
    f. The feet are pointed at an angle and close together. _____
    (g.) The arms hang comfortably at the sides. _____

23. Which of the following indicate correct care or technique for a patient who is using crutches? Select all that apply.
    a. The patient leans on the axillae to support his or her weight. _____
    (b.) Both crutches are transferred to one hand when preparing to sit. _____
    c. Crutches are placed 1 foot to the front and side of the feet. _____
    (d.) The patient has a non–weight-bearing left leg and is using a three-point gait. _____
    (e.) The unaffected leg is advanced first when the patient goes up the stairs. _____

24. Patients who are on prolonged bed rest need to be repositioned at least every _2_ hours.

25. a. When transferring patients who are able to assist from the bed to a chair, the chair should be positioned:
    toward strong side @ 45° angle towards bed
    b. Identify the steps, in order, for the use of a mechanical lift.

26. Logrolling a patient in bed requires at least _3_ caregivers to perform.

27. A nurse observes a patient and notes that there is limited range of motion in a few areas. This could be the result of:
    Inflammation, arthritis, altered nerve supply

28. The patient, who has some mobility in the upper arms and legs, needs to be moved up in bed. What should the nurse do to reduce friction when moving the patient?
    Patient assistance + use drawsheet

29. Half of all back pain is associated with:
    manual lifting

30. Improper positioning of patients in bed can lead to:
    pressure ulcers + contractures

31. What position is contraindicated for a patient who is obese or has a respiratory condition?
    prone

32. A mechanical device that is used for specific repetitive joint exercise is a:
    CPM machine
    Continuous passive motion

Select the best answer for each of the following questions:

33. A patient is able to bear weight on one foot. The crutch walking gait that the nurse teaches this patient is the:
    1. two-point gait.
    2. swing-through gait.
    3. three-point alternating gait.
    4. four-point alternating gait.

34. A nurse is working with a patient who is able only to minimally assist the nurse in moving from the bed to the chair. The nurse must help the patient stand. The correct technique for lifting the patient to stand and pivot to the chair is to:
    1. keep the legs straight.
    2. maintain a wide base with the feet.
    3. keep the stomach muscles loose.
    4. support the patient away from the body.

35. A nurse is assisting a patient who has been prescribed total bed rest to perform range-of-motion exercises. The nurse performs the exercises by:
    1. hyperextending the joints.
    2. working from proximal to distal joints.
    3. flexing the joints beyond where slight resistance is felt.
    4. providing support for joints distal to the joint being exercised.

36. A patient has experienced an injury to his lower extremity. The orthopedist has prescribed the use of crutches and a four-point gait. The nurse instructs the patient using this gait to:
    1. move the right foot forward first.
    2. move both crutches forward together.
    3. move the right foot and the left crutch together.
    4. move the right foot and the right crutch together.

37. The patient had a cerebrovascular accident (CVA/stroke) with resultant left hemiparesis. The nurse is instructing the patient on the use of a cane for support during ambulation. The nurse instructs the patient to:
    1. use the cane on the right side.
    2. use the cane on the left side.
    3. move the left foot forward first.
    4. move the right foot forward first.

38. A patient is admitted to the rehabilitation facility for physical therapy after an automobile accident. To conduct an assessment of the patient's body alignment, the nurse should begin by:
    1. observing the patient's gait.
    2. putting the patient at ease.
    3. determining the level of activity tolerance.
    4. evaluating the full extent of joint range of motion.

39. An average-size female patient who resides in the extended care facility requires assistance to ambulate down the hall. The nurse has noticed that the patient has some weakness on her right side. The nurse assists this patient to ambulate by:
    1. standing at her left side and holding the patient's arm.
    2. walking in front of her and having her hold on to her waist.
    3. standing behind her and encircling one arm around the patient's waist.
    4. standing at her right side and using a gait belt.

40. A patient has a cast on the right foot and is being discharged home. Crutches will be used for ambulation, and the patient has stairs to manage to enter the house and to get to the bedroom and bathroom. The nurse observes the patient using the correct technique in using the crutches on the stairs when the patient:
    1. advances the crutches first to ascend the stairs.
    2. uses one crutch for support while going up and down.
    3. uses the banister or wall for support when descending the stairs.
    4. advances the affected leg after moving the crutches when descending the stairs.

41. A patient is getting up to ambulate for the first time since a surgical procedure. While ambulating in the hallway, the patient complains of severe dizziness. The nurse should first:
    1. call for help.
    2. lower the patient gently to the floor.
    3. lean the patient against the wall until the episode passes.
    4. support the patient and move quickly back to the room.

42. One of the expected benefits of exercise is:
    1. decreased diaphragmatic excursion.
    2. decreased cardiac output.
    3. increased fatigue.
    4. decreased resting heart rate.

43. A nurse selects which of the following for maintaining dorsiflexion of a patient?
    1. Pillows
    2. Foot boots
    3. Bed boards
    4. Trochanter rolls

44. A nurse recognizes that the position that is contraindicated for a patient who is at risk for aspiration is:
    1. Fowler's.
    2. lateral.
    3. Sims'.
    4. supine.

45. A patient had total hip replacement surgery and requires careful postoperative positioning to maintain the legs in abduction. The nurse will obtain a:
    1. foot boot.
    2. trapeze bar.
    3. bed board.
    4. wedge pillow.

46. The patient is placed in bed in Fowler's position. To prevent external rotation of the hips, the nurse uses:
    1. foot boots.
    2. trochanter rolls.
    3. leg splints.
    4. side rails.

47. The first step in initiating an exercise program for a patient is to:
    1. select the equipment.
    2. design the fitness program.
    3. schedule time during the day.
    4. seek approval from the health care prescriber.

STUDY GROUP QUESTIONS

- What are body mechanics?
- How is body movement regulated by the musculoskeletal and nervous systems?
- What general changes occur in the body's appearance and function throughout growth and development?
- How can body mechanics be influenced by pathological conditions?
- What patient assessment data should be obtained regarding body mechanics?
- What is activity tolerance?
- How can proper body mechanics be promoted for patients in different health care settings?
- What safety measures should be implemented before patient transfers and ambulation?
- What are the proper procedures for range-of-motion exercises, transfers, positioning, and ambulation?
- How should a patient be instructed to use assistive devices, such as canes, walkers, and crutches?

STUDY CHART

Create a study chart to describe how to *Safely Use Assistive Devices for Ambulation* which identifies the nursing actions and patient instruction required to reduce possible hazards for the following devices: gait belt, cane, walker, crutches.

28 Safety

CASE STUDIES

1. You will be accompanying the visiting nurse to the home of a family with two young children who are ages 2 and 4 years.
   a. What general assessment information should be obtained regarding home safety during the visit?
   b. What specific safety observations should be made because there are two young children residing in the home?

2. A patient with diabetes mellitus is living at home and needs to take daily insulin injections.
   a. What are some of the precautions that this patient should take to avoid pathogen transmission and maintain safety?

3. You are currently working in a long-term care facility. There are a number of patients who are recognized as being at risk for falls. A restraint-free environment is desired.
   a. What specific interventions may be implemented to prevent falls and provide for patient safety without the use of restraints?

CHAPTER REVIEW

Complete the following:

1. Identify an example of a problem that may be encountered if a basic human need of a safe environment is not met.

2. Provide an example of a possible physical hazard that may be found in the home.

3. For older adults:
   a. Identify at least three (3) physiological changes that increase the risk of accidents for older adults.
   b. Indicate at least two (2) areas that should be included in teaching the older adult about:
      (1) Driving safety
      (2) Home environment safety

4. For each of the following, identify a nursing intervention that may be implemented to prevent injury and promote patient safety.
   a. Falls
   b. Patient-inherent accidents
   c. Procedure-related risks
   d. Equipment-related risks

5. The Centers for Medicare and Medicaid Services (CMS) have identified that payment will be denied for events that are not present on admission but occur during hospitalization. Which of the following are included in the listing of these "never events"? Select all that apply.
   a. Air embolism _____
   b. Blood transfusion _____
   c. Patient falls _____
   d. Wrong medication administered _____
   e. Surgical site infection _____
   f. Stage III pressure ulcer _____

6. Immunity that occurs as a result of injection of weakened or dead organisms and modified toxins is called:

7. For each of the following age groups, identify an example of a potential safety hazard.
   a. Infant, toddler, preschooler
   b. School-age child
   c. Adolescent
   d. Adult
   e. Older adult

8. During an assessment, a nurse determines that a patient with a high risk for injury is an individual experiencing:

9. For each of the following potential bioterrorist methods, identify a possible agent that may be used.
   a. Biological
   b. Chemical
   c. Radiological

10. There is a greater risk for poisoning as a result of finding multiple medications in the home of an older adult.
    True _____ False _____

11. An example of safety instruction for a school-age child would be:

12. The primary goal when using restraints (safety reminder devices) is to:

13. A restraint is indicated for a patient in the hospital. Which of the following are correct for the use of restraints? Select all that apply.
    a. Obtain renewals for restraint orders every 72 hours. _____
    b. Evaluate the patient at least every 2 hours. _____
    c. Pad the skin under the restraint. _____
    d. Remove the restraint at least every 2 hours. _____
    e. At least two fingers should fit under the secured restraint. _____
    f. Tie the restraint ends with a knot. _____
    g. Attach the restraint ties to the side rails. _____

14. Side rails may be used at any time to keep a patient in bed.
    True _____ False _____

15. An older adult patient who often forgets to take medication or does not remember if it was taken may benefit from a(n):

16. Identify an example of a medication safety strategy that is used in a health care agency.

17. For the following areas, identify a specific environmental adjustment that should be made to promote safety.
    a. Tactile deficit
    b. Visual deficit

18. Identify an example of an intervention that may be implemented as an alternative to patient restraint.

19. An example of a nursing diagnosis associated with patient safety concerns is:

20. Carbon monoxide poisoning can occur in the home.
    a. Identify the signs and symptoms associated with low concentrations.
    b. What safety measure is necessary to prevent exposure?

21. Explain the "Speak Up" campaign.

22. What resources/agencies are available for patient safety standards?

23. What are the leading causes of falls in the (a) home and (b) health care agency?

24. Information about chemical substances in the health care workplace can be found in:

25. The parents of an adolescent are concerned about possible substance abuse. What signs, symptoms, and behaviors are indicative of this problem?

26. For disaster management, hospitals are required to have what resources in place?

27. The application of physical restraints may be delegated to nursing assistive personnel.
    True _____ False _____

28. Identify the meaning of the following for fire management:
    R -   P -
    A -   A -
    C -   S -
    E -   S -

29. Match the type of fire extinguisher with the form of fire.
    Type A, Type B, Type C
    a. Grease fire _____
    b. Electrical fire _____
    c. Paper fire _____

30. The nurse notices that the plug for the infusion pump makes a spark when it is plugged into the wall socket. The nurse should:

31. Identify at least one (1) Patient Safety Goal identified by The Joint Commission for the following:
    a. Hospitals
    b. Home care

32. Place the steps for the Timed Get Up and Go Test in order:
    a. Stand still momentarily _____
    b. Sit down _____
    c. Walk 10 feet (3 meters) (in a line) _____
    d. Turn around _____
    e. Stand up from the armchair _____
    f. Walk back to chair _____
    g. Turn around _____

    What is an abnormal result for the test?

33. Indicate safety measures for the following:
    a. Use of home oxygen
    b. Food preparation

34. For the following patient scenario, identify the assessment findings that the nurse should focus on to prevent patient injuries.

    Upon entering the patient's home, the visiting nurse observed that the patient was wearing slippers with no back (slip-ons). The patient stated that she seemed always to leave her glasses somewhere. There were piles of newspapers and other items cluttering the floor around the living room chairs. The lighting in the stairway was less than 60 watts and there were throw rugs on the wood floors in the halls. When looking through the medicine cabinet with the patient, the nurse noted that some medications were expired. The patient admitted to falling once when getting up during the night to go to the bathroom.

Select the best answer for each of the following questions:

35. The nurse recognizes the importance of teaching the patient who is using oxygen at home that the leading cause of burns and fires is:
    1. smoking.
    2. the use of heating blankets.
    3. the misuse of the stove.
    4. damage to the oxygen tank.

36. An older adult patient is being discharged home. The patient will be taking furosemide (Lasix) on a daily basis. A specific consideration for this patient is:
    1. exposure to the sun.
    2. food consumption when taking the medication.
    3. the location of the bathroom.
    4. financial considerations for long-term care.

37. While walking through a hallway in the extended care facility, a nurse notices smoke coming from a wastebasket in a patient's room. Upon closer investigation, the nurse identifies that there is a fire that is starting to flare up. The nurse should first:
    1. extinguish the fire.
    2. remove the patient from the room.
    3. contain the fire by closing the door to the room.
    4. turn off all of the surrounding electrical equipment.

38. A patient is newly admitted to the hospital and appears to be disoriented. There is a concern for the patient's immediate safety. The nurse is considering the use of restraints to prevent an injury. The nurse recognizes that the use of restraints in a hospital requires:
    1. a physician's order.
    2. the patient's consent.
    3. a family member's consent.
    4. agreement among the nursing staff.

39. A nurse is completing admission histories for newly admitted patients to the unit. The nurse is aware that the patient with the greatest risk of injury:
    1. is 84 years of age.
    2. uses corrective lenses.
    3. has a history of falls.
    4. has arthritis in the lower extremities.

40. A child has ingested a poisonous substance. The parent is instructed by the nurse to:
    1. take the child to the hospital immediately.
    2. call the poison control center.
    3. take the child to the pediatrician.
    4. administer 30 mL of emetic.

41. A restraint that may be used to prevent an adult patient from pulling on and removing tubes or an IV is a(n):
    1. vest restraint.
    2. jacket restraint.
    3. extremity restraint.
    4. mummy restraint.

42. An older adult patient in the extended care facility has been wandering outside of the room during the late evening hours. The patient has a history of falls. The nurse intervenes initially by:
    1. placing an abdominal restraint on the patient during the night.
    2. keeping the light and the television on in the patient's room all night.
    3. reassigning the patient to a room close to the nursing station.
    4. having the family members check on the patient during the night.

43. A parent with three children has gone to the outpatient clinic. The children range in age from 2½ to 15 years old. A nurse is discussing safety issues with the parent. The nurse evaluates that further teaching is required if the parent states:
    1. "I have spoken to my teenager about safe sex practices."
    2. "I make sure that my child wears a helmet when he rides his bicycle."
    3. "My 8-year-old is taking swimming classes at the local community center."
    4. "Now my 2½-year-old can finally sit in the front seat of the car with me."

44. A bacteria that is spread through inadequate preparation or storage of food is:
    1. *Streptococcus.*
    2. *Candida.*
    3. *Listeria.*
    4. *Hepatitis B.*

STUDY GROUP QUESTIONS

- What are the basic human needs regarding safety?
- What are some physical hazards and how can they be reduced or eliminated?
- What developmental changes and abilities predispose individuals to accidents or injury?
- What additional risk factors may affect an individual's level of safety?
- What risks exist in a health care agency, and how can they be prevented?
- What safety measures and patient teaching should be implemented in different health care settings?
- What are the procedures for the correct use of side rails and restraints?
- How can a nurse avoid the use of patient restraints?
- What assessment information should be obtained regarding patient/family safety?
- How can a nurse assist patients and families in reducing or eliminating safety hazards?

29 Hygiene

CASE STUDIES

1. Your clinical experience is scheduled to be on a medical unit. It will be your responsibility to provide instruction to a patient who has just been diagnosed with diabetes mellitus.
   a. What specific information on hygienic care will be included for the patient's teaching session?

2. An older adult patient residing in an extended care facility requires assistance with hygienic care.
   a. What developmental changes are considered when assisting this patient to meet hygienic needs?

CHAPTER REVIEW

Match the description/definition in Column A with the correct term in Column B.

	Column A	Column B
e	1. Inflammation of the skin characterized by abrupt onset with erythema, pruritus, pain, and scaly oozing lesions	a. Abrasion
i	2. Thickened portion of the epidermis, usually flat and painless, on the undersurface of the foot or hand	b. Without teeth
h	3. Inflammation of the tissue surrounding the nail	c. Plantar wart
a	4. Scraping or rubbing away of the epidermis, resulting in localized bleeding	d. Xerosis
f	5. Keratosis caused by friction and pressure from shoes, mainly on toes	e. Contact dermatitis
c	6. Fungating lesion that appears on the sole of the foot	f. Corn
j	7. Loss of hair	g. Gingivitis
b	8. Edentulous	h. Paronychia
g	9. Inflammation of the gums	i. Callus
d	10. Abnormal drying of the skin	j. Alopecia

Complete the following:

11. Identify at least three (3) factors that contribute to a hygiene self-care deficit.
    diminished mobility, pain, mental illness, socioeconomic status

12. What modifications are done when providing hygienic care to a patient with dementia?

    In bed approach with no rinse soap

13. Which of the following techniques are appropriate for diabetic foot care? Select all that apply.
    a. Soaking the feet _____
    b. Rubbing the feet vigorously to dry them _____
    c. Walking barefoot to toughen the feet _____
    d. Applying lotion for dryness _____
    e. Wearing clean, white cotton socks _____
    f. Using a heating pad to warm the feet _____
    g. Applying a mild antiseptic to small cuts _____
    h. Avoiding elastic stockings _____

14. A nurse-initiated treatment for a skin rash is:

warm soak

15. When cleansing a patient's eyes, the nurse should use:

just water

16. The nurse recognizes that the skin goes through changes throughout the life span. Which of the following are accurate statements regarding the characteristics of the skin? Select all that apply.
    a. Neonatal skin is thinner. _____ *(circled)*
    b. The sebaceous glands become active during the toddler years. _____
    c. Young adult skin should be elastic, firm, and smooth. _____ *(circled)*
    d. The sweat glands are fully functional at puberty. _____ *(circled)*
    e. Skin thickens progressively with aging. _____
    f. Lubrication from the skin glands diminishes over time. _____ *(circled)*

17. For hygienic care, the nurse applies the ethical principle of autonomy, which means that the nurse should:

Allow patient to do as much as they are able

18. When is a standing shower contraindicated for a patient?

history of falls, fatigue or weakness

19. For the patient with a nursing diagnosis of *Activity Intolerance*, how can hygienic care be affected?

rest periods + repositioning during care

20. Identify ways that the nurse can promote healthy skin for the patient.

Assessment + reporting of changes + abnormalities in skin

21. True/False:
    a. Cotton-tipped applicators should be used to remove earwax.
       True _____   False _X_
    b. A 5- to 10-minute bath can add moisture to the skin of an older adult.
       True _X_   False _____

22. The nurse wants to help the patient to have healthy teeth and gums. Which of the following recommendations should be made to the patient? Select all that apply.
    a. Change the toothbrush every 6 to 8 months. _____
    b. Use a soft-bristle toothbrush with a straight handle. _____ *(circled)*
    c. Floss at least once each day. _____ *(circled)*
    d. Brush the teeth at least once each day. _____
    e. Use a toothbrush cover to protect the bristles. _____

23. Evidence-based practice indicates that this product is more effective than soap in reducing the bacteria found in washbasins:

Chlorhexidine gluconate 4%

24. The patient's eyeglasses should be kept:

in a case in the drawer of the bedside table

25. Ear irrigation is contraindicated in the presence of:

eardrum, perforated tympanic membrane

26. Asepsis is maintained during linen changes when the nurse:

linens away from uniform, soiled linens in laundry bin

27. Provide an example of how the nurse prepares a comfortable environment for the patient in the health care facility:

room temp, lighting, quiet, clean

28. Identify physiological conditions that may place a patient at risk for impaired skin integrity.

Vascular insufficiency, diabetes, incontinence

29. How does the use of a commercial "bag bath" differ from a regular patient bed bath?

No rinsing required

30. Identify a safety measure that is implemented when providing a tub bath for a patient.

assess for mobility, non slip mat, check on them

31. How may patients' cultural background influence their hygienic care practices?

frequency of showering

32. A nurse notes that a young adult patient has acne of the face and back. What care should be provided?

oil free cosmetics + diet change

33. Identify at least three guidelines for patient bathing and skin care.

mild cleanser, warm water, no force, Rom exercises

34. What patients may require special oral hygiene?

unconscious + artificial airways

35. Place the steps of the bed bath in the correct order:
    a. Back _7_
    b. Arms _2_
    c. Face _1_
    d. Abdomen _4_
    e. Legs _5_
    f. Perineal area _6_
    g. Chest _3_

36. Identify safety measures that should be implemented during oral care for an unconscious patient.

Check for gag reflex, suction to prevent aspiration

37. What is the procedure for irrigation of the ear?

38. Before providing nail care for a patient who is not diabetic, the nurse should:

    Soak for 10 minutes

39. During the bath, the nurse assesses the patient carefully. There are signs of vascular insufficiency in the lower extremities. This is determined based upon finding:

    No hair growth, infection, thick nails

40. What special considerations are included for the hygienic care of the older adult?

    Skin is more fragile, use warm water + mild soap

41. For the patient who uses a hearing aid, which are the appropriate instructions for the nurse to provide to the patient? Select all that apply.
    a. Check for whistling sounds _____
    b. Wear the hearing aid continuously _____
    c. Store the hearing aid in a warm, heated place _____
    d. Use alcohol to clean the hearing aid _____
    e. Check the battery while the hearing aid is in the ear _____
    f. Remove the battery if the hearing aid is not going to be used for a day or two _____

Select the best answer for each of the following questions:

42. A nurse is caring for an older adult patient in an extended care facility. The patient wears dentures, and the nurse delegated their care to the nursing assistant. The nurse instructs the assistant that the patient's dentures should be:
    1. cleaned in hot water.
    2. left in place during the night.
    3. brushed with a soft toothbrush.
    4. wrapped in a soft towel when not worn.

43. A nurse determines, after completing an assessment, that an expected outcome for a patient with impaired skin integrity will be that the:
    1. skin remains dry.
    2. skin has increased erythema.
    3. skin tingles in areas of pressure.
    4. skin demonstrates increased diaphoresis.

44. A patient has been hospitalized following a traumatic injury. The nurse is now able to provide hair care for the patient. The nurse includes:
    1. using hot water to rinse the scalp.
    2. cutting away matted or tangled hair.
    3. using the fingernails to massage the patient's scalp.
    4. applying peroxide to dissolve blood in the hair and then rinsing with saline.

45. While completing a patient's bath, a nurse notices a red, raised skin rash on the patient's chest. The next step for the nurse to take is to:
    1. moisturize the skin with lotion.
    2. wash the area again with hot water and soap.
    3. discuss proper hygienic care with the patient.
    4. assess for any other areas of inflammation.

46. A nurse is planning patient assignment with a nursing assistant. In delegating the morning care for a patient, the nurse expects the assistant to:
    1. cut the patient's nails with scissors.
    2. use soap to wash the patient's eyes.
    3. wash the patient's legs with long strokes from the ankle to the knee.
    4. place the unconscious patient in high-Fowler's position to provide oral hygiene.

47. A patient is receiving chemotherapy and is experiencing stomatitis. To promote comfort for this patient, a nurse recommends that the patient use:
    1. a firm toothbrush.
    2. normal saline rinses.
    3. a commercial mouthwash.
    4. an alcohol and water mixture.

48. For a patient with dry skin, a nurse should:
    1. apply moisturizing lotion.
    2. use hot water for bathing.
    3. obtain a dehumidifier.
    4. wash the skin frequently.

49. Use of an electric razor is specifically indicated for a patient who is being treated with:
    1. diuretics.
    2. antibiotics.
    3. anticoagulants.
    4. narcotic analgesics.

50. When making an occupied bed, the first step for a nurse is to:
    1. cover the patient with a bath blanket.
    2. position the patient on the far side of the bed.
    3. explain the procedure to the patient.
    4. adjust the height of the bed to waist level.

51. The nurse is providing information to a group of parents. Which of the following statements provides accurate information about the teeth?
    1. Permanent teeth are in place at 13 years of age.
    2. Wisdom teeth erupt in the 35 and older age group.
    3. The first permanent teeth come in at around 3 years of age.
    4. Teething occurs after the child reaches 1½ to 2 years old.

52. The nurse manager is evaluating a new staff member's patient care. Which of the following interventions demonstrates correct technique?
    1. Placing the bedpan on the overbed table
    2. Returning extra linens from the patient's room to the linen cart
    3. Using side rails all the time to keep the patient safely in bed
    4. Moving the bed up to change the linen and reposition the patient

STUDY GROUP QUESTIONS

- What hygienic care measures are necessary for the integumentary system?
- What factors may influence a patient's hygienic care practices?
- How do growth and development influence hygienic care needs?
- What are the patient teaching needs for hygienic care across the life span?
- What assessments of the integumentary system are necessary to determine integumentary alterations and hygienic care needs?
- What are the correct procedures for providing hygienic care and a comfortable environment for patients?
- How does a patient's self-care ability influence the provision of hygienic care?
- How is physical assessment integrated into the provision of hygienic care?
- What actions should be taken if a patient refuses hygienic care?

30 Oxygenation

CASE STUDY

1. You are the nurse in an outpatient clinic in which a 32-year-old woman receives ongoing medical treatment. She tells you that she has had asthma since she was a young child. While speaking with the patient, you notice that she is exhibiting mild wheezing and a productive cough. She appears slightly pale.
   a. What additional assessment questions should be asked of this patient?
   b. Identify a possible nursing diagnosis for this patient.
   c. What nurse-initiated actions may be taken at this time?
   d. Identify general information that should be included in patient teaching for promoting oxygenation.

CHAPTER REVIEW

Match the description/definition in Column A with the correct term in Column B.

	Column A	Column B
c	1. Collapse of alveoli, preventing exchange of oxygen	a. Hypoxia
d	2. Tachypnea pattern of breathing associated with metabolic acidosis	b. Pneumothorax
e	3. Need to sit upright to breathe easier	c. Atelectasis
b	4. Collection of air in the pleural space	d. Kussmaul respiration
i	5. Bloody sputum	e. Orthopnea
a	6. Inadequate tissue oxygenation at the cellular level	f. Hemothorax
g	7. Amount of blood in the ventricles at the end of diastole	g. Preload
f	8. Collection of blood in the pleural space	h. Afterload
h	9. Resistance of ejection of blood from the left ventricle	i. Hemoptysis
j	10. Difficulty breathing, sensation of breathlessness	j. Dyspnea

Complete the following:

11. The average resting heart rate for an adult is _____ beats per minute.

12. Chest movement is affected by what conditions?

13. Identify whether the following signs and symptoms are associated with left ventricular or right ventricular heart failure:
    a. Distended neck veins _____
    b. Ankle edema _____
    c. Pulmonary congestion _____
    d. Increased arterial blood pressure _____

14. Which of the following may cause hyperventilation? Select all that apply.
    a. Anxiety _____
    b. Fever _____
    c. Severe atelectasis _____
    d. Head injury _____
    e. Excessive administration of oxygen _____

15. Provide an example of a physiological alteration or problem that may result in each of the following:
    a. Decreased oxygen-carrying capacity
    b. Decreased inspired oxygen concentration
    c. Hypovolemia
    d. Increased metabolic rate

16. A premature infant has a deficiency of _____ and is at risk for hyaline membrane disease.

17. An example of a controllable risk factor for cardiopulmonary disease is:

18. Which of the following pathophysiological changes in the heart and lungs occur with aging? Select all that apply.
    a. Thinning of the ventricular wall of the heart _____
    b. SA node becoming fibrotic from calcification _____
    c. Increased elastin in the arterial vessel walls _____
    d. Increased chest wall compliance and elastic recoil _____

e. Decreased alveolar surface area _____
f. Increased responsiveness of central and peripheral chemoreceptors _____
g. Decreased number of cilia _____
h. Increased respiratory drive _____

19. A patient awakes in a panic and feels as though she is suffocating. This is noted by the nurse as:

20. A musical, high-pitched lung sound that may be heard on inspiration or expiration is:

21. Identify the following two cardiac rhythms:
    a.

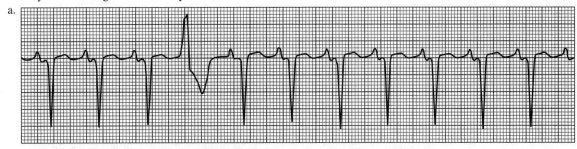

    b.

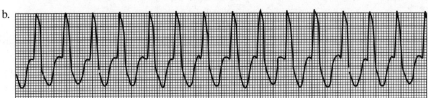

22. Briefly define the following abnormal chest wall movements:
    a. Retraction
    b. Paradoxical breathing

23. Which type of asepsis is used for tracheal suctioning?

24. Continuous bubbling in the chest tube water-seal chamber indicates:

25. Identify an example of a nursing intervention for promotion of each of the following:
    a. Dyspnea management
    b. Patent airway
    c. Lung expansion
    d. Mobilization of secretions

26. Identify the following types of oxygen delivery systems and the flow rate for each:
    a.

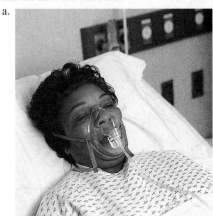

b.

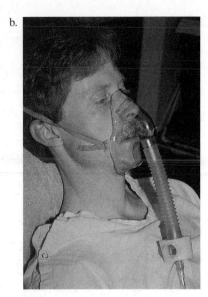

27. Identify the following for tuberculin (Mantoux) testing:
    a. A skin test is administered on a patient's:
    b. The test is read after _____ hours.
    c. A reddened, flat area is a(n) _____ reaction.
    d. The patient received a BCG vaccination, so the tuberculin skin test will most likely be:
       Positive _____   Negative _____

28. For chest percussion, vibration, and postural drainage:
    a. Chest percussion is contraindicated for a patient with:
    b. Vibration is used only during:
    c. The position for a 2-year-old for postural drainage is:

29. For continuous positive airway pressure (CPAP):
    a. CPAP is used for:
    b. The usual pressure setting is:
    c. A disadvantage of CPAP is:
    d. How is BiPAP different from CPAP?

30. For home oxygen therapy:
    a. It is indicated when the patient has an SaO_2 value of:
    b. What safety measures should be implemented when oxygen is used in the home?

31. The interventions in CPR are:
    C -
    A -
    B -

32. Defibrillation is recommended within _____ (time) for an out-of-hospital sudden cardiac arrest and within _____ (time) for an inpatient.

33. a. The prevalence of atrial fibrillation increases with age and is the leading contributing factor for stroke in the older adult.
       True _____ False _____
    b. Care of chest tubes can be delegated to a nursing assistant.
       True _____ False _____

34. The patient has oxygen via a nasal cannula. What specific nursing care should be provided for this patient?

35. For the nursing diagnosis *Ineffective Airway Clearance related to the presence of tracheobronchial secretions,* identify a patient outcome and a nursing intervention to assist the patient to meet the outcome.

36. Which of the following are appropriate interventions for patient suctioning? Select all that apply.
    a. Performing pharyngeal suctioning before tracheal suctioning _____
    b. Avoiding routine use of normal saline instillations when suctioning _____
    c. Applying suction for 30 seconds at a time _____
    d. Suctioning during the insertion and removal of the tube _____
    e. Allowing 1 to 2 minutes between suction passes _____
    f. Providing regular suctioning every 1 to 2 hours around the clock _____

37. Cardiac output is the result of the stroke volume × _____.

38. For a patient with hypoxia:
    a. What are the signs and symptoms?
    b. What treatment is anticipated?

39. Identify a possible nursing diagnosis for a patient with anemia.

40. Provide examples of dietary risks that may influence cardiopulmonary status and oxygenation.

41. The most effective positioning for a patient with cardiopulmonary disease is:

42. A method to encourage voluntary deep breathing for a postoperative patient is the use of an:

43. Identify at least two environmental or occupational hazards that may affect an individual's cardiopulmonary functioning:

44. Cardiac dysrhythmias may be caused by:

45. The nurse anticipates that atrial fibrillation will be treated with:

46. To reduce the incidence of ventilator associated pneumonia (VAP), the nurse will implement:

47. The nurse anticipates that treatment for hyperventilation will include:

48. Place the following steps for in-line suctioning in the correct sequence. The nurse has already positioned the patient and performed hand hygiene.
    a. Reassess pulmonary status. _____
    b. Insert the catheter until resistance is felt. _____
    c. Hyperoxygenate the patient. _____
    d. Withdraw the catheter, applying suction. _____
    e. Repeat the procedure, if indicated. _____
    f. Pick up the catheter enclosed in the plastic sheath. _____

49. Identify the areas on the chest tube system illustration below.

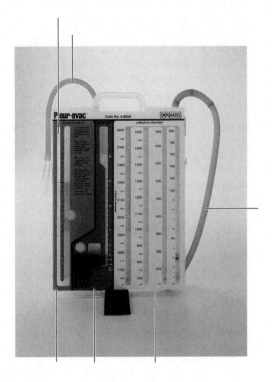

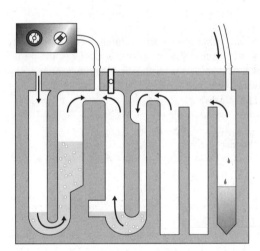

50. Identify the appropriate care for a patient with a closed chest tube drainage system in place. Select all that apply.
    a. Clamp the chest tube when the patient ambulates. _____
    b. Milk the tube for the patient who has just had thoracic surgery. _____
    c. Instruct the patient to inhale if the tube disconnects. _____
    d. Report more than 100 mL of sanguinous drainage after the patient is more than 8 hours postoperative. _____
    e. Keep the drainage unit upright. _____

51. Identify at least three (3) pathologies that reduce chest wall expansion.

52. Signs and symptoms of a myocardial infarction in women include:

53. What factors contribute to respiratory problems in infants and young children?

54. Which of the following are lifestyle factors that contribute to poor cardiopulmonary status? Select all that apply.
    a. Having a diet low in protein _____
    b. Participating in a daily exercise regimen _____
    c. Drinking significant amounts of alcohol _____
    d. Being a construction worker _____
    e. Having a high-stress job _____

55. An early sign that the patient's chronic cardiopulmonary disease is worsening is: _____.

56. The patient becomes breathless and tired during the physical exam. The nurse should:

57. Nebulization is used in the administration of what types of medications?

58. A Yankauer suction catheter is used for _____ _____ suction.

59. Positioning for the patient with right-sided atelectasis will be on the left or right side?

60. What medication is contraindicated for a patient with asthma?

61. Caution is used when administering oxygen to patients with chronic lung disease because:

62. Individuals have gone to the health fair to receive their free influenza vaccine. The nurse briefly discusses the medical backgrounds of the patients. The influenza vaccine will be withheld from the following individuals. Select all that apply.
   a. HIV-positive man _____
   b. Older adult woman _____
   c. Man with chronic arthritis _____
   d. Woman with a hypersensitivity to eggs _____
   e. Woman with a history of Guillain-Barré syndrome _____

Select the best answer for each of the following questions:

63. A patient has a chest tube in place to drain bloody secretions from the chest cavity. When caring for a patient with a chest tube, a nurse should:
   1. keep the drainage device above chest level.
   2. clamp the chest tube when the patient is ambulating.
   3. have the patient cough if the tubing becomes disconnected.
   4. leave trapped fluid in the tubing and estimate the amount.

64. A nurse is making a home visit to a patient who has emphysema (chronic obstructive pulmonary disease [COPD]). Specific instruction to control exhalation pressure for this patient with an increased residual volume of air should include:
   1. coughing.
   2. deep breathing.
   3. pursed-lip breathing.
   4. diaphragmatic breathing.

65. A patient has been admitted to a medical center with a respiratory condition and dyspnea. A number of medications are prescribed for the patient. For a patient with this difficulty, the nurse should question the order for:
   1. steroids.
   2. mucolytics.
   3. bronchodilators.
   4. narcotic analgesics.

66. After a patient assessment, the nurse suspects hypoxemia. This is based on the nurse finding that the patient is experiencing:
   1. restlessness.
   2. bradypnea.
   3. bradycardia.
   4. hypotension.

67. A patient has experienced some respiratory difficulty and is placed on oxygen via nasal cannula. A nurse assists the patient with this form of oxygen delivery by:
   1. changing the tubing every 4 hours.
   2. assessing the nares for breakdown.
   3. inspecting the back of the mouth q8h.
   4. securing the cannula to the nose with nonallergic tape.

68. A patient is being seen in an outpatient medical clinic. A nurse has reviewed the patient's chart and finds that there is a history of a cardiopulmonary abnormality. This is supported by the nurse's assessment of the patient having:
   1. scleral jaundice.
   2. reddened conjunctivae.
   3. symmetrical chest movement.
   4. clubbing of the fingertips.

69. A 65-year-old patient is seen in a physician's office for a routine annual checkup. As part of the physical examination, an ECG is performed. The ECG reveals a normal P wave, P-R interval, and QRS complex and a heart rate of 58 beats per minute. The nurse evaluates this finding as:
   1. sinus tachycardia.
   2. sinus bradycardia.
   3. sinus dysrhythmia.
   4. supraventricular bradycardia.

70. A patient is admitted to a medical center with a diagnosis of left ventricular congestive heart failure. A nurse is completing the physical assessment and is anticipating finding that the patient has:
   1. liver enlargement.
   2. peripheral edema.
   3. pulmonary congestion.
   4. jugular neck vein distention.

71. A patient has just returned to the unit after abdominal surgery. A nurse is planning care for this patient and is considering interventions to promote pulmonary function and prevent complications. The nurse:
    1. teaches the patient leg exercises to perform.
    2. asks the physician to order nebulizer treatments.
    3. demonstrates the use of a flow-oriented incentive spirometer.
    4. informs the patient that his secretions will need to be suctioned.

72. A nurse manager is evaluating the care that is provided by a new staff nurse during the orientation period. One of the patients requires nasotracheal suctioning, and the nurse manager determines that the appropriate technique is used when the new staff nurse:
    1. places the patient in the supine position.
    2. prepares for a clean or nonsterile procedure.
    3. suctions the oropharyngeal area first and then moves to the nasotracheal area.
    4. applies intermittent suction for 10 seconds while the suction catheter is being removed.

73. Chest tubes have been inserted into a patient after thoracic surgery. In working with this patient, a nurse should:
    1. coil and secure excess tubing next to the patient.
    2. clamp off the chest tubes except during respiratory assessments.
    3. milk or strip the tubing every 15 to 30 minutes to maintain drainage.
    4. remove the tubing from the connection to check for adequate suction.

74. A patient is being discharged home with an order for oxygen prn. In preparing to teach the patient and family, a priority for the nurse is to provide information on the:
    1. use of the oxygen delivery equipment.
    2. physiology of the respiratory system.
    3. use of PaO_2 levels to determine oxygen demand.
    4. length of time that the oxygen is to be used by the patient.

75. In discriminating types of chest pain that a patient may experience, a nurse recognizes that pain associated with inflammation of the pericardial sac is noted by the patient experiencing:
    1. knifelike pain to the upper chest.
    2. constant, substernal pain.
    3. pain with inspiration.
    4. pain aggravated by coughing.

76. A nurse is checking a patient who has a chest tube in place and finds that there is constant bubbling in the water-seal chamber. The nurse should:
    1. tighten loose connections.
    2. leave the chest tube clamped.
    3. raise the tubing above the level of the insertion site.
    4. prepare the patient for the removal of the tube.

77. The patient is admitted with a diagnosis of COPD. The appropriate oxygen delivery method for this patient is a:
    1. simple face mask with 5 to 8 L/min (50%) O_2.
    2. Venturi mask with 8 L/min (35% to 40%) O_2.
    3. nasal cannula with 1 to 2 L/min (28%) O_2.
    4. partial nonrebreather mask with 6 to 10 L/min (80%) O_2.

78. A nurse is completing a physical assessment of a patient with a history of a cardiopulmonary abnormality. A finding associated with hyperlipidemia is the patient having:
    1. cyanosis.
    2. xanthelasma.
    3. petechiae.
    4. ecchymosis.

79. During patient assessment, which of the following is an expected sign of hypoxemia?
    1. Pale conjunctivae
    2. Central cyanosis
    3. Dependent edema
    4. Splinter hemorrhages

STUDY GROUP QUESTIONS

- How do the anatomy and physiology of the cardiovascular and respiratory systems promote oxygenation?
- What physiological factors affect oxygenation?
- How do growth and development influence oxygenation?
- How do behavioral and environmental factors influence oxygenation?
- What are some common alterations in cardiovascular and pulmonary functioning?
- How are the critical thinking and nursing processes applied to patients having difficulty with oxygenation?
- What assessment information should be obtained to determine the patient's oxygenation status?
- What findings usually are seen in a patient who has inadequate oxygenation?
- How can the nurse promote oxygenation for patients in the health promotion, acute care, and restorative care settings?
- What specific measures and procedures should be implemented by the nurse to manage dyspnea, maintain a patent airway, mobilize secretions, and expand the lungs?
- What should be included in patient/family teaching for promotion and maintenance of oxygenation?
- What safety measures should be implemented for the use of oxygen in the home?

31 Sleep

CASE STUDIES

1. A middle-aged adult patient has gone to a physician's office to obtain a prescription for a "sleeping pill" because she has been having difficulty either falling or staying asleep. You are completing the initial nursing assessment and discover that the patient is recently divorced and trying to juggle extensive work and child care responsibilities.
   a. Identify a possible nursing diagnosis and outcome for this patient.
   b. Indicate nursing interventions and teaching areas for this patient.

2. A nurse has just been moved to the night shift in the hospital and starts to experience difficulty in getting to sleep when he gets home. He is finding it harder to focus at work.
   a. What can be done to assist the nurse in adapting to the change in his work schedule and sleep pattern?

CHAPTER REVIEW

Match the description/definition in Column A with the correct term in Column B.

	Column A	Column B
_____	1. Cessation of breathing for periods of time during sleep	a. Cataplexy
_____	2. A decrease in the amount, quality, and consistency of sleep	b. Sleep deprivation
_____	3. Awaking at night to urinate	c. Circadian rhythm
_____	4. Sudden muscle weakness during intense emotions	d. Parasomnia
_____	5. Difficulty falling or staying asleep	e. Sleep
_____	6. 24-hour day/night cycle	f. Sleep apnea
_____	7. Disorder that produces abnormal behavior or emotions	g. Insomnia
_____	8. Excessive sleepiness during the day	h. Nocturia
_____	9. A recurrent, altered state of consciousness that occurs for sustained periods.	i. Narcolepsy

Complete the following:

10. Provide examples of factors that may affect sleep.

11. Which of the following are appropriate nursing interventions to assist the older adult patient to achieve adequate sleep? Select all that apply.
    a. Altering the daily sleep and wake times _____
    b. Encouraging the patient to stay in bed even if not feeling sleepy _____
    c. Limiting the patient's caffeine intake in the late afternoon or evening _____
    d. Lowering the head of the bed as flat as possible _____
    e. Encouraging increased fluid intake 2 to 4 hours before sleep _____

    f. Avoiding use of sedatives and hypnotics, if possible _____
    g. Encouraging daytime naps of 1 to 2 hours _____
    h. Providing social activities and exercise _____

12. Identify a way in which a nurse can promote a restful environment in the acute care setting.

13. It is expected that during sleep the heart rate will decrease by 10 beats per minute from the daytime average rate.
    True _____ False _____

14. Very few older adults experience sleep problems.
    True _____ False _____

15. Normal sleep cycles usually last _____ (time) and are followed by _____ sleep.

16. Identify at least two nursing interventions that may be implemented related to a patient's sleep:
    a. Comfort measures
    b. Safety measures

17. A nurse tells a patient to include what information in a sleep diary?

18. What are the best types of bedtime snacks for promoting sleep?

19. A nurse recommends to the parents of a newborn that the best way to position the child for sleep is on his/her:

20. Identify at least one patient outcome related to sleep.

21. For sleep disturbances:
    a. What physical and behavioral problems may occur when individuals have an insufficient amount of sleep?

    b. What are the safety considerations for patients with narcolepsy, EDS, sleep deprivation, and/or nocturia?

22. Use of technology, such as cell phones, close to bedtime can lead to changes in sleep and excessive daytime sleepiness. True _____ False _____

23. What is the value of REM sleep?

24. Central sleep apnea is frequently seen in patients who have which pathological conditions?

25. Identify at least two questions to ask to assess a patient's sleep habits.

26. For a patient with chronic insomnia, the nurse should:

27. For the patient with obstructive sleep apnea, identify the recommendations for health promotion. Select all that apply.
    a. Weight loss _____
    b. Use of benzodiazepines _____
    c. Change of bedtime routine _____
    d. Use of analgesics _____
    e. Elevating the head of the bed _____

Select the best answer for each of the following questions:

28. Individuals experience changes in their sleep patterns as they progress through the life cycle. A nurse assesses that a patient is experiencing bedtime fears, restlessness during the night, and nightmares. These behaviors are associated with:
    1. infants.
    2. toddlers.
    3. preschoolers.
    4. school-age children.

29. A nurse is making rounds during the night to check on patients. When she enters one of the rooms at 3:00 AM, she finds that the patient is sitting up in a chair. The patient tells the nurse that she is not able to sleep. The nurse should first:
    1. obtain an order for a hypnotic.
    2. assist the patient back to bed.
    3. provide a glass of warm milk and a back rub.
    4. ask about activities that have previously helped her sleep.

30. A nurse is working on a pediatric unit at the local hospital. A 4-year-old boy is admitted to the unit. To assist this child to sleep, the nurse:
    1. reads to him.
    2. teaches him relaxation activities.
    3. allows him to watch TV until he is tired.
    4. has him get ready for bed very quickly, without advance notice.

31. A patient is found to be awakening frequently during the night. There are a number of medications prescribed for this patient. The nurse determines that the medication that may be creating this patient's particular sleep disturbance is the:
    1. narcotic.
    2. beta blocker.
    3. antidepressant.
    4. antihistamine.

32. A nurse suspects that a patient may be experiencing sleep deprivation. This suspicion is validated by the nurse's finding that the patient has:
    1. increased reflex response.
    2. blurred vision.
    3. cardiac arrhythmia.
    4. increased response time.

33. A nurse is working in a sleep clinic that is part of the local hospital. In preparing to work with patients with different sleep needs, the nurse understands that:
    1. bedtime rituals are most important for adolescents.
    2. regular use of sleeping medications is appropriate.
    3. warm milk before bedtime may help a patient sleep.
    4. individuals are most easily aroused from sleep during stages 3 and 4.

34. A nurse is visiting a patient in his home. While completing a patient history and home assessment, the nurse finds that there are many prescription medications kept in the bathroom cabinet. In determining possible areas that may influence the patient's sleep patterns, the nurse looks for a classification of medication that may suppress the patient's rapid eye movement (REM) sleep. The nurse looks in the cabinet for a:
   1. diuretic.
   2. stimulant.
   3. beta blocker.
   4. nasal decongestant.

35. A newborn is taken to a pediatrician's office for the first physical exam. The parents ask the nurse when they can expect the baby to sleep through the night. The nurse responds that, although there may be individual differences, infants usually develop a nighttime pattern of sleep by the age of:
   1. 6 weeks.
   2. 3 months.
   3. 6 months.
   4. 10 months.

36. A nurse is working with older adults in the senior center. A group is discussing problems with sleep. The nurse recognizes that older adults:
   1. take less time to fall asleep.
   2. are more difficult to arouse from sleep.
   3. have a significant decline in stage 4 sleep.
   4. require more sleep than middle-aged adults.

37. A patient with congestive heart failure is being discharged from the hospital to her home. The patient will be taking a diuretic daily. The nurse recognizes that, with this drug, the patient may experience:
   1. nocturia.
   2. nightmares.
   3. reduced REM sleep.
   4. increased daytime sleepiness.

38. During a home visit, a nurse discovers that the patient has been having difficulty sleeping. To assist the patient to achieve sufficient sleep, an appropriate question the nurse might ask is:
   1. "Do you keep your bedroom completely dark at night?"
   2. "Do you nap enough during the day?"
   3. "Why don't you eat something right before you go to bed?"
   4. "What kinds of things do you do right before bedtime?"

39. A patient has gone to the sleep clinic to determine what may be creating his sleeping problems. In addition, his partner is having sleep pattern interruptions. If this patient is experiencing sleep apnea, the nurse may expect the partner to identify that the patient:
   1. snores excessively.
   2. talks in his sleep.
   3. is very restless.
   4. walks in his sleep.

40. A nurse anticipates that the patient who is in non–rapid eye movement (NREM) stage 1 sleep is:
   1. easily aroused.
   2. completely relaxed.
   3. having vivid, full-color dreams.
   4. experiencing significantly reduced vital signs.

41. A nurse is working with a patient who has a history of respiratory disease. This patient is expected to demonstrate:
   1. longer time falling asleep.
   2. decreased NREM sleep.
   3. increased awakenings in the early morning.
   4. need for extra pillows for comfort.

42. To help promote sleep for a patient, a nurse recommends:
   1. exercise about 2 hours before bedtime.
   2. intake of a large meal about 3 hours before bedtime.
   3. drinking alcoholic beverages at bedtime.
   4. napping frequently during the afternoon.

43. An expected treatment for sleep apnea is:
   1. biofeedback.
   2. full body massage.
   3. administration of hypnotics.
   4. continuous positive airway pressure (CPAP).

44. As sleep aids, medications that are considered relatively safe to use are:
   1. nonbenzodiazepines.
   2. barbiturates.
   3. psychotropics.
   4. antihistamines.

45. An expected observation of a patient in REM sleep is:
   1. possible enuresis.
   2. sleepwalking.
   3. loss of skeletal muscle tone.
   4. easy arousal from external noise.

46. A parent asks the nurse what the appropriate amount of sleep is for her 11-year-old child. The nurse responds correctly by informing the parent that children in this age group should average:
   1. 14 hours per night.
   2. 12 hours per night.
   3. 10 hours per night.
   4. 7 hours per night.

47. Parents ask the nurse about having their child sleep in their bed with them. The nurse's best response is to:
   1. discourage the practice.
   2. identify that the child will probably sleep more soundly with them.
   3. recommend that lots of soft bedding be used to protect the child.
   4. indicate that there are risks associated with this practice.

STUDY GROUP QUESTIONS

- What is sleep?
- What are the physiological processes involved in sleep?
- How is sleep regulated by the body?
- What are the functions of sleep?
- What purpose do dreams serve?
- What are the normal requirements and patterns of sleep across the life span?
- What factors may influence sleep?
- What are some common sleep disorders and nursing interventions?
- What information should be included in a sleep history?
- How are the critical thinking and nursing processes applied with patients experiencing insufficient sleep or rest?
- What measures may be implemented by the nurse to promote sleep for patients/families?
- What information should be included in patient/family teaching for the promotion of rest and sleep?

STUDY CHART

Create a study chart to describe *Sleep Patterns Across the Life Span*, which identifies the sleep patterns and needs for infants, toddlers, preschoolers, school-age children, adolescents, adults, and older adults.

32 Pain Management

CASE STUDIES

1. A patient is going to be using a PCA pump with a morphine infusion after surgery.
   a. What assessments must be made before and while the patient uses the pump?
   b. What medications are usually prescribed for PCA?
   c. What information is needed in the teaching plan for this patient?

2. You are admitting a patient who is in labor. She tells you that this is her second child and that she had a "hard time having the first one because the pain was just horrible."
   a. What are the possible expectations of this patient?
   b. In applying the QSEN competency of patient-centered care, what nursing interventions do you include for this patient?

CHAPTER REVIEW

Match the description/definition in Column A with the correct term in Column B.

	Column A	Column B
h	1. Local anesthesia, with minimal sedation, given between the vertebrae	a. Pain
a	2. Unpleasant, subjective sensory and emotional experience	b. Analgesic
d	3. Extends from the point of injury to another body area	c. Exacerbation
g	4. Can cause the fight-or-flight response of the general adaptation syndrome	d. Radiating pain
e	5. Rapid onset, lasts briefly	e. Acute pain
c	6. Increase in the severity of symptoms	f. Chronic pain
b	7. Classification of medication used for pain relief	g. Superficial pain
f	8. Prolonged, varying in intensity	h. Epidural infusion

Complete the following:

9. Identify and briefly describe the four (4) physiological processes of pain.

10. The gate control theory of pain suggests that pain can be reduced through the use of:

11. Which of the following are physiological responses to acute pain as a result of sympathetic stimulation? Select all that apply.
    a. Decreased respiratory rate _____
    b. Increased heart rate _____
    c. Peripheral vasodilation _____
    d. Increased blood glucose level _____
    e. Diaphoresis _____
    f. Pupil constriction _____
    g. Decreased blood pressure _____

12. For a patient with chronic pain, identify the following:
    a. Associated symptoms
    b. An example of a lifestyle response to chronic pain

13. Identify two responses that an infant or child could have to pain.

14. The single most reliable indicator of pain is the:

15. Using the PQRSTU assessment guide, identify nursing interventions for the following.
    a. Quality
    b. Region
    c. Timing

16. Identify how a nurse may assess the level of pain for the following patients.
    a. Toddler

    b. Person for whom English is a second language

    c. Person with dementia

17. a. To determine the location of a patient's pain, a nurse should ask the patient to:
    b. The patient indicates that the discomfort is located in the right side of the abdomen. Provide an example of how the pain experience could be appropriately documented for this patient.

18. A pain rating of _____ on a scale of 0 to 10 is an emergency and requires immediate action.

19. For a patient who experiences discomfort upon ambulation or during a dressing change, a nurse should plan to:

20. An example of how a nurse may individualize a patient's treatment for pain is:

21. Which of the following are correct statements regarding transcutaneous electrical nerve stimulation (TENS)? Select all that apply.
    a. It is an invasive procedure. _____
    b. It requires a health care provider's order. _____
    c. Electrodes are applied directly onto skin. _____
    d. Controls are adjusted until the patient feels a buzzing sensation. _____
    e. It can be very expensive. _____

22. Which of the following medications are indicated for the treatment of mild to moderate pain? Select all that apply.
    a. Ibuprofen (Motrin) _____
    b. Morphine _____
    c. Codeine _____
    d. Fentanyl _____
    e. Acetaminophen (Tylenol) _____
    f. Propoxyphene (Darvon) _____

23. Identify two examples of nonpharmacological interventions that may be implemented to relieve pain.

24. An example of an adjuvant medication that may be used in conjunction with an analgesic to manage a patient's pain is:

25. The usual dosage of on-demand morphine in the PCA is:

26. Complete the following about analgesics.
    a. A priority nursing intervention specifically for the patient with an epidural analgesic infusion is:
    b. A priority nursing assessment for all patients before and while receiving analgesics is:

27. Identify an intervention that a nurse should implement to adapt or alter the environment to promote a patient's comfort:

28. A patient who may experience phantom pain is someone who has:

29. The term for patient-controlled oral analgesia is: _____.

30. Whenever possible, the best way to evaluate the effectiveness of pain management is to: _____.

31. The ABCDE approach to pain assessment and management is:
    A
    B
    C
    D
    E

32. Concomitant symptoms associated with pain include:

33. Identify whether the following statements are true or false.
   a. Nurses can allow their own misconceptions about or interpretations of the pain experience to affect their willingness to intervene for their patient.
      True ✕ False _____
   b. The degree and quality of pain are related to the patient's definition of pain.
      True ✕ False _____
   c. When patients are experiencing pain, they will not hesitate to inform you.
      True _____ False ✕
   d. Fatigue decreases a patient's perception of pain.
      True _____ False ✕
   e. A nurse should provide descriptive words for a patient to assist in assessing the quality of the pain.
      True ✕ False _____
   f. Pain assessment can be delegated to assistive personnel.
      True _____ False ✕
   g. Large doses of opioids for the terminally ill patient will hasten the onset of death.
      True _____ False ✕
   h. Health care providers initially order higher doses than needed for patients with cancer pain.
      True ✕ False _____
   i. The Joint Commission (TJC) has a standard that requires health care workers to assess all patients for pain.
      True ✕ False _____
   j. Pain is a normal part of aging.
      True _____ False ✕
   k. Nurses should anticipate that higher doses of oral opioids will be ordered after patients are converted from the IV form.
      True ✕ False _____
   l. The least invasive pain management therapy should be tried first.
      True ✕ False _____

Select the best answer for each of the following questions:

34. A patient is experiencing pain that is not being managed by analgesics given by the oral or intramuscular routes. Epidural analgesia is initiated. The nurse is alert for a complication of this treatment and observes the patient for:
   1. diarrhea.
   2. hypertension.
   3. urinary retention.
   4. an increased respiratory rate.

35. A patient had a laparoscopic procedure this morning and is requesting a pain medication. The nurse assesses the patient's vital signs and decides to withhold the medication based on the finding of:
   1. temperature = 99° F, rectally.
   2. pulse rate = 90 beats per minute, regular.
   3. respirations = 9 per minute, shallow.
   4. blood pressure = 130/80 mm Hg, consistent with prior reading.

36. A nurse is working with an older adult population in the extended care facility. Many of the patients experience discomfort associated with arthritis and have analgesics prescribed. In administering an analgesic medication to an older adult patient, the nurse should:
   1. give the medication when the pain increases in severity.
   2. combine opioids for a greater effect.
   3. use the IM route whenever possible.
   4. give the medication before activities or procedures.

37. One of the patients that a nurse is working with on an outpatient basis at the local clinic has rheumatoid arthritis. The patient has no known allergies to any medications, so the nurse anticipates that the physician will prescribe:
   1. amitriptyline.
   2. butorphanol.
   3. indomethacin. NSAID
   4. morphine.

38. An adolescent has been carried to the sidelines of the soccer field after experiencing a twisted ankle. The level of pain is identified as low to moderate. The nurse observes that the patient has:
   1. pupil constriction.
   2. diaphoresis.
   3. a decreased heart rate.
   4. a decreased respiratory rate.

39. A nurse on the pediatric unit is finding that it is sometimes difficult to determine the presence and severity of pain in very young patients. The nurse recognizes that toddlers may be experiencing pain when they have:
   1. an increased appetite.
   2. a relaxed posture.
   3. an increased degree of cooperation.
   4. disturbances in their sleep patterns.

40. A patient on the oncology unit is experiencing severe pain associated with his cancer. Although analgesics have been prescribed and administered, the patient is having "breakthrough pain." The nurse anticipates that his treatment will include:
   1. the use of a placebo.
   2. experimental medications.
   3. an increase in the opioid dose.
   4. administration of medications every hour.

41. A patient is experiencing pain that is being treated with a fentanyl transdermal patch. The nurse advises this patient to:
   1. avoid exposure to the sun.
   2. change the patch site every 2 hours.
   3. apply a heating pad over the site.
   4. expect immediate pain relief when the patch is applied.

42. A patient is experiencing severe pain and has been placed on a morphine drip. During the patient's assessment, the nurse finds that the patient's respiratory rate is 6 breaths per minute and shallow. The nurse anticipates that the patient will receive:
    1. naloxone. — Narcan for overdose in emergency situation
    2. morphine.
    3. incentive spirometry.
    4. no additional treatment for this expected response.

43. An assessment tool that has the patient select words from a list that most accurately reflect his/her pain severity is the:
    1. Brief Pain Inventory (BPI).
    2. Visual Analog Scale (VAS).
    3. Verbal Descriptor Scale (VDS).
    4. Critical Care Pain Observation Tool (CCPOT).

44. A nurse is working for an oncology unit in the medical center. All of the patients experience pain that requires management. The nurse should visit first with the patient who is also exhibiting signs of:
    1. anxiety.
    2. fatigue.
    3. distraction.
    4. depression.

45. For a patient with a consistent level of discomfort, the most effective pain relief is achieved with administration of analgesics:
    1. PRN.
    2. every 3 to 4 hours.
    3. every 12 hours.
    4. around the clock.

46. A nurse anticipates that the patient with visceral pain will describe the pain as:
    1. sharp.
    2. cramping.
    3. burning.
    4. shooting.

47. Which of the following orders would the nurse question for the patient who has an epidural infusion for pain relief?
    1. Use of pulse oximetry
    2. Tubing changes every 24 hours
    3. An order for a sedative
    4. Use of fentanyl in the infusion

48. Because of the possible cardiovascular and neurological effects, which of the following analgesic orders for an older adult patient should be questioned?
    1. Acetaminophen
    2. Aspirin
    3. Ibuprofen
    4. Propoxyphene

STUDY GROUP QUESTIONS

- How may a nurse use a holistic approach to assist a patient in achieving comfort?
- What is pain?
- What are the physiological components of the pain experience?
- How may a patient respond, physiologically and behaviorally, to a pain experience?
- What factors influence the pain experience?
- How are acute and chronic pain different?
- How should a nurse assess a patient's pain?
- How may a patient characterize pain?
- What nonpharmacological measures may be used to relieve pain?
- What interventions may a nurse implement to promote comfort and relieve pain?
- What pharmacological measures are available for pain relief?
- How is a back rub/massage performed to achieve an optimum effect?
- What actions should a nurse take if comfort or pain relief measures are not effective?
- What information should be included in patient/family teaching for pain control or relief?

STUDY CHART

Create a study chart to describe the *Factors Influencing Pain and Comfort* that identifies how age, sex, culture, meaning of pain, and previous experience of a patient alter the pain experience.

33 Nutrition

CASE STUDIES

1. You are working with a patient who is being discharged from the acute care unit after a heart attack (myocardial infarction). The patient's primary care provider has prescribed medical nutrition therapy with a diet that is low in sodium and saturated fat. The patient comes from a family in which food plays an important role in traditional culture practices.
   a. What do you need to know about the patient and the family to assist in dietary planning?
   b. How can you assist this patient to meet the prescribed dietary requirements?

2. A pregnant woman is at the medical office for a prenatal checkup. What nutritional recommendations should be provided to this patient?

3. You are working in a home care agency and have a large older adult patient population. In planning care, what nutritional considerations should be taken into account for these patients?

4. As an occupational health nurse, you are concerned with positive health behaviors for the employees. You have noticed that some of the workers are overweight.
   a. Identify the nursing diagnosis and general goals based upon your observation.
   b. What should you include in a teaching plan to promote nutritional health for the employees?

CHAPTER REVIEW

Match the description/definition in Column A with the correct term in Column B.

Column A	Column B
_____ 1. Increase in blood glucose level	a. Anabolism
_____ 2. Breakdown of food products into smaller particles	b. Hypoglycemia
_____ 3. Production of more complex chemical substances through the synthesis of nutrients	c. Digestion
	d. Anthropometry
_____ 4. All biochemical and physiological processes by which the body maintains itself	e. Catabolism
_____ 5. Organic substances in food that are present in small amounts and act as coenzymes in biochemical reactions	f. Nutrients
	g. Minerals
_____ 6. Inorganic elements that act as catalysts in biochemical reactions	h. Metabolism
_____ 7. Substances necessary for body functioning	i. Hyperglycemia
_____ 8. Breakdown of complex body substances into simpler substances	j. Vitamins
_____ 9. Decrease in blood glucose level	
_____ 10. Measurement of size and makeup of body at specific sites	

Complete the following:

11. Identify an example of a nutrition objective from *Healthy People 2020*.

12. For vitamins:
    a. Which vitamin is synthesized by the body?
    b. What are the fat-soluble vitamins?
    c. Identify an example of an antioxidant vitamin.

13. Identify whether the following represent carbohydrates, proteins, or fats.
    a. Starches _____
    b. Meats _____
    c. Linoleic acid _____
    d. Fiber _____
    e. 9 kcal/g of energy _____
    f. Amino acids _____
    g. Fruits _____

14. For patients with alterations in bowel elimination, identify which type of fiber should be recommended:
    a. Prevention of diarrhea: _____
    b. Prevention of constipation: _____

15. What information can you provide to an individual at a health fair who is interested in general nutritional guidelines?

16. Provide an example of an alternative dietary pattern.

17. What are the roles of minerals in the body?

18. Describe the functions of water in the body.

19. For each area of nutritional assessment, identify specific elements to pursue with the patient.
    a. Food and nutrient intake
    b. Physical examination
    c. Anthropometric measurements

20. Which of the following are indicators of malnutrition? Select all that apply.
    a. Listlessness _____
    b. Straight arms and legs _____
    c. Some fat under the skin _____
    d. Paresthesia _____
    e. Loss of ankle reflexes _____
    f. Rapid heart rate _____
    g. No palpable masses _____
    h. Apathy _____
    i. Dry, scaly skin _____
    j. Reddish-pink mucous membranes _____
    k. Spongy gums with marginal redness _____
    l. Surface papillae present on the tongue _____
    m. Pale conjunctivae _____
    n. Corneal xerosis _____
    o. Firm, pink nails _____
    p. Calf tenderness and tingling _____

21. A nurse calculates a patient's body mass index (BMI) by dividing the weight in kilograms by the height in square meters. If the patient weighs 180 pounds and is 6 feet tall, what is the BMI?

22. A neurogenic cause of dysphagia is:

    A myogenic cause is:

23. A common sign or symptom of food-borne illnesses is:

24. A nurse on an acute care unit is concerned about the patient's appetite.
    a. What are the stressors in the environment that have an impact upon a patient's nutritional intake?
    b. Identify at least two interventions that should be implemented by the nurse to promote the patient's appetite.

25. Identify the interventions that a nurse should implement for the patient who is experiencing dysphagia.

26. An advantage of enteral nutrition over parenteral nutrition is that enteral nutrition:

27. Regarding enteral tube feedings:
    a. What are the contraindications to nasogastric tube placement?
    b. The most serious complication of tube feedings is:
    c. To avoid this complication, the nurse should:
    d. Displacement of a jejunostomy tube can lead to:
    e. The nasogastric tube becomes clogged. The nurse should:
    f. Intermittent nasogastric feeding tubes are clamped/closed to prevent:
    g. The method of choice for long-term enteral feeding for the patient who has not had upper GI surgery is:

28. On the food label pictured, what is/are the possible concerns?

```
┌─────────────────────────────────────────┐
│            Nutrition Facts               │
│  Serving Size: 1/2 cup (114 g)           │
│  Servings Per Container: 4               │
│  ─────────────────────────────────────── │
│  Amount per Serving                      │
│  ─────────────────────────────────────── │
│  Calories 260                            │
│  Calories from Fat 120                   │
│  ═══════════════════════════════════════ │
│                        % Daily Value*    │
│  Total Fat 13 g              20%         │
│    Saturated Fat 5 g         25%         │
│    Trans Fat 0 g                         │
│  Cholesterol 30 mg           10%         │
│  Sodium 660 mg               28%         │
│  Total Carbohydrate 31 g 11%             │
│    Dietary Fiber 0 g          0%         │
│    Sugars 5 g                            │
│  Protein 5 g                             │
│  ─────────────────────────────────────── │
│  Vitamin A 4%      •    Vitamin C 1%     │
│  Calcium 15%       •    Iron 4%          │
│  *Percents (%) of a Daily Value are based on │
│  a 2,000 calorie diet. Your Daily Values may │
│  vary higher or lower depending on your  │
│  calorie needs.                          │
│                      2,000    2,500      │
│   Nutrient          calories  calories   │
│  Total Fat          <65 g     <80 g      │
│   Saturated Fat     <20 g     <25 g      │
│  Cholesterol        <300 mg   <300 mg    │
│  Sodium             <2,400 mg <2,400 mg  │
│  Total Carbohydrate 300 g     375 g      │
│   Dietary Fiber     25 g      30 g       │
│  1 g Fat = 9 calories                    │
│  1 g Carbohydrate = 4 calories           │
│  1 g Protein = 4 calories                │
└─────────────────────────────────────────┘
```

29. Identify foods that are choking hazards for toddlers.

30. What are the contributing factors to adolescent obesity and nutritional deficiencies?

31. The pH of the gastric aspirate for a patient who has been fasting is:

32. A parenteral nutrition formula that is hyperosmolar (greater than 10% dextrose) should be administered through a(n) _____ venous line.

33. A patient will be receiving parenteral nutrition (PN). Identify the following:
    a. The main reason for use of PN:
    b. A major nursing goal for the patient receiving PN:
    c. A nursing intervention to assist the patient in the prevention of metabolic complications related to PN therapy:
    d. Guidelines and precautions for lipid infusions:

34. Identify a dietary measure that should be implemented for a patient without teeth or with ill-fitting dentures.

35. A screening tool for older adults is the Mini Nutritional Assessment (MNA). Select all of the following correct statements about this tool.
    a. It is an 18-item tool. _____
    b. There are four sections to complete. _____
    c. The sections are divided into screening and assessment items. _____
    d. A score above 20 indicates a positive nutritional assessment. _____
    e. Anthropometric measures are required for the screening. _____

36. Indicate whether the following statements are true or false.
    a. Infants require more protein than adults.
       True _____ False _____
    b. Childhood obesity is five times higher than it was 30 years ago.
       True _____ False _____
    c. Unsaturated fatty acids have a minimal effect on blood cholesterol.
       True _____ False _____

37. What is the purpose of the ChooseMyPlate program?

38. What interventions should be implemented for a patient who is receiving enteral feedings? Select all that apply.
    a. Keep the head of the bed elevated to 30 to 45 degrees. _____
    b. Withhold the feeding if the residual is 50 to 100 mL. _____
    c. Tube placement is confirmed by monitoring the pH of aspirate. _____
    d. Gastric residual volume is measured daily. _____
    e. Continuous feedings are administered through an infusion pump. _____
    f. Tubing should be flushed with 200 mL of water before and after each feeding. _____

39. To decrease cholesterol levels, the best type of fatty acid intake is:

40. Complete a brief narrative documentation example that includes the following:
    10 Fr nasogastric tube, left side insertion, verification of placement, patient tolerance of procedure

41. The nurse is going to provide a continuous enteral feeding. Place the following steps in the correct order. Note: Certain steps have been completed, such as hand hygiene.
   a. Label the bag. _____
   b. Verify the order. _____
   c. Pour the feeding into the gravity bag. _____
   d. Bring the formula to room temperature. _____
   e. Check the expiration date on the formula. _____
   f. Connect the tubing to the gravity bag. _____
   g. Open the clamp and hang the bag on an IV pole. _____

42. What items are included in the Subjective Global Assessment (SGA)?

Select the best answer for each of the following questions:

43. A nurse is working with a patient who requires an increase in complete proteins in the diet. The nurse recommends:
   1. milk.
   2. cereals.
   3. legumes.
   4. vegetables.

44. A nurse is talking with a community resident who has gone to the health fair. The resident tells the nurse that he takes a lot of extra vitamins every day. Because of the greater potential for toxicity, the resident is advised not to exceed the dietary guidelines for:
   1. vitamin A.
   2. vitamin B_1.
   3. vitamin B_{12}.
   4. folic acid.

45. A nurse is working with a patient who is a lactovegetarian. The food that is selected as appropriate for this dietary pattern is:
   1. fish.
   2. milk.
   3. eggs.
   4. poultry.

46. A patient states that he does not eat fish anymore. An appropriate follow-up question by the nurse is which of the following?
   1. "Why don't you like fish?"
   2. "What caused you to lose interest in fish?"
   3. "Does fish make you feel ill in some way?"
   4. "Aren't you aware that fish is a valuable source of nutrients?"

47. A nurse is preparing to insert a nasogastric tube for enteral feedings. The nurse recognizes that this intervention is used when the patient:
   1. has a gag reflex.
   2. is not able to chew foods.
   3. is slow to eliminate food.
   4. is not able to ingest foods.

48. A nurse is preparing the enteral feeding for a patient who has a nasogastric tube in place. The most effective method that the nurse can use to check for placement of a nasogastric tube is to:
   1. perform a pH analysis of aspirated secretions.
   2. measure the visible tubing exiting from the nose.
   3. inject air into the tube and auscultate over the stomach.
   4. place the end of the tube into water and observe for bubbling.

49. A female patient who has gone to a family planning center is taking an oral contraceptive. This patient should increase vitamin B_6 and niacin intake. The nurse recommends that the patient consume more:
   1. tomatoes.
   2. whole grains.
   3. citrus fruits.
   4. green, leafy vegetables.

50. A patient tells the nurse that she is a vegan. Which of the following vitamin supplements is needed to promote health for this patient?
   1. Niacin
   2. Vitamin C
   3. Thiamine
   4. Vitamin B_{12}

51. A nurse is assigned to make home visits to a number of patients. Of the patients that the nurse visits, the patient with the greatest risk of a nutritional deficiency is the patient with:
   1. decreased metabolic requirements.
   2. an alteration in dietary schedule.
   3. a body weight that is 5% over the ideal weight.
   4. a weight loss of 3% within the past 6 months.

52. After surgery, a patient is having her dietary intake advanced. After a period of NPO, the patient is placed on a clear liquid diet. What food does the nurse request for the patient?
   1. Milk
   2. Soup
   3. Custard
   4. Popsicles

53. While completing an assessment during a home visit, a nurse discovers that the patient has a history of congestive heart failure and is taking digoxin 0.25 mg daily. Being aware that medications may influence the patient's dietary patterns, the nurse is alert to the patient experiencing:
   1. anorexia.
   2. gastric distress.
   3. an alteration in taste.
   4. an alteration in smell.

54. A patient on the unit has an enteral tube in place for feedings. When the nurse enters the room, the patient says that he is experiencing cramps and nausea. The nurse should:
    1. cool the formula.
    2. remove the tube.
    3. use a more concentrated formula.
    4. decrease the administration rate.

55. Which of the following statements made by the parent of an infant indicates the need for additional teaching?
    1. "I'll wait to give the baby regular cow's milk until he is a year old."
    2. "I'll start with cereal as the first solid food that I give to the baby after about 4 months."
    3. "I'll add a little honey to the baby's bottle to help him digest the formula."
    4. "When he can have them, I'll wait a few days in between giving the baby any new foods."

56. For the family that cans food at home, there is a need for specific instruction about ways to prevent:
    1. botulism.
    2. E. coli.
    3. salmonella.
    4. listeriosis.

57. The individual with the highest percentage of water in the body is a(n):
    1. infant.
    2. obese patient.
    3. lean patient.
    4. older adult.

58. A patient with a gastrostomy has an excessive residual volume of 200 mL. The nurse should:
    1. request an order for a chest x-ray.
    2. alter the type of feeding being given.
    3. request an order for an antidiarrheal agent.
    4. return the contents to the stomach.

59. A nurse is monitoring a patient's laboratory reports. Which of the following, if decreased, is indicative of anemia?
    1. BUN level
    2. Creatinine level
    3. Albumin level
    4. Hemoglobin level

60. A nurse is instructing the family of a patient who is on an National Dysphagia Diet Task Force (NDDTF) dysphagia puree diet to include:
    1. mashed potatoes.
    2. moistened breads.
    3. well-cooked noodles.
    4. soft fruits.

61. A nurse recognizes that a patient on a low cholesterol diet requires additional teaching if he indicates that he eats which of the following?
    1. oatmeal.
    2. pastries.
    3. dried fruits.
    4. green peppers.

62. A realistic weight loss goal for the patient who is overweight is:
    1. 1 pound per week.
    2. 3 pounds per week.
    3. 5 pounds per week.
    4. 7 pounds per week.

63. To prevent the presence of E. coli in food, a nurse specifically instructs a patient and family to:
    1. carefully can foods at home.
    2. boil shellfish completely.
    3. cook ground beef well.
    4. keep dairy products refrigerated.

64. A nurse is visiting a patient in the home and notes that additional teaching is required if the patient is observed:
    1. cooking poultry to 180° F.
    2. thawing frozen foods at room temperature.
    3. discarding all foods that may be spoiled.
    4. cleaning the inside of the refrigerator with bleach.

65. Tube feedings are ordered for a patient with a nasogastric tube. Unless the agency specifies otherwise, the nurse should:
    1. dilute the feedings with water.
    2. infuse the feedings over the course of 1 to 2 hours.
    3. begin with 150 to 250 mL at a time.
    4. increase feedings by 100 to 150 mL per feeding every 8 hours.

66. Which one of the following foods is avoided by the patient on a gluten-free diet?
    1. Cow's milk
    2. Oatmeal
    3. Canned fruit
    4. Coffee

67. The patient is receiving continuous enteral nutrition via a nasogastric tube and begins to vomit. The nurse should:
    1. slow down the feeding.
    2. remove the tube.
    3. aspirate remaining gastric content.
    4. place the patient in side-lying position.

68. During the insertion of a nasogastric tube, the unit nurse manager is observing the new nurse graduate. Correction is required when the new nurse:
    1. has the patient flex the head after the tube passes the nasopharynx.
    2. rotates the tube 180 degrees during the insertion.
    3. encourages the patient to swallow as the tube moves along.
    4. advances the tube during patient inspiration.

STUDY GROUP QUESTIONS

- What are the basic principles of nutrition?
- What body processes are involved in the intake, use, and elimination of foods?
- What are the six major nutrients, their purposes, and their food sources?
- What are the current recommendations for daily nutritional intake?
- How do nutritional needs change across the life span?
- How does culture/ethnicity influence dietary intake?
- What are some common alternative food patterns?
- How should a nurse assess a patient's nutritional status?

- What patients are at a greater risk for nutritional deficiencies?
- What nursing diagnoses may be appropriate for patients with nutritional alterations?
- How does a nurse assist patients to meet nutritional needs in the health promotion, acute care, and restorative care settings?
- What special diets may be prescribed for individuals?
- What are the nursing procedures for implementation of enteral and parenteral nutrition?
- What guidelines and precautions should be considered by a nurse in assisting a patient with enteral or parenteral nutrition?
- What general information should be included for patients/families for promotion or restoration of an adequate nutritional intake?

STUDY CHART

Create a study chart to describe the six nutrients that identifies the uses of each in the body and their food sources: carbohydrates, proteins, lipids, vitamins, minerals, and water.

34 Urinary Elimination

CASE STUDIES

1. A patient is going to the medical center for an intravenous pyelogram (IVP).
   a. What nursing assessments and patient teaching should be completed before this test is performed?
   b. What are the nurse's responsibilities for the patient after an IVP?

2. You will be working with unlicensed assistive personnel in an extended care setting.
   a. What urinary care may be safely delegated by a nurse?

3. On an acute care unit, a patient is to have her catheter removed. The primary nurse tells you that all that is necessary is to "cut it, wait for the balloon to deflate, and pull it out."
   a. How will you proceed with this catheter removal?

4. A clean-voided or midstream urine specimen is required from a male patient. He is able to perform activities of daily living, including hygienic care.
   a. How will you teach this patient to obtain the specimen?

5. A patient had surgery and an incontinent urinary diversion was created.
   a. What are the special needs of this patient and the interventions that you will implement?

CHAPTER REVIEW

Match the description/definition in Column A with the correct term in Column B.

Column A	Column B
_____ 1. Accumulation of urine in the bladder because of inability to empty bladder completely	a. Urgency
	b. Hematuria
_____ 2. Painful or difficult urination	c. Oliguria
_____ 3. Difficulty in initiating urination	d. Retention
_____ 4. Volume of urine remaining in the bladder after voiding	e. Nocturia
_____ 5. Feeling the need to void immediately	f. Frequency
_____ 6. Voiding large amounts of urine	g. Dysuria
_____ 7. Urination, particularly excessive, at night	h. Residual urine
_____ 8. Presence of blood in the urine	i. Hesitancy
_____ 9. Voiding very often	j. Polyuria
_____ 10. Diminished urinary output in relation to fluid intake	

Complete the following:

11. An example of a noninvasive procedure that may be used to examine the urinary system is:

12. What are the indications for the use of intermittent and indwelling urinary catheterization?

13. What positions may be used for catheterization of a female patient?

14. a. The recommended daily fluid intake for dilution of urine, promotion of micturition, and flushing the urethra of microorganisms is:

    b. The minimum urinary output for an adult is _____ per hour.

15. Provide an example of how each of the following factors may influence urination:

    a. Sociocultural
    b. Fluid intake
    c. Pathological conditions
    d. Medications

16. Identify how the following pathological conditions can influence urination:

    a. Arthritis
    b. Diabetes mellitus
    c. Prostate enlargement

17. a. The type of urinary incontinence that results from increased intraabdominal pressure with leakage of a small amount of urine is called:

    b. The treatment for this type of incontinence includes:

18. Which of the following are the expected characteristics of a normal urine specimen? Select all that apply.

    a. pH 10 _____
    b. Protein 4 mg _____
    c. Presence of glucose _____
    d. Specific gravity 1.2 _____
    e. Amber color _____

19. What is a priority when managing a patient's condom catheter?

20. To maintain a patient's dignity and self-esteem when assisting with urinary elimination, the nurse makes sure to:

21. Manual compression of the bladder is called:

22. Which of the following statements are correct for urinary diversions? Select all that apply.

    a. A ureterostomy is a continent diversion. _____
    b. Continent diversions have pouches created to store urine. _____
    c. Patients with urinary diversions need special clothing and have activity restrictions. _____

23. For a patient on strict intake and output, identify how urinary output can be measured.

24. Identify a method that a nurse may implement to stimulate a patient to void:

25. To assist a patient to start and stop the urine stream, a nurse instructs the patient that a way to strengthen the pelvic floor muscles is by performing:

26. Identify the distance of catheter insertion:

    a. Female adult patient:
    b. Male adult patient:

27. Which of the following are appropriate techniques for indwelling catheter care? Select all that apply.

    a. Keep the drainage bag below the level of the bladder. _____
    b. Provide perineal care daily. _____
    c. Cleanse in a direction toward the urinary meatus. _____
    d. Attach the drainage bag to the side rail of the bed. _____
    e. Open the connection at the drainage bag to obtain a urine specimen. _____
    f. Avoid having any dependent loops of tubing. _____
    g. Drain all urine in the bag before patient ambulation or exercise. _____
    h. For the immobile patient, empty the drainage bag every 24 hours. _____

28. To prevent nocturia, a nurse instructs a patient to:

29. Identify how the mobility status of an older adult may influence urination.

30. Which of the following are expected signs or symptoms for a patient with acute onset urinary retention? Select all that apply.

    a. Tenderness over the symphysis pubis _____
    b. Hematuria _____
    c. Diaphoresis _____
    d. Oliguria _____
    e. Dysuria _____
    f. Incontinence _____

31. How can urinary infection be prevented or reduced for a patient with an indwelling catheter?

32. Which of the following statements are correct regarding a cystoscopy? Select all that apply.
    a. The procedure may be performed under general anesthesia. _____
    b. Fluids are restricted before and during the procedure. _____
    c. Antibiotics are often administered intravenously. _____
    d. An informed consent is not required. _____
    e. Bowel preparation is performed the evening before the test. _____
    f. The patient is NPO if the test is performed with local anesthesia. _____
    g. Bed rest is usually indicated immediately after the test. _____
    h. Bloody or cloudy urine may be observed after the test. _____
    i. Fluid intake is encouraged after the test is completed. _____

33. During a physical assessment, what techniques are used to:
    a. determine the presence of a kidney infection?
    b. assess the bladder?

34. Identify the following for a bladder scanner:
    a. Use:
    b. When to measure:

35. Identify the characteristic of the urine for a patient with:
    a. daily administration of furosemide (Lasix): _____
    b. liver disease: _____
    c. urinary tract infection: _____

36. Urinary specimens for analysis should be sent to the laboratory within _____ hours of collection.

37. Place the following steps for a clean-catch specimen in the correct order:
    a. Void in the toilet. _____
    b. Provide instruction to the patient. _____
    c. Void in a sterile urine cup. _____
    d. Cleanse the urinary meatus. _____
    e. Stop the urine stream. _____

38. The patient is going to have a computerized axial tomography (CT) scan to identify the possible presence of calculi. Identify the following:
    a. Preparation before the test:
    b. Care after the test:

39. The nurse observes that the patient has some problems with hygiene. To prevent a UTI, the nurse instructs the patient to:

40. Identify the correct urinary catheter (single, double, or triple-lumen) to use for each of the following interventions:
    a. Indwelling catheter with bladder irrigation:
    b. Intermittent catheterization:
    c. Indwelling catheter:

41. What are the responsibilities of the nurse after the removal of a urinary catheter?

42. Identify the following for a suprapubic catheter:
    a. Purpose of insertion:
    b. Nursing care:

43. The patient has an incontinent urinary diversion and requires care of the stoma. Place the nursing actions in the correct order:
    a. Apply the pouch and press firmly into place. _____
    b. Cleanse the skin around the stoma. _____
    c. Remove the protective backing from the adhesive surface on the pouch. _____
    d. Measure the stoma. _____
    e. Cut an opening in the pouch. _____

44. What types of medications are used to treat urgency urinary incontinence?

45. Which of the following foods can irritate the bladder and contribute to urgency? Select all that apply.
    a. Caffeinated beverages _____
    b. Breads _____
    c. Fish _____
    d. Spicy foods _____
    e. Cheese _____
    f. Citrus foods _____

46. Self-catheterization by the patient is done with clean technique.
    True _____ False _____

47. Timed voiding is based upon a fixed schedule and not on the patient's urge to void.
    True _____ False _____

48. The nurse is teaching the patient how to prevent UTIs. Identify the information that should be included in the instruction. Select all that apply.
    a. Cleanse the perineum from back to front. _____
    b. Void before and after sexual intercourse. _____
    c. Wear nylon underwear. _____
    d. Avoid bubble baths. _____
    e. Drink coffee or tea regularly. _____
    f. Try to empty the bladder completely with each voiding. _____

49. Identify at least four measures that the nurse should employ to reduce the chance of a catheter associated urinary tract infection (CAUTI).

50. What are three possible questions to ask the patient to determine if there are any urinary symptoms present?

51. In the photo, what intervention is needed to have appropriate urinary drainage?

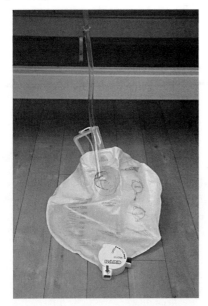

52. What lumen would be used to inflate the catheter balloon?

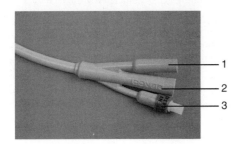

Select the best answer for each of the following questions:

53. The nurse recognizes that an intervention for a patient with stress incontinence is instruction regarding:
    1. use of a mobility aid.
    2. intermittent catheterization.
    3. pelvic muscle exercises.
    4. antimuscarinic medications.

54. The nurse is going to be catheterizing an average-size 9-year-old boy. The appropriate catheter size for this child is:
    1. 5 to 6 FR.
    2. 8 to 10 FR.
    3. 12 to 14 FR.
    4. 15 to 17 FR.

55. For the nursing diagnosis *Functional Urinary Incontinence,* the difficulty is related to the patient's:
    1. inability to completely empty the bladder.
    2. lack of sensation of a full bladder.
    3. difficulty in getting out of the chair and going to the toilet.
    4. pressure during coughing or sneezing.

56. For the patient who has had a continent urinary reservoir created, the nurse instructs the patient that there will be a need to:
    1. catheterize the pouch 4 to 6 times/day.
    2. eliminate urine through the intestine.
    3. use the Valsalva maneuver to empty the pouch through the urethra.
    4. restrict the intake of fluids.

57. The nurse is going to explain to new parents about toilet training. The parents are informed that early onset of a child's control of voluntary voiding does not occur until the age of:
    1. 6 months old.
    2. 12 months old.
    3. 18 months old.
    4. 4 years old.

58. A patient on the medical unit is scheduled to have a 24-hour urine collection to diagnose a urinary disorder. The nurse should:
    1. note the start time on the container.
    2. have the patient void while defecating.
    3. start with the first voiding sample from the patient.
    4. continue with the test if a specimen is flushed away.

59. One of a nurse's assigned patients is experiencing urgency urinary incontinence (UI). The nurse anticipates a medication that may be ordered for this difficulty is:
    1. propantheline.
    2. oxybutynin.
    3. bethanechol.
    4. phenylpropanolamine.

60. Several patients in a long-term care unit have indwelling urinary catheters in place. A nurse is delegating catheter care to the nursing assistant. The nurse includes instruction in:
    1. using lotion on the perineal area.
    2. disinfecting the first 2 to 3 inches of the catheter every 2 hours.
    3. ensuring that the drainage bag is secured to the side rail.
    4. cleansing about 4 inches along the length of the catheter, proximal to distal.

61. For a renal ultrasound, the patient is instructed to:
    1. not eat or drink for 8 hours before.
    2. have a full bladder.
    3. complete bowel cleansing.
    4. not do anything out of his/her routine, because there is no special preparation for this procedure.

62. Prevention of infection is a patient outcome that is identified for a patient with a urinary alteration and an indwelling catheter. The nurse assists the patient to attain this outcome by:
   1. emptying the drainage bag daily.
   2. draining all urine after the patient ambulates.
   3. performing perineal care q8h and prn.
   4. opening the drainage system only at the connector points to obtain specimens.

63. A patient being seen at a urologist's office suffers from urge incontinence. The nurse anticipates that treatment for this difficulty will include:
   1. biofeedback.
   2. catheterization.
   3. anti-muscarinic drug therapy.
   4. electrical stimulation.

64. A nurse notes that there is an order on a patient's record for a sterile urine specimen. The patient has an indwelling urinary catheter. The nurse will proceed to obtain this specimen by:
   1. withdrawing the urine from a urinometer.
   2. opening the drainage bag and removing urine.
   3. disconnecting the catheter from the drainage tubing.
   4. using a syringe to withdraw urine from the catheter port.

65. A patient had a laparoscopic procedure in the morning and is having difficulty voiding later that day. Before initiating invasive measures, the nurse intervenes by:
   1. administering a cholinergic agent.
   2. applying firm pressure over the perineal area.
   3. increasing the patient's daily fluid intake to 3000 mL.
   4. rinsing the perineal area with warm water.

66. To determine the possibility of a renal problem, a patient is scheduled to have an intravenous pyelogram (IVP). Immediately after the procedure, a nurse will need to evaluate the patient's response and be alert to:
   1. an infection in the urinary bladder.
   2. an allergic reaction to the contrast material.
   3. urinary suppression from injury to kidney tissues.
   4. incontinence from paralysis of the urinary sphincter.

67. A unit manager is evaluating the care that has been given to a patient by a new nursing staff member. The manager determines that the staff member has implemented an appropriate technique for clean-voided urine specimen collection if:
   1. fluids were restricted before the collection.
   2. sterile gloves were applied for the procedure.
   3. the specimen was collected after the initial stream of urine had passed.
   4. the specimen was placed in a clean container and then placed in the utility room.

68. A patient at the urology clinic is diagnosed with reflex incontinence. This problem was identified by the patient's statement of experiencing:
   1. a constant dribbling of urine.
   2. an urge to void and not enough time to reach the bathroom.
   3. an uncontrollable loss of urine when coughing or sneezing.
   4. no urge to void and being unaware of bladder fullness.

69. A female patient has an order for urinary catheterization. A nursing student will be evaluated by the instructor on the insertion technique. The student is identified as implementing appropriate technique if:
   1. the catheter is advanced 7 to 8 inches.
   2. a new cotton ball or swab is used for each wipe when cleansing the urethral meatus.
   3. the catheter is reinserted if it is accidentally placed in the vagina.
   4. both hands are kept sterile throughout the procedure.

70. A patient is diagnosed with prostate enlargement. The nurse is alert to a specific indication of this problem when finding that the patient has:
   1. chills.
   2. cloudy urine.
   3. polyuria.
   4. bladder distention.

71. Stress incontinence is associated with:
   1. irritation of the bladder.
   2. neurological trauma.
   3. alcohol or caffeine ingestion.
   4. coughing or sneezing.

72. For patients with diabetes mellitus, a nurse anticipates that the patients will experience:
   1. dribbling.
   2. hesitancy.
   3. polyuria.
   4. hematuria.

73. A nurse recognizes that one of the specific purposes of intermittent catheterization is for:
   1. prevention of obstruction.
   2. assessment of residual urine.
   3. urinary drainage during surgical procedures.
   4. recording of output for comatose patients.

74. A nurse notes that there is no urine in a drainage bag since it was emptied 1½ hours ago. The nurse should first:
   1. remove the catheter.
   2. provide additional fluids.
   3. check for kinks or bends in the tubing.
   4. apply external pressure on the patient's bladder.

75. The best way to remove urine from a patient's skin is for the nurse to use:
    1. alcohol.
    2. mild soap.
    3. an antibacterial agent.
    4. a hydrogen peroxide mix.

76. A nurse manager is observing a new nurse staff member provide care for a patient with a condom catheter. The manager determines that correction and additional instruction are required for the new employee if the staff nurse is observed:
    1. draping the patient and exposing only the genitalia.
    2. attaching the urinary drainage bag to the lower bed frame.
    3. using adhesive tape to secure the catheter to the patient's penis.
    4. clipping the hair at the base of the penile shaft.

77. A patient who is taking phenazopyridine needs to be instructed that a specific side effect of this medication is that:
    1. the urine will turn orange.
    2. there will be an increased urinary frequency.
    3. back pain will be moderately severe.
    4. occasional dizziness may be experienced.

78. A nurse anticipates that a treatment option for a patient with functional incontinence will include:
    1. catheterization.
    2. bladder training.
    3. electrical stimulation.
    4. hormone replacement.

STUDY GROUP QUESTIONS

- What is the normal anatomy and physiology of the urinary system?
- What factors may influence urination?
- What are some common urinary elimination problems, their causes, and patient signs and symptoms?
- How do growth and development influence urinary function and patterns?
- How can urinary drainage be surgically altered, and why would an alteration be necessary?
- What measures may be implemented to prevent infection in the urinary tract?
- How does a nurse assess a patient's urinary function/elimination?
- What noninvasive and invasive procedures may be used to determine urinary function?
- What diagnostic tests are used to determine the characteristics of urine?
- What are the expected characteristics of urine?
- What nursing interventions are appropriate for promoting urination in the health care and home care settings?
- What information should be included in teaching patients/families about promotion of urination and prevention of infection?

35 Bowel Elimination

CASE STUDIES

1. You have arranged with your instructor and the home care agency to visit a 76-year-old woman. In completing your initial assessment, the patient tells you that she has been having difficulty over the past 2 years in "moving her bowels." She takes you to the bathroom, where she shows you a collection of over-the-counter laxatives and enemas. The patient also tells you that, since the death of her husband, she does not do a lot of cooking, relying on sandwiches and prepared foods.
   a. Based on this information, identify a nursing diagnosis, patient goal(s)/outcomes, and nursing interventions related to bowel elimination.

2. A patient is scheduled to have a colonoscopy performed.
   a. Identify the patient teaching that is provided before the procedure.

CHAPTER REVIEW

Match the description/definition in Column A with the correct term in Column B.

Column A

_____ 1. Propulsion of food through the gastrointestinal (GI) tract

_____ 2. Agent used to empty the bowel

_____ 3. Artificial opening in the abdominal wall

_____ 4. Dilated rectal veins

_____ 5. Blood in the stool

Column B

a. Stoma

b. Hemorrhoids

c. Peristalsis

d. Melena

e. Cathartic

Complete the following:

6. Constipation in the older adult is usually the result of:

7. What types of patients should be cautioned against straining during defecation and why?

8. a. A common cause of diarrhea in health care facilities is:
   b. This common occurrence can be prevented by:
   c. If persistent diarrhea occurs, a patient is at risk for:

9. The most frequently reported GI complaints are:

10. Provide an example of the effect that fecal incontinence can have on an individual:

11. Which of the following factors will interfere with bowel elimination and decrease peristalsis? Select all that apply.
   a. Slower esophageal emptying _____
   b. Eating raw vegetables _____
   c. Immobilization _____
   d. Consumption of lean meats _____
   e. Anxiety _____
   f. Emotional depression _____
   g. Abdominal surgery _____
   h. Use of antibiotics _____
   i. Food allergies _____
   j. Parkinson's disease _____
   k. Use of narcotic analgesics _____
   l. Drinking fruit juices _____
   m. Tube feedings _____

12. Discuss how a patient's cultural background may influence care for elimination needs.

13. Identify a risk factor for colon cancer.

14. Identify two nursing interventions for a patient who is experiencing:
    a. Constipation
    b. Diarrhea

15. Provide an example of how each of the following factors influences bowel elimination:
    a. Positioning
    b. Pregnancy
    c. Diagnostic tests
    d. Diet
    e. Personal habits

16. How can a nurse promote comfort for a patient with hemorrhoids?

17. Identify at least three areas included in a GI assessment.

18. Enema administration:
    a. What is the correct position for an adult patient to receive an enema?
    b. The enema tube is inserted as follows:
       Adult: _____ inches or _____ cm
       Child: _____ inches or _____ cm
    c. The height of the bag for a regular adult enema should be _____ inches or _____ cm above the level of the anus.
    d. An enema that is used to treat patients with hyperkalemia is:
    e. A hypertonic enema works by:
    f. A commonly used over-the-counter hypertonic enema is:

    g. For a soapsuds enema, the only appropriate soap to use is:

    h. Provision of "enemas until clear" means:

    i. After administration of an enema, what assessments should be made?

19. The nurse anticipates that which of the osmotic laxatives could be prescribed for patients experiencing constipation: Select all that apply.
    a. Lactulose _____
    b. Loperamide _____
    c. Sorbitol _____
    d. Magnesium hydroxide _____
    e. Bisacodyl _____
    f. Polyethylene glycol _____

20. How is the QSEN competency for patient-centered care incorporated into the care of a patient with elimination needs?

21. A patient receiving tube feedings may experience diarrhea as a result of:

22. Identify what should be included in a focused assessment of a patient's bowel function.

23. What surgical procedures are anticipated for patients with:
    a. colorectal cancer?
    b. diverticulitis?

24. Which of the following are correct practices that should be included in the teaching plan for a patient with an ostomy? Select all that apply.
    a. Using creams around the peristomal skin _____
    b. Emptying the pouch when it is one-third to one-half full _____
    c. Washing the peristomal skin with a detergent soap _____
    d. Using sterile technique _____
    e. Anticipating a significant amount of bleeding _____
    f. Changing the entire pouching system daily _____
    g. Using the same manufacturer's flange and pouch _____
    h. Cutting the pouch opening approximately $1/16$ to $1/8$ inch larger than the stoma _____
    i. Applying a skin barrier around the stoma _____

25. Which of the following fecal characteristics are expected findings? Select all that apply.
    a. Yellow infant's stool _____
    b. A defecation frequency greater than three times per day for an adult _____
    c. White stool _____
    d. Tarry stool _____
    e. Soft, formed stool _____
    f. 150 mg/day average amount of stool _____

26. Before giving a patient a bedpan, the nurse should:

27. Select which of the following interventions may be delegated to assistive personnel.
    a. Digital removal of an impaction _____
    b. Enema administration _____
    c. Ostomy pouching _____
    d. Assisting the patient to use the bedpan _____

28. When determining placement of the nasogastric tube, the nurse expects that, if the tube is in the stomach, the gastric pH will be:

29. a. *Clostridium difficile* is transmitted by:
    b. Transmission of *C. difficile* can be prevented or reduced by:

30. Identify a positive outcome for a patient who has a colostomy.

31. Normal defecation in the acute or long-term care environment may be promoted by:

32. Nasogastric tube irrigation is usually done with _____ mL of _____ (solution). Suction applied to the NG tube is usually _____.

33. Place the following steps for nasogastric tube insertion in the correct order:
    a. Have the patient drink water and swallow. _____
    b. Perform hand hygiene. _____
    c. Auscultate for bowel sounds. _____
    d. Insert the tube past the nasopharynx. _____
    e. Prepare the equipment. _____
    f. Measure the distance to insert the tube. _____
    g. Ask the patient to talk. _____
    h. Identify the patient. _____
    i. Position the patient in high Fowler's. _____
    j. Lubricate the tube. _____

Select the best answer for each of the following questions:

34. For a patient with a nasogastric tube who has a painful, distended abdomen, the first most appropriate action by the nurse is to:
    1. remove the tube.
    2. irrigate the tube.
    3. pull the tube out farther.
    4. notify the supervisor.

35. A patient expresses a feeling of mild cramping during the administration of a saline enema. The nurse should first:
    1. discontinue the procedure.
    2. change the solution.
    3. lower the bag to slow the infusion.
    4. allow the solution to cool.

36. The patient begins to cough during the insertion of the nasogastric tube. The nurse should:
    1. remove the tube.
    2. lower the head of the bed.
    3. check the back of the throat.
    4. advance the tube further.

37. A nurse observes a nursing assistant carrying out bowel retraining with a patient in the extended care facility. The nurse identifies that the assistant implements an incorrect procedure when:
    1. allowing the patient adequate time in the bathroom.
    2. taking the patient to the bathroom at regular times throughout the day.
    3. pulling the curtain around the patient while on the commode.
    4. restricting fluids with breakfast and lunch meals.

38. For patients who have been prescribed extended bed rest, the prolonged immobility may result in reduced peristalsis and fecal impaction. A nurse is alert to one of the first signs of an impaction when the patient experiences:
    1. headaches.
    2. abdominal distention.
    3. overflow diarrhea.
    4. abdominal pain with guarding.

39. A patient has been admitted to an acute care unit with a diagnosis of biliary disease. When assessing the patient's feces, the nurse expects that they will be:
    1. bloody.
    2. pus filled.
    3. black and tarry.
    4. white or clay colored.

40. The nurse is documenting the appearance of the colostomy stoma. The term for a stoma that is above the abdominal skin level is:
    1. budded.
    2. flush.
    3. retracted.
    4. edematous.

41. A nurse is preparing to administer an enema to a 7-year-old child. When assembling the equipment, the nurse will prepare an enema of:
    1. 100 to 250 mL of fluid.
    2. 300 to 500 mL of fluid.
    3. 600 to 800 mL of fluid.
    4. 800 to 950 mL of fluid.

42. A nurse recognizes that the greatest challenge for skin care will be for a patient with a(n):
    1. ileostomy.
    2. sigmoid colostomy.
    3. descending ostomy.
    4. ileoanal pouch.

43. A nurse evaluates that a patient has normal bowel sounds by auscultating all four quadrants and finding:
    1. 4 sounds per minute.
    2. 15 sounds per minute.
    3. 40 sounds per minute.
    4. no bowel sounds after 1 minute.

44. A nurse instructs a patient who is taking an iron supplement that his stool may be:
    1. red and liquid.
    2. pale and frothy.
    3. mucus filled.
    4. black and tarry.

45. A nurse is caring for a patient with a Salem sump tube for gastric decompression. Which of the following actions by the nurse requires correction?
    1. Clamping off the blue lumen or air vent
    2. Using clean technique to insert the tube
    3. Anchoring the tube to the patient's gown
    4. Keeping the nares lubricated

46. A nurse recognizes that the intake of mineral oil to promote bowel elimination interferes with the absorption of:
    1. vitamin A.
    2. vitamin B_6.
    3. vitamin C.
    4. niacin.

47. Further follow-up is required if a patient informs the nurse that he regularly uses:
    1. Fleet enemas.
    2. tap water enemas.
    3. castile soap enemas.
    4. normal saline enemas.

48. During a digital removal of a fecal impaction, a nurse notes that the patient has bradycardia. The nurse should:
    1. provide oxygen.
    2. discontinue the procedure.
    3. turn the patient on the right side.
    4. instruct the patient to take rapid, deep breaths.

49. In the teaching plan for a patient who will be having a fecal occult blood test, which of the following foods should be noted for producing a false negative result?
    1. Fish
    2. Pasta
    3. Vitamin C
    4. Whole grain bread

50. The nurse is aware that a test for fecal ova and parasites requires:
    1. performing the test 3 times while the patient is NPO.
    2. keeping the sample at room temperature or warming.
    3. using a chemical fixative for the sample.
    4. saving the sample for 3 to 5 days.

STUDY GROUP QUESTIONS

- What is the normal anatomy and physiology of the gastrointestinal system?
- How is bowel elimination influenced by the process of growth and development?
- What are some common bowel elimination problems?
- How are continent and incontinent bowel diversions/ostomies different?
- What is included in the nursing assessment of a patient to determine bowel elimination status?
- What diagnostic tests may be used to determine the presence of bowel elimination disorders?
- How are the critical thinking and nursing processes applied to situations in which patients are experiencing alterations in bowel elimination?
- What nursing interventions may be implemented to promote bowel elimination and comfort for patients in the health promotion, acute care, and restorative care settings?
- What information should be included in the teaching plan for patients/families with regard to promotion and/or restoration of bowel elimination?

STUDY CHART

Create concept maps with nursing diagnoses, related assessment data, and nursing interventions for the following: constipation, diarrhea, and incontinence.

36 Immobility

CASE STUDIES

1. A patient has just gone to the rehabilitation facility. She has been immobilized with a spinal cord injury from an automobile accident. You are aware of the physical hazards of immobility, but her withdrawn behavior is your concern now.
   a. What can you do to prevent the possible psychological and emotional effects of the patient's period of immobility?

2. A patient will be getting out of bed for the first time after having surgery and receiving general anesthesia.
   a. What actions should be taken by the nurse to promote the patient's safety?

3. You are the nurse in a long-term care facility and your assignment includes several older adult patients who are immobile.
   a. What actions should be taken specifically for this older adult population?

CHAPTER REVIEW

Match the descriptions/definitions in Column A with the correct term in Column B.

	Column A	Column B
i	1. Characterized by bone resorption	a. Renal calculi
e	2. Temporary decrease in blood supply to an organ or tissue	b. Diuresis
d	3. Capacity to maneuver around freely	c. Hypostatic pneumonia
j	4. Permanent plantar flexion	d. Mobility
c	5. Lung inflammation from stasis or pooling of secretions	e. Ischemia
b	6. Increased urine excretion	f. Atelectasis
f	7. Collapse of alveoli	g. Thrombus
h	8. Bathing, dressing, eating	h. Activities of daily living
a	9. Calcium stones in the kidney	i. Disuse osteoporosis
g	10. Accumulation of platelets, fibrin, clotting factors, and cellular elements attached to the interior wall of an artery or vein	j. Footdrop

Complete the following:

11. The objectives or advantages of bed rest are:

12. Identify at least three pathological influences on mobility.

13. Which of the following pathophysiological changes occur with immobility? Select all that apply.
    a. Increased basal metabolic rate _____
    b. Decreased gastrointestinal motility _____
    c. Orthostatic hypotension _____
    d. Increased appetite _____
    e. Increased oxygen availability _____
    f. Hypercalcemia _____
    g. Increased lung expansion _____
    h. Decreased cardiac output _____
    i. Increased dependent edema _____
    j. Decreased stressors _____
    k. Increased urinary stasis _____
    l. Decreased passive behaviors _____

14. An example of a fluid and electrolyte imbalance that may occur with prolonged immobility is:

15. An example of a common behavioral change that may be observed in an immobilized patient is:

16. A nurse anticipates that a patient on prolonged bed rest will have a heart rate that is faster by _____%.

17. Virchow triad is related to _____, and the three associated problems are:

18. With an immobilized child, the nurse's focus is on:

19. An important concept when working with patients who are immobilized is to maintain the patient's autonomy. The nurse can accomplish this by:

20. Identify at least one major change that may occur in each of the following body systems as a result of immobility and a nursing intervention to prevent or treat the change.
   a. Cardiovascular system

   b. Respiratory system

   c. Integumentary

   d. Gastrointestinal

   e. Urinary

   f. Musculoskeletal

21. Using the algorithm for patient transfers, the appropriate intervention for a patient who is cooperative, has upper body strength, but cannot bear full weight should be: _____

22. What areas are included in a focused assessment of patient mobility?

23. Identify for each of the following illustrations what range-of-joint-motion (ROJM) exercise is being performed:

   a.

b.
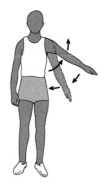

c.
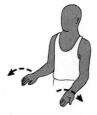

d.
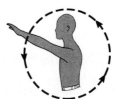

e.
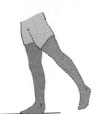

24. To evaluate muscle atrophy, a nurse should:

25. Where should a nurse check for edema in an immobilized patient?

26. For an immobilized patient, identify the usual frequency of assessment for the following:
   a. Respiratory status
   b. Anorexia
   c. Urinary elimination
   d. Intake and output
   e. Anthropometric measurements

27. Specific ROJM exercises to prevent thrombophlebitis include:

28. For a patient who will have antiembolic stockings:
    a. The contraindications for their use are:
    b. How often are they are removed?
    c. A nurse makes sure that the stockings are NOT:
    d. Application of the stockings may be delegated to an unlicensed nursing assistant.
    True _____ False _____

29. Which of the following actions are correct for the use of a sequential compression device? Select all that apply.
    a. The back of the patient's ankle and knee are aligned with markings on the sleeve. _____
    b. A hand width is left between the sleeve and the patient's skin. _____
    c. The sleeve and device are removed once daily. _____
    d. The unit is observed through one complete cycle after application. _____

30. a. A medication that is used to reduce the risk of thrombophlebitis is:
    b. It is usually given every _____ hours by the _____ route.

31. An immobilized patient is experiencing shortness of breath and chest pain. The nurse suspects a pulmonary emboli. Which of the following independent or nurse-initiated actions should be taken immediately? Select all that apply.
    a. Administering heparin _____
    b. Placing the patient in an upright position _____
    c. Drawing arterial blood gases _____
    d. Administering fluids _____
    e. Checking the patient's oxygen saturation _____

32. For a patient who is at risk for falls, which assessment should be used?

33. For a patient who had a cerebrovascular accident (CVA, or stroke) with right-sided hemiplegia, identify how the patient can be involved in joint exercise.

34. Identify at least two measures to prevent pressure ulcers.

35. Identify a nursing diagnosis for a patient who is immobilized.

Select the best answer for each of the following questions:

36. After a CVA (stroke) a patient is prescribed prolonged bed rest. During assessment, the nurse is especially alert to the presence of:
    1. an increased joint ROM.
    2. an increased hemoglobin level.
    3. an increased muscle mass.
    4. a unilateral increase in calf circumference.

37. An older adult patient had a fractured hip repaired 2 days ago. The patient is having more difficulty than expected in moving around, and the nurse is concerned about possible respiratory complications. In assessing the patient for possible atelectasis, the nurse expects to find:
    1. a decreased respiratory rate.
    2. wheezing on inspiration.
    3. asymmetrical breath sounds.
    4. rubbing sounds during inspiration and expiration.

38. For a patient who has been placed in a spica (full body) cast, the nurse remains alert to possible changes in the cardiovascular system as a result of immobility. The nurse may find that the patient has:
    1. hypertension.
    2. tachycardia.
    3. hypervolemia.
    4. an increased cardiac output.

39. A possible complication for a patient who has been prescribed prolonged bed rest is thrombus formation. For the nurse to assess the presence of this serious problem, the nurse should:
    1. attempt to elicit Chvostek sign.
    2. palpate the temperature of the feet.
    3. measure the patient's calf and thigh diameters.
    4. observe for hair loss and skin turgor in the lower legs.

40. A patient was prescribed extended bed rest after abdominal surgery. The patient now has an order to be out of bed. The nurse should first:
    1. assess respiratory function.
    2. obtain the patient's blood pressure measurement.
    3. ask if the patient feels light-headed.
    4. assist the patient to the edge of the bed.

41. A patient has been placed in skeletal traction and will be immobilized for an extended period of time. The nurse recognizes that there is a need to prevent respiratory complications and intervenes by:
    1. suctioning the airway every hour.
    2. changing the patient's position every 4 to 8 hours.
    3. using oxygen and nebulizer treatments regularly.
    4. encouraging deep breathing and coughing every hour.

42. Patients who are immobilized in health care facilities require that their psychosocial needs be met along with their physiological needs. A nurse recognizes a patient's psychosocial needs when telling the patient the following:
    1. "The staff will limit your visitors so that you will not be bothered."
    2. "We will help you get dressed so you look more like yourself."
    3. "We can discuss the routine to see if there are any changes that we can make with you."
    4. "A roommate can sometimes be a real bother and very distracting. We can move you to a private room."

43. A patient is transferred to a rehabilitation facility from the medical center after a CVA (stroke). The CVA resulted in severe right-sided paralysis, and the patient is very limited in mobility. To prevent the complication of external hip rotation for this patient, the nurse uses a:
   1. footboard.
   2. bed board.
   3. trapeze bar.
   4. trochanter roll.

44. A patient who has deep vein thrombosis is at risk for:
   1. atelectasis.
   2. pulmonary emboli.
   3. orthostatic hypotension.
   4. hypostatic pneumonia.

45. The equipment that is used on a bed to assist a patient to raise the torso is a:
   1. sandbag.
   2. bed board.
   3. trapeze bar.
   4. wedge pillow.

46. For exercise, which of the following is appropriate for an immobilized older adult?
   1. Gradual, extended warm-ups
   2. Rapid transitions and movements
   3. Sustained isometric exercises of at least a minute
   4. Slowing of exercise rate in the presence of angina or breathlessness

47. If all of the following are prescribed, the best nursing strategy for the prevention of renal calculi is:
   1. administration of diuretics.
   2. provision of a high-fiber diet.
   3. insertion of a urinary catheter.
   4. offering of 2 liters of fluid per day.

48. A nurse is instructing a patient on joint range of motion and performance of shoulder abduction. The nurse correctly instructs the patient to:
   1. raise the arm straight forward.
   2. move the arm in a full circle.
   3. move the arm until the thumb is turned inward and toward the back.
   4. raise the arm to the side to a position above the head.

49. To prevent plantar flexion, a nurse will obtain:
   1. trochanter rolls.
   2. foot boots.
   3. sandbags.
   4. hand splints.

50. A nurse is instructing a patient on ROJM and performance of forearm supination. The nurse correctly instructs the patient to:
   1. move the palm toward the inner aspect of the forearm.
   2. turn the lower arm and hand so the palm is up.
   3. straighten the elbow by lowering the hand.
   4. touch the thumb to each finger of the hand.

51. A patient has weakness to the upper and lower extremities and has been on bed rest for several days. Which of the following actions performed by the new staff nurse requires correction?
   1. Performing passive ROJM exercises
   2. Having the patient do as much of the bath as possible
   3. Massaging the lower extremities
   4. Assisting the patient to different positions every 1½ hours

52. A patient is being instructed to perform dorsiflexion of the foot. The nurse observes the patient's ability to:
   1. turn the foot and leg toward the other leg.
   2. move the foot so the toes point upward.
   3. turn the sole of the foot medially.
   4. straighten and spread the toes of the foot.

53. The nurse is applying a sequential compression device on the immobilized patient. Which of the following actions is appropriate?
   1. Make sure the red light is on so the unit will run.
   2. Remove the device after 2 to 3 days.
   3. Check for function after 10 or more complete cycles.
   4. Fit 2 fingers between the patient's leg and the device sleeve.

STUDY GROUP QUESTIONS

- What are the basic concepts of mobility?
- What is immobility?
- How is bed rest used therapeutically?
- What physiological changes may occur throughout the body as a result of immobility?
- What psychosocial and developmental changes may occur as a result of immobility?
- What assessments should be made by a nurse to determine the effect of immobility on the patient?
- What nursing interventions should be implemented to prevent or treat the effects of immobility?

37 Skin Integrity and Wound Care

CASE STUDY

1. You are a student nurse assigned to provide care to a patient in an extended care facility. While assisting the patient from the bed to the shower chair, you notice reddened areas on her sacral region and on both elbows and heels. The skin on these areas is intact, but the redness does not go away.
   a. Identify a nursing diagnosis, patient goal/outcomes, and nursing interventions related to this patient's assessment data.

CHAPTER REVIEW

Match the description/definition in Column A with the correct term in Column B.

	Column A	Column B
_____	1. Localized collection of blood under the tissues	a. Induration
_____	2. Separation of wound layers with protrusion of visceral organs	b. Approximate
_____	3. Wound edges come together	c. Abrasion
_____	4. Superficial loss of dermis	d. Laceration
_____	5. Pressure exerted against the skin when the patient is moved	e. Dehiscence
_____	6. Hardening of tissue resulting from edema or inflammation	f. Granulation tissue
_____	7. Removal of devitalized tissue	g. Hematoma
_____	8. Torn, jagged damage to dermis and epidermis	h. Evisceration
_____	9. Separation of skin and tissue layers	i. Debridement
_____	10. Red, moist tissue consisting of blood vessels and connective tissue	j. Shearing force

Complete the following:

11. Mark the areas on the body that are common sites for pressure ulcer development.

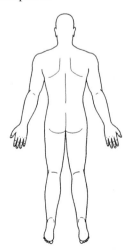

12. Identify the following stages of pressure ulcer development:

a.

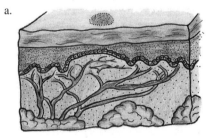

b.

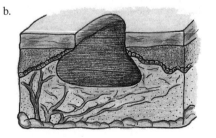

13. Provide an example of an external and internal contributing factor for pressure ulcer formation.

14. Patients in what age groups are at the highest risk for sensitivity to heat and cold applications?

15. The major change in an older adult's skin that contributes to pressure ulcer development is:

16. Identify the following related to wound healing.
    a. A clean surgical wound with little tissue loss heals by:

    b. A severe laceration or chronic wound heals by:

17. Identify if the following statements are true or false.
    a. Wounds that are kept moist for several days heal faster than those that are kept dry.
       True _____ False _____
    b. Specimens for wound cultures should be taken from wound areas with clean, healthy skin.
       True _____ False _____

18. Identify a complication of wound healing that is assessed by the nurse in the following examples.
    a. Separation of the layers of the skin with serosanguineous drainage noted
    b. Bluish swelling or mass at the site
    c. Fever, general malaise, and increased white blood cell (WBC) count
    d. Green, odorous local drainage
    e. Decreased blood pressure, increased pulse rate, increased respirations
    f. Visceral organs protruding through abdominal wall
    g. Wound edges swollen, painful, with redness extending from the edges outward

19. a. Assessment of a pressure ulcer includes:

    b. Identify the methods or indicators that are used for assessing darkly pigmented skin.

20. Identify an example of how each of the following factors influences wound healing.
    a. Age
    b. Obesity
    c. Diabetes
    d. Immunosuppression

21. Match each of the following types of wound drainage with its correct description.

Drainage	Description
a. Serous	1. Pale, more watery, with plasma and red blood cells
b. Sanguineous	2. Thick, yellow, green, or brown with organisms and white blood cells
c. Serosanguineous	3. Clear, watery plasma
d. Purulent	4. Fresh bleeding

22. Provide at least one nursing intervention that should be implemented to prevent pressure ulcer formation specifically related to:
    a. Pressure reduction
    b. Skin care

23. Arrange the steps for obtaining a wound culture in correct order.
    a. When tip is saturated, insert into appropriate sterile container. _____
    b. Complete lab slip providing clinical data, which includes wound site, time collected, and prior antibiotics. _____
    c. Moisten swab with normal saline. _____
    d. While applying pressure, rotate applicator within 1 to 2 cm² of clean wound tissue (try to draw out tissue fluid). _____
    e. Clean wound surface 1 cm² with an antiseptic solution. _____

24. A patient with a dirty penetrating wound is asked by the nurse whether a _____ injection has been received within the last 10 years.

25. Identify how the nurse determines whether a wound is healing.

26. A patient who is sitting out of bed in a chair and requires assistance to move around should be limited to _____ hours sitting and should be repositioned every _____ hour(s).

27. A nurse can reduce friction or shear by:

28. Nursing care of an abrasion or laceration includes:

29. For use of a negative pressure wound therapy system:
    a. The purpose of the therapy is to:
    b. The tube is attached to:
    c. The dressing that is used for this system is:
    d. What should be done if the patient verbalizes an increase in discomfort with this treatment?

30. For wound irrigation, identify the following that are considered as safe guidelines.
    a. Syringe size
    b. Needle gauge
    c. psi
    d. The syringe should be held how far above the wound?
    e. During an irrigation, the nurse notes sanguineous return. The nurse should:
    f. It is noted that there is retained debris in the wound. The nurse should:

31. Identify what is pictured in the following illustrations:

    a.

    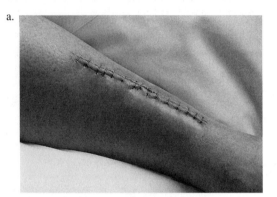

    b.

    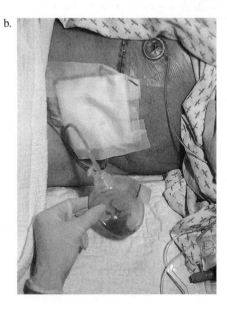

32. Which of the following are correct nursing interventions for elastic bandages? Select all that apply.
    a. Placing the body part to be bandaged in anatomical position _____
    b. Applying a bandage to an extremity from proximal to distal _____
    c. Positioning pins or knots toward the wound _____
    d. Overlapping turns by one half to two thirds the width of the bandage _____
    e. Assessing circulation once daily _____

33. Identify the steps in caring for a traumatic wound.

34. Specify whether the following effects are a result of heat (H) therapy, cold (C) therapy, or both.
    a. Vasoconstriction _____
    b. Decreased blood viscosity _____
    c. Increased tissue metabolism _____
    d. Decreased muscle tension _____
    e. Increased capillary permeability _____

35. a. Provide an instance in which the application of heat is contraindicated.
    b. Provide an instance in which the application of cold is contraindicated.

36. The usual duration of time for the application of heat or cold is:

37. Which of the following are correct for the application of heat or cold? Select all that apply.
    a. Providing a timer or clock so the patient may help time the application _____
    b. Allowing the patient to adjust the temperature setting _____
    c. Placing the patient in a position that prevents movement away from the temperature source _____
    d. Maintaining the temperature as hot or cold as the patient is able to tolerate _____
    e. Applying a heating pad or cold pack directly to the skin _____
    f. Adding hotter solution to a soak to maintain temperature while the patient remains immersed _____
    g. Keeping the rest of the patient draped or covered while receiving treatment _____

38. Using the Braden Scale, what is this patient's risk for pressure ulcer development?

		Score
Sensory	Very limited	_____
Moisture	Occasionally	_____
Activity	Chairfast	_____
Mobility	Very limited	_____
Nutrition	Probably inadequate	_____
Friction/Shear	Potential problem	_____
	Total Score	_____
	Patient Risk	_____

142

39. Which of the following are correct for application of a moist dressing? Select all that apply.
    a. Wringing out excess moisture from the dressing _____
    b. Pouring the solution directly onto the dressing in the wound _____
    c. Loosely packing sinus tracks or dead spaces in the wound _____
    d. Avoiding the use of secondary dressings _____
    e. Using Montgomery ties or straps perpendicular to the wound _____

40. a. Nonblanchable hyperemia is:
    b. This assessment signifies:
    c. When nonblanchable hyperemia is assessed, the stage is reversible if pressure is relieved.
    True _____ False _____

41. Which of the following are correct actions for a postoperative dressing? Select all that apply.
    a. Routinely changing the dressing soon after the procedure _____
    b. Reinforcing saturated dressings _____
    c. Providing the patient with an analgesic 30 minutes before the dressing change _____
    d. Expecting inflammation of the wound edges for at least a week after the surgery _____
    e. Noting the amount, color, consistency, and odor of wound drainage _____

42. A patient will need to continue to perform dressing changes when he is discharged to his home. Identify the necessary nursing assessments/evaluations before the patient's discharge.

43. Topical skin care for a patient should include: Select all that apply.
    a. Massaging reddened areas _____
    b. Examining the skin at least daily _____
    c. Using a mild cleansing agent _____
    d. Keeping the head of the bed at greater than a 30-degree angle _____
    e. Applying a moisture-barrier product _____
    f. Repositioning the patient in the chair every 3 hours _____

44. The usual wound care in the home environment is performed by the patient or family using sterile technique.
    True _____ False _____

45. Match the following wounds with the type of dressing that is most appropriate.

    Wounds
    1. Occlusive, forming a gel with the wound surface, they protect the wound from contaminants _____
    2. Best for wounds with moderate drainage, deep wounds, undermining, and tunnels, moist or dry _____
    3. Semipermeable to oxygen. Used as a primary dressing in wounds with minimal tissue loss that have very little wound drainage _____

    Dressings
    a. Gauze
    b. Transparent film
    c. Hydrocolloid

46. The correct way to remove old tape from the skin is to:

47. How can the nurse reduce discomfort during dressing changes?

48. Describe the correct application of a sling.

49. The desired temperature for a cold soak is _____.

Select the best answer for each of the following questions:

50. To avoid pressure ulcer development for an immobilized patient at home, a nurse recommends a surface to use on the bed. A surface type that is low-cost and easy to use in the home is a(n):
    1. foam overlay surface.
    2. air overlay surface.
    3. air fluidized surface.
    4. low air loss surface.

51. For a patient in the extended care facility who has a nursing diagnosis of *Impaired Physical Mobility*, a nurse will implement:
    1. massage of reddened skin areas.
    2. movement of the patient in the chair every 3 hours.
    3. maintenance of a position while in bed at 30 degrees or lower.
    4. placement of plastic absorptive pads directly beneath the patient.

52. A patient has experienced a traumatic injury that will require applications of heat. The nurse implements the treatment based on the principle that:
   1. long exposures help the patient develop tolerance to the procedure.
   2. the foot and the palm of the hand are the most sensitive to temperature.
   3. patient response is best to minor temperature adjustments.
   4. patients are more tolerant to temperature changes over a large body surface area.

53. A severely overweight patient has returned to the unit after having major abdominal surgery. When the nurse enters the room, it is evident that the patient has moved or coughed and the wound has eviscerated. The nurse should immediately:
   1. assess vital signs.
   2. contact the physician.
   3. apply light pressure on the exposed organs.
   4. place sterile towels soaked in saline over the area.

54. A patient with a knife protruding from his upper leg is taken into the emergency department. A nurse is waiting for the physician to arrive when a newly hired nurse comes to assist. The nurse delegates the new staff member to do all of the following as soon as possible except:
   1. assess vital signs.
   2. remove the knife to cleanse the wound.
   3. wrap a bandage around the knife and injured site.
   4. apply pressure to the surrounding area to stop bleeding.

55. A nurse is assessing a patient's wound and notices that it has very minimal tissue loss and drainage. There are a number of dressings that may be used according to the protocol on the unit. The nurse selects:
   1. gauze.
   2. alginate.
   3. negative pressure wound therapy.
   4. transparent film.

56. A nurse is completing an assessment of the patient's skin integrity and identifies that an area is a full-thickness wound with damage to the subcutaneous tissue. The nurse identifies this stage of ulcer formation as:
   1. Stage I.
   2. Stage II.
   3. Stage III.
   4. Stage IV.

57. A patient has a large wound to the sacral area that requires irrigation. The nurse explains to the patient that irrigation will be performed to:
   1. decrease scar formation.
   2. decrease wound drainage.
   3. remove debris from the wound.
   4. improve circulation in the wound.

58. A nurse is working with an older adult patient in an extended care facility. While turning the patient, the nurse notices that there is a reddened area on the patient's coccyx. The nurse implements skin care that includes:
   1. soaking the area with normal saline.
   2. cleaning the area with mild soap, drying, and applying a protective moisturizer.
   3. washing the area with an astringent and painting it with povidone-iodine solution.
   4. applying a dilute solution of hydrogen peroxide and water and using a heat lamp to dry the area.

59. A patient has a wound to the left lower extremity that has minimal exudates and collagen formation. The nurse identifies the healing phase of this wound as:
   1. primary intention.
   2. proliferative phase.
   3. secondary intention.
   4. inflammatory phase.

60. After neurosurgery, a nurse assesses the patient's bandage and finds that there is fresh bleeding coming from the operative site. The nurse describes this drainage to the surgeon as:
   1. serous.
   2. purulent.
   3. sanguineous.
   4. serosanguineous.

61. A patient has a surgical wound on the right upper aspect of the chest that requires cleansing. The nurse implements appropriate aseptic technique by:
   1. opening the cleansing solution with sterile gloves.
   2. moving from the outer region of the wound toward the center.
   3. cleaning the wound twice and discarding the swab.
   4. starting at the drainage site and moving outward with circular motions.

62. A nurse is working in a physician's office and is asked by one of the patients when heat or cold should be applied. In providing an example, the nurse identifies that cold therapy should be applied for the patient with:
   1. a newly fractured ankle.
   2. menstrual cramping.
   3. an infected wound.
   4. degenerative joint disease.

63. A patient will require the application of a binder to provide support to the abdomen. When applying the binder, the nurse uses the principle that:
   1. the binder should be kept loose for patient comfort.
   2. the patient should be sitting or standing when it is applied.
   3. the patient must maintain adequate ventilatory capacity.
   4. the binder replaces the need for underlying bandages or dressings.

64. A nurse is aware that malnutrition places a patient at a greater risk for tissue damage. The patient with the greatest risk is the individual who:
    1. experienced a 7% weight loss in 4 months.
    2. is between 45 and 60 years of age.
    3. has an albumin level of 5 mg/100 mL.
    4. has a transferrin level of 120 mg/dL.

65. The agent that is most effective and safest for cleaning a granular wound is:
    1. acetic acid.
    2. normal saline.
    3. povidone-iodine.
    4. hydrogen peroxide.

66. A nurse is working with a patient who has a stage III, clean ulcer with significant exudate. The nurse anticipates that which of the following dressings will be used?
    1. Composite film dressing
    2. Transparent dressing
    3. Calcium alginate dressing
    4. Gauze dressing

67. For a patient's optimal nutritional intake that will promote formation of new blood vessels and collagen synthesis, the nurse plans to teach the patient to include a sufficient intake of:
    1. fats.
    2. proteins.
    3. carbohydrates.
    4. fat-soluble vitamins.

68. The nurse notices that the skin surrounding a wound appears macerated. The nurse should:
    1. obtain a wound culture.
    2. monitor lab results.
    3. turn the patient more frequently.
    4. select a different dressing.

STUDY GROUP QUESTIONS

- What are pressure ulcers and what contributes to their development?
- Where are pressure ulcers most likely to develop?
- What are the stages of pressure ulcer development?
- What are the classifications of wounds?
- How do wounds heal?
- What are the possible complications of wound healing?
- How do pressure ulcers affect health care costs?
- What tools may be used to predict patients' risks for pressure ulcer development?
- What should be included in the nursing assessment of patients to determine their risk for pressure ulcer development?
- How are wounds managed in emergency and nonemergency health care settings?
- What types of drainage may be seen in wounds?
- How are wound cultures obtained?
- How can the nurse prevent pressure ulcer development?
- What nursing interventions may be implemented to treat pressure ulcers and wounds?
- What are the procedures for dressing changes and wound care?
- What criteria are used in the selection of dressings and sutures or staples?
- What are the principles involved in heat and cold therapy, including patient safety?
- What information should be included in patient/family teaching for prevention and treatment of pressure ulcers, wound care, and use of heat and cold therapy?

38 Sensory Alterations

CASE STUDIES

1. You are making a home visit to a patient with diabetes mellitus who is losing his eyesight (diabetic retinopathy).
   a. What interventions may be implemented with the patient to assist in maintaining adequate sensory stimulation?
   b. How can you promote a safe environment for him?

2. You have been assigned to care for a patient in the intensive care unit (ICU).
   a. What sensory alterations may this patient experience?
   b. How can you prevent the occurrence of these alterations or reduce their impact?

CHAPTER REVIEW

Complete the following:

1. Identify other terms for the following.
   a. Sight:
   b. Hearing:
   c. Taste:
   d. Smell:
   e. Touch:
   f. Position sense:

2. Identify one of the major diseases that can lead to visual impairment.

3. Provide the correct term for each of the following:
   a. A buildup of earwax in the external auditory canal
   b. Hearing loss associated with aging
   c. Opacity of the lens resulting in blurred vision
   d. Decreased salivary production or dry mouth
   e. Intermittent hearing loss, vertigo, tinnitus, and pressure in the ears

4. Identify how the following factors may influence sensory function:
   a. Age: older adulthood
   b. Medications
   c. Smoking
   d. Environment

5. How can a nurse evaluate a patient's vision and hearing during routine interactions or care?

6. For visual and hearing impairments in children:
   a. A common cause of blindness is:
   b. What information should be included when teaching parents about eyesight safety?
   c. Common causes of hearing impairment are:

7. Orientation to the environment for a patient with a sensory deficit should include:

8. Identify a way that a nurse can modify sensory stimulation in the health care environment.

9. A nurse may communicate with a hearing-impaired patient by:

10. For a patient with cataracts, the nurse anticipates which of the following signs and symptoms? Select all that apply.
    a. Cloudy vision _____
    b. Eye pain _____
    c. Glare _____
    d. Burning sensation _____
    e. Poor night vision _____
    f. Double vision _____

11. Indicate how a nurse may assist patients with the following deficits to adapt their home environments for safety:
    a. Hearing deficit
    b. Diminished sense of smell
    c. Diminished sense of touch

12. Identify a possible nursing diagnosis and goal/outcome for a patient with a sensory deficit.

13. In relation to screening for sensory deficits:
    a. Provide an example of a general screening that is conducted to determine visual and/or auditory deficits.
    b. The recommendation of frequency for hearing screenings is:

14. Which of the following are appropriate in promoting sensory stimulation in the home environment? Select all that apply.
    a. Reducing glare by using sheer curtains on windows _____
    b. Using pale colors on surfaces _____
    c. Serving bland foods with similar textures _____
    d. Using a pocket magnifier _____
    e. Introducing fragrant flowers _____
    f. Playing recorded music with high-frequency sound _____

15. A patient has gone to the local walk-in emergency center with flu-like symptoms. After seeing the physician, the patient shows the nurse the prescriptions the physician has written. The patient should be informed that ototoxicity may occur with the administration of which of the following medications? Select all that apply.
    a. Furosemide _____
    b. Vitamin C _____
    c. Acetaminophen _____
    d. Erythromycin _____
    e. Cough suppressant with codeine _____
    f. Aspirin _____

16. Identify at least one rationale for why a patient may not use his or her hearing aid.

17. A patient with a diminished tactile sense may be assisted with hygiene and grooming by:

18. What are the signs and symptoms associated with Ménière's disease?

19. The nurse is caring for a patient with a hearing aid. What is included in the care for this patient and the assistive device?

20. Behaviors that are specific for an adult with a visual impairment include: Select all that apply.
    a. Poor coordination _____
    b. Rocking _____
    c. Squinting _____
    d. No reaction to being touched _____
    e. Accidental falls _____
    f. Increase in appetite _____

21. Identify community resources where a patient with a sensory impairment may be referred.

22. The occupational health nurse wants to promote safety for the employees. What general safety measures may be implemented by the nurse in a work environment?

23. Provide an example of a patient who may experience sensory deprivation.

Select the best answer for each of the following questions:

24. An expected outcome for a patient with an auditory deficit should include:
    1. minimizing use of affected sense(s).
    2. preventing additional sensory losses.
    3. promoting the patient's acceptance of dependency.
    4. controlling the environment to reduce sensory stimuli.

25. A nurse is working with patients at the senior day care center and recognizes that changes in sensory status may influence the older adult's eating patterns. For patients who are experiencing changes in their dietary intake, the nurse will assess for:
    1. presbycusis.
    2. xerostomia.
    3. vestibular ataxia.
    4. peripheral neuropathy.

26. Parents arrive at the pediatric clinic with their 1½-year-old child. The parents ask the nurse if there are signs that may indicate that the child is not able to hear well. The nurse explains to the parents that they should be alert to the child:
    1. awakening to loud noises.
    2. responding reflexively to sounds.
    3. having delayed speech development.
    4. remaining calm when unfamiliar people approach.

27. A nurse is assessing a patient for a potential gustatory impairment. This may be indicated if the patient has a(n):
    1. weight loss.
    2. blank look or stare.
    3. increased sensitivity to odors.
    4. period of excessive clumsiness or dizziness.

28. Which of the following is a priority safety measure in the acute care environment for a patient with a sensory deficit?
    1. Encouraging the family to visit the patient
    2. Referring the patient to a support group
    3. Determining the patient's medical history
    4. Orienting the patient to the surroundings

29. A responsive patient had eye surgery, and patches have been temporarily placed on both eyes for protection. The evening meal has arrived, and the nurse will be assisting the patient. In this circumstance, the nurse should:
    1. feed the patient the entire meal.
    2. encourage family members to feed the patient.
    3. allow the patient to be totally independent and feed himself.
    4. orient the patient to the locations of the foods on the plate and provide the utensils.

30. After a cerebrovascular accident (CVA, or stroke), a patient is found to have receptive aphasia. The nurse may assist this patient with communication by:
    1. obtaining a referral for a speech therapist.
    2. using a system of simple gestures and repeated behaviors.
    3. providing the patient with a letter chart to use to answer questions.
    4. offering the patient a notepad and pen to write down questions and concerns.

31. A patient has been diagnosed with glaucoma. The nurse anticipates that the patient will report a history of:
    1. severe redness and itching of the eyes.
    2. cloudy and blurred vision.
    3. painless loss of peripheral vision.
    4. dark spaces blocking forward vision and distortion of lines.

32. A mother is taking her newborn for his first physical examination. She expresses concern because during her pregnancy she may have been exposed to an infectious disease, and the baby's hearing could be affected. The nurse inquires if the patient was exposed to:
    1. rubella.
    2. pneumonia.
    3. tuberculosis.
    4. a urinary tract infection.

33. For a patient with a hearing deficit, the best way for the nurse to communicate is to:
    1. approach the patient from the side.
    2. use visible facial expressions.
    3. shout or speak very loudly to the patient.
    4. repeat the entire conversation if it is not totally understood.

34. The school nurse recognizes that the most common type of visual disorder in children is:
    1. glaucoma.
    2. retinal detachment.
    3. nearsightedness.
    4. macular degeneration.

35. Because of the possibility of diminished independence for the patient with sensory losses, an important and specific ethical standard for the nurse to follow is the preservation of:
    1. autonomy.
    2. fidelity.
    3. justice.
    4. nonmaleficence.

STUDY GROUP QUESTIONS

- What are the human senses and their functions?
- What factors influence sensory function?
- What are some common sensory alterations?
- What types of patients are at risk for developing sensory alterations?
- How should a nurse assess a patient's sensory function?
- What behaviors or changes in lifestyle patterns or socialization may indicate a sensory alteration?
- How can a nurse promote sensory function and prevent injury and isolation in the health promotion and acute and restorative care settings?
- What screening processes are used to determine the presence of sensory alterations?
- How may the family/significant others be involved in the care of a patient with a sensory alteration?
- What information should be included in patient/family teaching for promotion of sensory function and prevention of injury?

39 Surgical Patient

CASE STUDIES

1. Your patient is scheduled to have extensive abdominal surgery with a large midline incision.
   a. How can you assist this patient to promote respiratory function postoperatively?

2. A patient is having outpatient surgery.
   a. How may preoperative teaching be conducted and what information should be included?
   b. The patient does not appear to have an understanding of the surgery or possible complications. What should you do?

3. While completing the preoperative checklist, you discover that a patient's temperature is 101° F.
   a. What action should be taken?

4. A patient insists that his good luck medallion must go with him everywhere, even to surgery.
   a. What should you do?
   b. What personal items or prosthetics should be accounted for before surgery?

5. A patient had laparoscopic surgery on his right knee and is going to be discharged to his home. His wife and young children have visited often during his hospital stay.
   a. What general information do you need to prepare the patient and the family for the discharge?

6. A patient has come into the ambulatory surgery center in the hospital for hernia repair. Upon admission to the PACU, the patient's oxygen saturation is 88% and he is not easy to arouse. There is no evidence of bleeding on the lower right abdominal dressing and no distention.
   a. What should you do for this patient in the PACU?
   b. After 3 hours, the patient has still not had any urinary output. What options are available?

CHAPTER REVIEW

Match the description/definition in Column A with the correct term in Column B.

	Column A	Column B
g	1. Performed on the basis of the patient's choice; not essential for health	a. Palliative surgery
c	2. Involves extensive reconstruction or alteration in body parts; poses risks to well-being	b. Transplant surgery
a	3. Relieves or reduces intensity of disease symptoms; will not produce cure	c. Major surgery
f	4. Must be done immediately to save life or preserve function of body part	d. Ablative surgery
h	5. Surgical exploration that allows physician to confirm medical status; may involve removal of body tissue for analysis	e. Cosmetic surgery
e	6. Performed to improve personal appearance	f. Emergency surgery
d	7. Amputation or removal of diseased body part	g. Elective surgery
b	8. Performed to replace malfunctioning organs or structures	h. Diagnostic surgery

Complete the following:

9. a. In relation to the operative experience, a patient who smokes cigarettes is at a greater risk for:
    b. Postoperative care for this patient requires more aggressive:

10. a. Identify a medical condition that may increase a patient's surgical risk.
    b. Malignant hyperthermia is associated with:
    c. The pregnant patient is at greater risk because of:

11. Identify an example of how changes in each of the following body systems place the older adult patient at risk during surgery.
    a. Cardiovascular
    b. Pulmonary
    c. Renal
    d. Neurological

12. Obesity places a patient at greater risk for surgery as a result of:

13. Identify a consideration for surgical patients who are taking the following medications:
    a. Insulin
    b. Antibiotics
    c. NSAIDs

14. Provide two examples of information that is usually included in preoperative teaching.

15. For preoperative screening, identify a routine screening test that may be ordered for a patient.

16. Identify the commonly used types of preoperative medications.

17. Identify two nursing diagnoses and related outcomes that may be formulated for a patient who will be having his or her first surgery.

18. The patient is going to receive general anesthesia for the surgical procedure. Specify the general NPO criteria for the following.
    a. No food or fluids _____ hours before surgery
    b. No meat or fried foods _____ hours before surgery

19. Identify the adverse effects associated with the following types of anesthesia.
    a. General anesthesia
    b. Regional anesthesia
    c. Local anesthesia
    d. Conscious sedation

20. Which of the following preoperative interventions are appropriate? Select all that apply.
    a. Completing bowel preparation before GI surgery _____
    b. Shaving the surgical site with a razor _____
    c. Providing antimicrobial soap for bathing _____
    d. Removing the patient's wig _____
    e. Leaving artificial fingernails intact _____
    f. Removing a hearing aid when the patient gets to the operating room (OR) _____

21. In the presurgical care unit (PSCU) and OR, how is verification done to determine:
    a. Right patient
    b. Right frame of mind of the patient
    c. Preparation for surgery

22. Identify whether the following tasks are responsibilities of the circulating nurse (C) or scrub nurse (S).
    a. Completion of preoperative assessments/verification _____
    b. Application of sterile drapes _____
    c. Establishment of the intraoperative plan of care _____
    d. Calculation of blood loss and urinary output _____
    e. Provision of sterile equipment for the surgeon _____
    f. Documentation of the procedure _____
    g. Maintenance of the sterile field _____

23. For the following, identify a nursing intervention for intraoperative patient care.
    a. Prevention of injury
    b. Maintenance of patient's body temperature
    c. Prevention of infection

24. Identify a specific nursing intervention to prevent the following postoperative complications.
    a. Pulmonary stasis
    b. Venous stasis
    c. Wound infection
    d. Gastrointestinal stasis

25. Which of the following assessment findings for a patient in the postanesthesia care unit (PACU) signify that the patient is qualified to be discharged from the unit? Select all that apply.
    a. Oxygen saturation 96% _____
    b. Rales on auscultation _____
    c. Pulse rate 110 beats per minute _____
    d. Bilateral peripheral pulses _____
    e. Abdominal distention _____
    f. Response to verbal stimuli _____
    g. Sluggish hand grasp and pupillary response _____
    h. Quarter-size sanguineous spot maintained on incisional dressing _____
    i. 30 mL per hour urinary output _____

26. A nurse is aware that a patient should void within _____ hours after surgery. For the patient who has not voided, what should the nurse do?

27. After general anesthesia, postoperative oral intake usually begins with an order for _____ (diet).

28. With regard to postoperative wound healing and care, which of the following statements are correct? Select all that apply.
    a. The surgical dressing is changed after the patient leaves the PACU. _____
    b. Any visible drainage on the surgical dressing should be marked. _____
    c. The patient who has an order for an oral analgesic should be medicated 20 minutes before an uncomfortable dressing change. _____
    d. Redness, warmth, and edema should be expected at the incision site. _____
    e. Wound drainage should be measured once a day. _____
    f. The patient should be draped during a dressing change to minimize exposure. _____

29. a. The patient in the illustration is demonstrating the use of a(n):

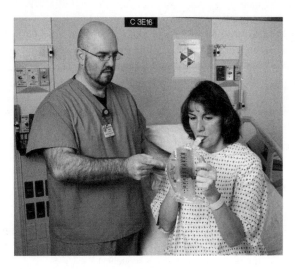

    b. This device is used to prevent:

30. For a patient who will be alert during a surgical procedure, what support should be provided by the nurse?

31. Identify examples of routine postoperative patient assessments and interventions.

32. What physical signs and symptoms are indicative of a latex allergy?

33. The American Society of Anesthesiologists recommends that postoperative analgesics be administered:

34. Indicate which of the following are appropriate interventions in the postanesthesia care unit (PACU). Select all that apply.
    a. Irrigating an existing N/G tube with normal saline _____
    b. Providing oral fluids _____
    c. Measuring I & O _____
    d. Yelling loudly to arouse the patient _____
    e. Checking for bleeding at the surgical site _____
    f. Administering analgesics _____

35. Research indicates that the use of preventive measures decreases the incidence of postoperative wound infection. Identify at least three (3) of those interventions.

36. What is included in the hand-off communication ANTICipate?

37. Identify two nursing diagnoses and a related outcome for each that may be formulated for a patient in the postoperative period.

Select the best answer for each of the following questions:

38. A nurse is starting the preparations for a patient who is having surgery tomorrow morning. The nurse prepares to have the consent form completed. The nurse recognizes that informed consent:
    1. is valid if the patient is disoriented.
    2. is signed by the patient after the administration of preoperative medications.
    3. indicates that the patient is aware of the procedure and its possible complications.
    4. requires that the nurse provide information about the surgery before the consent can be signed.

39. A patient is taken to PACU after surgery. A nurse is assessing the patient and is alert to the indication of a postoperative hemorrhage if the patient exhibits:
    1. restlessness.
    2. warm, dry skin.
    3. a slow, steady pulse rate.
    4. a decreased respiratory rate.

40. A nurse is checking the vital signs of a patient who had major surgery yesterday. The nurse discovers that the patient's temperature is slightly elevated. This finding is usually indicative of:
    1. a postoperative wound infection.
    2. an allergic response to latex.
    3. a response to the anesthesia.
    4. extensive neural damage.

41. A nurse is completing the preoperative checklist for a woman who will be having surgery. The nurse determines that the surgeon and anesthesiologist should be informed of which of the patient's laboratory results?
    1. Hemoglobin level: 10 g/dL
    2. Potassium level: 4.2 mEq/L
    3. Platelet count: 210,000/mm^3
    4. Prothrombin time: 11 seconds

42. A patient has received a spinal anesthetic during the surgical procedure. The nurse is alert to possible complications of the anesthetic and is assessing the patient for a:
    1. rash.
    2. headache.
    3. nephrotoxic response.
    4. hyperthermic response.

43. A patient is being evaluated for transfer from the PACU to the patient's unit. The nurse determines that the patient will be approved for transfer if the patient exhibits:
    1. increased wound drainage.
    2. pulse oximetry of 95%.
    3. respirations of 30 breaths per minute.
    4. nonpalpable peripheral pulses.

44. A patient is scheduled to have abdominal surgery later in the morning. At 9:00 AM, while completing the preoperative checklist, the nurse recognizes the need to contact the surgeon immediately. The nurse has identified that the patient:
    1. received an enema at 6:00 AM.
    2. admitted to recent substance abuse.
    3. ate a hamburger last evening at 6:00 PM.
    4. has bowel sounds in all four quadrants of the abdomen.

45. A patient is being positioned in the PACU after surgery. Unless contraindicated, the nurse should place the patient:
    1. prone.
    2. in high Fowler's.
    3. supine with arms across the chest.
    4. on the side with the face turned downward.

46. When a patient first arrives at PACU, the nurse will:
    1. provide oral fluids.
    2. allow the patient to sleep.
    3. provide a warm blanket.
    4. remove the urinary catheter.

47. A nurse is visiting a patient who had surgery 9 hours ago. The nurse asks if the patient has voided, and the patient responds negatively. At this time, the nurse:
    1. provides more oral fluids.
    2. inserts an IV and administers fluids.
    3. obtains an order for urinary catheterization.
    4. recognizes that this is a normal outcome.

48. During a patient assessment in the PACU, a nurse finds that the patient's operative site is swollen and appears tight. The nurse suspects:
    1. infection.
    2. hemorrhage.
    3. lymphedema.
    4. subcutaneous emphysema.

49. An immediate postoperative priority in providing nursing care for a patient is:
    1. airway patency.
    2. relief of pain.
    3. sufficient circulation to the extremities.
    4. prevention of wound infection.

50. A 54-year-old patient is scheduled to have a gastric resection. The nurse informs the surgeon preoperatively of the patient's history of:
    1. a tonsillectomy at age 10.
    2. employment as a telephone repair person.
    3. smoking two packs of cigarettes per day.
    4. taking acetaminophen for minor body aches.

51. A patient has been taking warfarin at home. The patient is going to be admitted for a surgical procedure, and the nurse anticipates that this prescribed medication will be:
    1. administered as usual.
    2. increased in dose immediately before the procedure.
    3. reduced in dose by half immediately before the procedure.
    4. discontinued at least 2 days before the procedure.

52. During the intraoperative phase, a nurse's responsibility is reflected in the statement:
    1. "I think that the patient requires more information about the procedure and its consequences."
    2. "There seems to be a missing sponge, so a recount must be done to see that all of the sponges were removed."
    3. "The patient has signed the request. I will prepare the medications and then get the record completed."
    4. "The patient appears reactive and stable. Dressing to wound is dry and intact. Analgesic administered per order."

53. A nurse is assisting a patient with postoperative exercises. The patient tells the nurse, "Blowing into this thing [incentive spirometer] is a waste of time." The nurse explains to the patient that the specific purpose of this therapy is to:
    1. stimulate the cough reflex.
    2. promote lung expansion.
    3. increase pulmonary circulation.
    4. directly remove excess secretions from the respiratory tract.

54. A patient is scheduled for surgery, and a nurse is completing the final areas of the preoperative checklist. After administering the preoperative medications, the nurse should:
    1. assist the patient to void.
    2. obtain the informed consent.
    3. prepare the skin at the surgical site.
    4. place the side rails up on the bed or stretcher.

55. At the ambulatory surgery center, a patient is having surgery using general anesthesia. The nurse will expect this patient to:
    1. ambulate immediately after being admitted to the recovery area.
    2. meet all of the identified criteria in order to be discharged home.
    3. remain in the phase I recovery area longer than a hospitalized patient.
    4. receive large amounts of oral fluids immediately entering the recovery area.

56. A nurse is preparing a patient for surgery and recognizes that the greatest risk of bleeding is for the patient with:
    1. diabetes mellitus.
    2. emphysema.
    3. thrombocytopenia.
    4. immunodeficiency syndrome.

57. A patient has a nasogastric tube in place after surgery and complains to the nurse of nausea. The nurse should first:
    1. remove the NG tube.
    2. provide oral fluids.
    3. move the patient side to side.
    4. irrigate the tube with normal saline.

58. Which of the following individuals is most at risk for postoperative wound infection?
    1. A pregnant patient
    2. A patient who smokes cigarettes
    3. A patient with poorly controlled diabetes
    4. A patient experiencing periods of sleep apnea

59. A patient's surgeon has previously discussed the procedure with the patient, but the patient has a few more questions. The best way for the nurse to approach this is to first:
    1. refer the patient back to the surgeon.
    2. determine what the patient has been told already.
    3. provide details of what the procedure will be like.
    4. get the consent form for the patient to read.

60. The nurse is alert for signs of a postoperative wound infection:
    1. within 24 hours of the surgery.
    2. 1 to 2 days after the surgery.
    3. 3 to 6 days after the surgery.
    4. 2 weeks after the surgery.

61. After surgery, the patient is suspected of having a pulmonary embolism. This is determined by the patient experiencing:
    1. restlessness, chills.
    2. dyspnea, sudden chest pain.
    3. hypotension, nausea.
    4. productive cough, crackles in the lungs.

STUDY GROUP QUESTIONS

- How are surgeries classified?
- What are some surgical risk factors, and why do they increase the patient's risk?
- How does the incision site influence a patient's recovery?
- How may previous surgical experiences influence the patient's expectations of surgery?
- What general information should be included in preoperative teaching?
- What is the purpose of the preoperative exercises that are explained and demonstrated to patients?
- What preoperative assessments should be made by a nurse?
- What are some common preoperative diagnostic tests that may be ordered for a patient?
- What nursing interventions are implemented in the preoperative care of patients?
- How does a nurse prepare and assist a patient in the acute care setting on the day of surgery?
- What are the roles of nurses in the operating room and in the recovery setting?
- What interventions are implemented to maintain patient safety and well-being in the operating room and postanesthesia care area?
- What nursing care is critical in the immediate postoperative stage?
- What are the similarities and differences between preanesthesia and postanesthesia care for patients in the acute care and ambulatory surgery settings?
- What general information should be included in postoperative teaching for patients/families in the acute care and ambulatory surgery settings?
- How may the family/significant other be involved in the patient's perioperative experience?

STUDY CHART

Create a study chart on Surgical Risk Factors that identifies how age, nutritional status, obesity, immunocompetence, fluid/electrolyte balance, and pregnancy may affect the patient's perioperative experience.

Answer Key

CHAPTER 1

Case Study

1. a. The preferred educational requirement for a nurse re-searcher is a doctoral degree, with at least a master's degree in nursing.
   b. To maintain this role, Mr. R. would need to continue his formal education in doctoral or postdoctoral study and/or participate in continuing education activities. In many states, continuing education hours are required to main-tain nursing licensure as an LPN/LVN, RN, and APRN.

Chapter Review

1. c
2. d
3. a
4. b
5. a. The NLN advances excellence in nursing education to prepare nurses to meet the needs of a diverse population in a changing health care environment.
   b. The purpose of the ANA is to improve standards of health and the availability of health care, to foster high standards for nursing, and to promote the professional development and general and economic welfare of nurses.
   c. The ICN promotes national associations of nurses, improves standards of nursing practice, seeks a higher status for nurses, and provides an international power base for nurses.
6. Career paths that a nurse can choose are clinical practice, education, research, management, administration, and even entrepreneurship.
7. Nurses and their professional organizations have lobbied for creating smoke-free environments and stronger anti-tobacco laws, setting up anti-gang coalitions, establishing safer en-vironments for walking and physical fitness in their com-munities, and advocating for breastfeeding.
8. The three components of nursing care are care, cure, and coordination.
9. Accurate statements about Nurse Practice Acts in the United States are a, c.
10. Four core roles for APRNs are clinical nurse specialist (CNS), nurse practitioner (NP), certified nurse midwife (CNM), and certified RN anesthetist (CRNA).
11. Essential skills for nurses include time management, thera-peutic communication, patient education, and compassion-ate implementation of psychomotor skills.
12. To become a nurse educator or advanced practice nurse, a master's or doctoral degree is required.

13. Continuing education involves formal, organized educa-tional programs offered by universities, hospitals, state nurses associations, professional nursing organizations, and educational and health care institutions. In-service edu-cation is instruction or training provided by a health care agency or institution designed to increase the knowledge, skills, and competencies of nurses and other health care professionals employed by the institution.
14. f
15. a
16. d
17. b
18. c
19. g
20. e
21. External influences on nursing include health care reform, demographic changes of the population, increasing num-bers of medically underserved, workplace issues, the nurs-ing shortage, and the threat of bioterrorism.
22. Workplace hazards that are faced by nurses include muscu-loskeletal injuries, such as back injury and repetitive motion disorders, and violence.
23. The use of genomics in health care allows providers to deter-mine how genomic changes contribute to patient conditions and influence treatment decisions such as assessment and symptom management and titration of medications based on a patient's response.
24. The QSEN competencies for patient-centered care are a and c.
25. The ANA Standards of Professional Performance include b, d, e, and g.
26. 4
27. 4
28. 1

CHAPTER 2

Case Studies

1. a. This is an individual entering her middle adult years who is experiencing stress in her personal and professional life. She is being called upon by her employer and her child to meet their expectations, and she believes that this does not allow her the time to meet her health needs. The symptoms of gastrointestinal distress may be a response to the pres-sures in her life.
   b. Initially the nurse may spend time with this patient to discuss the patient's personal feelings and needs. The patient may benefit from instruction in stress reduction and relaxation techniques, along with a review of time management. The nurse may investigate with her if there are support people at work and in the neighborhood to assist her in keeping up with her busy schedule. This

individual also may be assisted in making an appointment for medical follow-up to determine her current health status.

2. a. There are several factors that could influence Mr. G.'s ability to manage his illness, including other health issues that he may have, how he perceives the illness, his prior lifestyle and social activities, family support, financial security, emotional stability, and his ability to comprehend the treatment regimen.

   b. Mr. G. could demonstrate illness behaviors, such as
   - losing motivation to participate in his care
   - becoming depressed, angry, anxious, or withdrawn
   - overly seeking or avoiding health care providers
   - assuming a dependent role

   c. Mr. G.'s wife could also exhibit emotional responses, including fear of her husband's ability to maintain his normal activities (work, socialization) and/or her ability to assist him with his care. She could also become overly protective of him or critical of his ability to manage his treatment. His wife could perceive that she will have to take on a larger role in keeping the household going.

   d. The QSEN competency of safety is applied in Mr. G.'s situation by making sure that he knows about the disease, his treatment requirements, and the indications when assistance should be sought. For example, Mr. G. needs to know what affect the combination of exercise and insulin will have on his physiology so that he does not experience a situation that could lead to a loss of consciousness and an injury.

Chapter Review

1. e
2. d
3. g
4. c
5. b
6. f
7. a
8. False

9. Health promotion for an older adult may include
   - Helping to maintain function and independence and improve quality of life.
   - Encouraging older adults to participate in group activities.
   - Monitoring older patients for acute and chronic diseases.
   - Encouraging physical activity.

10. The order, from lowest to highest need, is Physiological, Safety, Love and Belongingness, Self-Esteem, and Self-Actualization.

11. a. External variable
    b. External variable
    c. Internal variable
    d. External variable

12. Positive health behaviors include immunizations, adequate sleep, exercise, and good nutrition.

13. Negative health behaviors include smoking, substance abuse, poor diet, and refusal to take medication or follow a treatment regimen.

14. The goals of *Healthy People 2020* are to (1) attain high-quality, longer lives, (2) achieve health equality, (3) create social and physical environments that promote good health, and (4) promote quality of life across all life states.

15. Answers a, c, e, and f are external variables.

16. 2
17. 3
18. 1
19. 2
20. 1
21. 3
22. 2
23. 4
24. 3
25. 1

CHAPTER 3

Case Studies

1. a. This patient could benefit from the services of a hospice organization for either home care and/or inpatient care, depending on the program.

2. a. As a nurse on a busy medical unit it is important to be aware of the patients' needs and expectations to form effective partnerships to enhance the level of nursing care given. Managed care organizations expect patients who are hospitalized to be cared for and discharged within a projected time period. Therefore, as the nurse manager on the unit, you will have to use resources efficiently to help your patients successfully recover and return home. You will want to consider how to work efficiently with the staff to assess patients' needs, provide care, and prepare the patients for discharge.

   b. The QSEN competency of teamwork and collaboration can be applied by fostering open communication with the staff, demonstrating respect for them, and encouraging them to be part of the decision-making processes on the unit. For example, as the unit manager, you could ask the nursing staff for their input on strategies that will improve services, such as transport of patients to the radiology department.

Chapter Review

1. f
2. j
3. b
4. g
5. a
6. i
7. d
8. c
9. h
10. e

11. Hospice

12. Discharge planning should begin the moment the patient enters the health care agency; the planning assists in the transition of the patient's care from one environment to the other (such as from the hospital to the home). The patient's ongoing needs are anticipated and identified, and necessary services/resources are coordinated before the patient's discharge.

13. Developments in technology influence many aspects of health care delivery. New types of equipment for patient monitoring, computerization, and electronic communication and record-keeping systems create a need for health care providers to be up to date.

14. Utilization review is designed for review of admissions, diagnostic testing, and treatments provided by physicians or health care providers to patients. The purpose is to identify and eliminate overuse of diagnostic and treatment services.

15. a. Primary
    b. Tertiary
    c. Restorative
    d. Restorative
    e. Continuing
    f. Preventative
    g. Primary
    h. Preventative
    i. Secondary
    j. Continuing
    k. Secondary
    l. Restorative

16. The role of the case manager is to coordinate efforts of all the disciplines to achieve the most efficient and appropriate plan of care for the patient. The focus of case management is on discharge planning.

17. Vulnerable populations include children and women, older adults, the mentally ill, and the homeless.

18. Access to health care options are found in selections a, e, and g.

19. Patient referrals include
    • Involving the patient and family in the process, including selecting the necessary referral
    • Explaining the service to be provided, the reason for the referral, and what to expect from the referral's services
    • Making a referral as soon as possible
    • Informing the care provider receiving the referral of as much information about the patient as possible to avoid duplication of effort and exclusion of important information
    • Determining what the referral discipline (e.g., physical therapy, social work, diet and nutrition, radiology) recommends for the patient's care, and incorporating this into the treatment plan as soon as possible

20. The Patient Protection and Affordable Care Act of 2010 focuses on the major goals of increasing access to health care services for all, reducing health care costs, and improving health care quality. Provisions in the law include insurance industry reforms that increase insurance coverage and decrease costs, increased funding for community health centers, increased primary care services and providers, and improved coverage for children (HealthReform.gov, 2010).

21. Areas addressed in the Minimum Data Set for Resident Assessment include
    • Resident's background
    • Cognitive, communication/hearing, and vision patterns
    • Physical functioning and structural problems
    • Mood, behavior, and activity pursuit patterns
    • Psychosocial well-being
    • Bowel and bladder continence
    • Health conditions
    • Disease diagnoses
    • Oral/nutritional and dental status
    • Skin condition
    • Medication use
    • Special treatments and procedures

22. Cost is one of the biggest drawbacks to an assisted-living facility.

23. Two systems stimulated through health care reform are Accountable Care Organizations (ACO) and Patient-Centered Medical Homes (PCMH).

24. Nursing centers provide the services in selections a, b, and d.

25. Quality and safety are demonstrated by health care agencies through The Joint Commission, Six Sigma, and Value Stream Mapping.

26. Accurate statements about a critical access hospital include b and d.

27. The National Database of Nursing Quality Indicators include
    • Patient falls
    • Patient falls with injury
    • Pressure ulcers—community acquired, hospital acquired, unit acquired
    • Staff mix
    • Nursing hours per patient day
    • RN surveys on job satisfaction and practice environment scale
    • RN education and certification
    • Pediatric pain assessment cycle

28. Globalization and the nursing shortage are related because, in an effort to provide high-quality care, health care institutions may recruit nurses from around the world to work in the United States. The movement of nurses away from their home country can leave that country with its own shortage. The hiring of nurses from other nations also can require American hospitals to better understand and work with nurses from different cultures and with different needs.

29. The National Priorities Partnership focuses on
    • Patient and Family Engagement—providing patient-centered, effective care
    • Population Health—bringing increased focus on wellness and prevention
    • Patient Safety—focusing on eliminating errors whenever and wherever possible
    • Care Coordination—providing patient-centered, high-value care
    • Palliative Care—providing appropriate and compassionate care for patients experiencing advanced illnesses
    • Overuse—focusing on waste reduction to achieve effective, affordable care
    • Health Information Technology—providing safer, better coordinated care through use of electronic medical records and other sources of information technology
    • Disparities—reducing disparities through provision of culturally competent care

30. The purpose of a Professional Standards Review Organization (PSRO) is to review the quality, quantity, and cost of health care services provided through Medicare and Medicaid.

31. 3
32. 2
33. 1
34. 4
35. 2
36. 3
37. 4
38. 1
39. 2

CHAPTER 4

Case Studies

1. a. There are a variety of physiological, psychological, and sociocultural problems that the older adult may have, including the following:
   Physiological: Heart disease, hypertension, arthritis, stroke (cerebral vascular accident), diabetes, sensory impairments (failing eyesight and hearing), cognitive impairments (Alzheimer's disease), cancer, malnutrition

Psychological: Depression, anxiety, substance abuse, dependence, other altered coping abilities, loss

Sociocultural: Finances, housing, separation from family

   b. The nurse should investigate what is already available for older adults. This information should be available at the local municipal building/center, library, and/or health department. If not already available, the nurse should look into the possibility of working with the local government, health department, and other members of the community to offer such services as the following: older adult day care; community activities (e.g., day trips and exercise groups) and transportation; health screenings; nutritional programs; in-person and telephone support groups; advice regarding security, financial, and housing concerns; and reduced or no-cost home maintenance assistance. Older adults should be encouraged, whenever possible, to become involved in activities that provide mutual satisfaction and stimulation, such as school programs where they can read to elementary school children or offer consultation to businesses in their area of expertise.

2. a. An assessment of the home environment should include
- Overall appearance:
  - Condition of walls, floors, windows, doors, ceilings
  - Cleanliness, presence of vermin
- Atmosphere: comfort, personal items
- Utilities: water, heating/cooling, lighting
- Neighborhood: safety, available resources (food, transportation, etc.)

   b. You will want to assess the patient's
- Overall physical status, including a general survey, vital signs, glucose level, and ability to perform ADLs
- Knowledge about diabetes and the care required, including therapeutic diet and medications
- Ability to manage the health care regimen physically, emotionally, cognitively, and financially
- Support systems: family, friends, local resources (clinics, pharmacies)

Chapter Review

1. The focus of community-based care is on health promotion, disease prevention, and restorative care.
2. Challenges for community-based nursing practice include increased sexually transmitted infections, pollution, new life-threatening diseases, lack of health care insurance, and underimmunization of infants.
3. The difference between public and community health nursing is that public health nursing focuses on the factors that influence health promotion and health maintenance needs of a population, while community health nursing focuses on the health care of individuals, families, and groups within the community.
4. Specific risks for vulnerable populations:
   a. Immigrant: Access to health care may be limited because of language barriers and lack of benefits, resources, and transportation. Some immigrant populations have specific health care risks such as hepatitis B, tuberculosis, and dental problems.
   b. Poor and homeless: People who live in poverty are more likely to live in dangerous environments, work in high-risk jobs, have less nutritious diets, and experience multiple stressors.

   Homeless patients are usually jobless, do not have the advantage of shelter, and must cope with finding a place to sleep at night and finding food. They may experience worsening chronic health problems because they do not get nutritious meals and have no place to store medications, if they can afford them. In addition, they lack a healthy balance of rest and activity.
   c. Mentally ill: Patients in the community are at a greater risk for abuse, assault, and injury. Many patients with pervasive mental illnesses are homeless or have poor housing and may lack the ability to maintain employment or to care for themselves.
   d. Older adult: There is a greater incidence of chronic disease and an increased need for health care services.
5. The role of the nurse in community-based practice is
   a. Case manager
   b. Educator/teacher
   c. Epidemiologist
6. The three components of a community are structure or locale, the people, and the social systems.
7. Interventions for a family with a member experiencing substance abuse include obtaining a drug use history; educating adults about safe drug storage and the risks for, drug-drug, drug-alcohol, and drug-food interactions; giving general information about drugs (e.g., drug name, purpose, side effects, dosage); instructing adults about pre-sorting techniques; counseling adults about substance abuse; promoting stress management to avoid the need for drugs or alcohol; and arranging for and monitoring detoxification if appropriate.
8. For a patient with Alzheimer's disease, interventions for the patient include maintaining high-level functioning, protection, and safety; encouraging human dignity; demonstrating to the primary family caregiver techniques to dress, feed, and toilet the patient; providing frequent encouragement and emotional support to the caregiver; acting as an advocate for the patient when dealing with respite care and support groups; protecting the patient's rights; providing support to maintain family members' physical and mental health; maintaining family stability; and recommending financial services if needed.
9. The potential safety hazards in the photo are: There is a wrinkled throw rug by her feet, along with an ottoman and other clutter that she could trip over. The folding table next to her is not steady enough to hold her weight, if she lost her balance. She uses a cane and may need the glasses (on the table) to see when she is ambulating. She appears to be wearing a medic alert necklace, which indicates that she may have other medical problems.
10. 3
11. 4
12. 1
13. 2

CHAPTER 5

Case Studies

1. a. A patient who does not appear to understand a procedure should not sign a consent form. The physician must be contacted to provide the information to the patient. The nurse's role in this situation is to witness the signing of the consent form only if the patient demonstrates an understanding of the procedure. Because the nurse will not be performing the procedure, it is not his or her responsibility to describe what will or will not be done during the surgery.

2. a. Any question of a written order should be clarified with the prescriber. You should not depend on the "guess" of another colleague, even if it is a supervisor.

   b. If the medication is administered according to the charge nurse's belief, and the order is not correct, then you are accountable for the result.

3. a. In an emergency situation, treatment may be provided to an individual without obtaining consent. If there is sufficient opportunity to obtain consent, the divorced parent who has legal custody of the child must be contacted.

4. a. You will have to investigate your state's statutes to determine what information is required to be reported for a colleague in a suspected substance abuse situation. In many states, the nurse is held accountable if he or she is knowledgeable about an impaired practitioner but does not report the situation to the Board of Nursing. In most instances, the situation is not acted on immediately; it is investigated further by the appropriate authorities.

5. a. Posting on social media sites, even when patients or colleagues are not specifically described, breaches a patient's trust and may be a form of lateral violence with respect to co-workers (ANA, 2011). This breach of confidentiality should be addressed with the staff member. It is important to know the employer's policies on the use of social media. The professional nurse has an obligation to report breaches of privacy and confidentiality.

   b. Inappropriate use of a patient's confidential information or image may be reported to the State Board of Nursing, and the nurse could face disciplinary charges (NCSBN, 2011).

Chapter Review

1. i	5. e	9. c
2. f	6. b	10. g
3. a	7. h	
4. j	8. d	

11. A nurse may avoid being liable by following the standards of care, providing competent care, communicating with other health care providers, documenting fully, and developing an empathetic rapport with patients.

12. Standards of care are defined in Nurse Practice Acts by boards of nursing, state and federal hospital licensing laws, professional and specialty organizations, and agency policies and procedures.

13. a. Informed consent requires that the patient
    - Understands the options and risks of the care provided
    - Has an opportunity to ask questions
    - Provides consent voluntarily
    - Is a competent adult

    b. The nurse is responsible for witnessing the patient's signature on the consent form and asking if he/she understands the procedure(s). If a patient denies understanding, or if it is suspected that he/she does not understand, then the physician or health care provider and nursing supervisor should be notified.

14. True

15. Professional negligence is termed malpractice.

16. The correct aspects of the Good Samaritan Law are choices b and c.

17. Verbal or telephone orders should be signed within 24 hours.

18. The two standards for determination of death are cardiopulmonary and whole brain.

19. False

20. The elements of malpractice are
    - The nurse owed a duty to the patient.
    - The nurse did not carry out the duty or breached the duty.
    - The patient was injured.
    - The patient's injury was caused by the nurse's failure to carry out that duty.

21. The coroner is notified if the patient's death is unforeseen or sudden or if the patient was not seen by a physician within 36 hours of death.

22. Felonies related to a Nurse Practice Act are b and c.

23. Advance directives act to instruct about withholding or withdrawing life-sustaining procedures in patients who are terminally ill.

24. Health care workers are required to report attempted suicide, rape, gunshot wounds, unsafe or impaired professional practice, child abuse, and certain communicable diseases.

25. Examples of preventable errors include patient falls, urinary tract infections, and pressure ulcers.

26. This is an apology statute.

27. Verdicts must be reported to the National Practitioner Data Bank (NPDB).

28. Examples of "never events" are a, b, and f.

29. Physical or chemical restraint requires a provider's order and careful oversight for appropriate use. They should only be used in emergency situations.

30. The Patient Self-Determination Act (1991) requires health care institutions to inquire whether a patient has created an advance directive, to give patients information on advance directives, and to document whether a patient states he or she has an advance directive.

31. The correct order for organ donation consent is: c, b, d, e, f, a.

32. HIPAA sets standards for the electronic exchange of private and sensitive health information.

33. Common sources of negligence are medication errors that result in injury to patients; IV therapy errors resulting in infiltration or phlebitis; burns to patients caused by equipment, bathing, or spills of hot liquids and foods; falls resulting in injury to patients; failure to use aseptic technique when required; errors in sponge, instrument, or needle counts in surgical cases, meaning an item was left in a patient; failure to give a report, or giving an incomplete report, to oncoming shift personnel; failure to adequately monitor a patient's condition; and failure to notify a health care provider of a significant change in a patient's status.

34. 2	38. 1	42. 1
35. 3	39. 2	43. 4
36. 4	40. 1	
37. 3	41. 4	

CHAPTER 6

Case Studies

1. a. **Step 1.** Is this an ethical dilemma?

   Review of scientific data does not resolve the patient's situation, his question is perplexing, and your response and his action will have a profound relevance for human concern.

   Step 2. Gather all the information relevant to the case.

   The patient is a 42-year-old man with severe multiple sclerosis who is unable to perform the simplest activities of daily living. He appears to be aware of his situation and is seeking an alternative to his present lifestyle. You are his home care nurse and are aware of the patient's situation.

   Step 3. Examine and determine one's own values on the issues.

   Use of the values' clarification process may assist you in determining your beliefs about assisted suicide and the quality and sanctity of life.

   Step 4. State the problem clearly.

   The patient has an interest in being "helped to die," and he has involved you in a possible dilemma by asking you to assist him in getting more information about this method.

   Step 5. Consider possible courses of action.

   You may or may not be able to assist the patient in his actual pursuit of an assisted suicide because of your beliefs. In addition, the legal view on assisted suicide varies from state to state and will have to be investigated before any action is taken by you or the home care agency. A discussion with your supervisor and colleagues may assist in determining a course of action. (You should inform the patient that you will be sharing this information with other members of the health team.) If the patient is intent on finding out about, and possibly pursuing, an assisted suicide, his family members (if available) may become involved.

   Step 6. Negotiate the outcome.

   Communication with the patient may determine whether there are other alternatives to the patient's plan. Work with the patient to consider all of the possibilities, but respect the patient's wish, even if it is to pursue assisted suicide.

   Step 7. Evaluate the action.

   The actions taken by the nurse and other members of the home care agency should be documented. Recognize that satisfaction with the outcome by the patient and the nurse may not be possible. There are no right or wrong answers to ethical questions. Evaluation is based on the effectiveness of working through the problem to a reasonable solution.

   b. The nurse in this situation should be the patient's advocate. The first step is to determine if the patient is truly intent on pursuing this alternative measure. If he really is interested, then the nurse may assist him in a number of ways. Information on assisted suicide may be obtained directly or indirectly for the patient. The nurse may not be able to

become involved but can be supportive of the patient's decision to investigate the procedure. There are legal and ethical considerations that may inhibit the nurse from having any involvement, in which case the patient should be referred to others who may support him in his actions.

2. a. You cannot copy or forward medical records without a patient's consent. Health care workers are not allowed to share health care information with others without specific patient consent. This includes laboratory results, diagnosis, and prognosis. In addition, family members or friends of the patient are not permitted access to the patient's personal health information without the patient's consent.

Chapter Review

1. f	4. b	7. e
2. g	5. c	8. d
3. h	6. a	9. i

10. Access to a patient's medical record requires the patient's consent.

11. End-of-life issues include "do not resuscitate" (DNR) or "allow natural death" (AND) orders, assisted suicide/euthanasia, living wills, and maintenance or removal of life-sustaining measures.

12. a. Deontology
    b. Feminist ethics
    c. Utilitarianism

13. a. Cost containment: not having enough staff or equipment with monetary cutbacks, having limitations on coverage and benefits, providing restricted hours and services
    b. Cultural sensitivity: accepting a patient's refusal of treatment (e.g., Christian Scientist's beliefs), recognizing the need for special diets or concern for the body of the deceased

14. Digital transmission can be an ethical concern because there could be a question of where the information is being sent and who is able to access the information. Photos, lab results, and other sensitive data must be kept safe from public scrutiny.

15. 4	18. 3	21. 2
16. 4	19. 4	
17. 4	20. 1	

CHAPTER 7

Case Studies

1. a. Using the PICO format, you may develop a question based on the following:

   P = Patient population of interest: home care patients, using this specific glucose monitor, who are having difficulty with the results and insulin management

   I = Intervention of interest: determination of whether the problem is patient or equipment related

   C = Comparison of interest: how the patients with other monitors are doing with their insulin management

   O = Outcomes: Home care patients will have confidence in the use and results of their blood glucose monitors.

Their insulin management will be effective in controlling their glucose.

   b. The trigger in this situation is problem focused.
2. a. Staff and patients on a surgical unit may be interested in the following areas for quality improvement:
   - Postoperative complications, such as the incidence of hemorrhage and infection
   - Patient response to pain management
   - Safety, including postoperative ambulation
   - Effectiveness of preoperative education
   - Ease of use and effectiveness of the preoperative checklist
   - Family involvement in care
   - Patient and family satisfaction with care

Chapter Review

1. c
2. d
3. a
4. b
5. Evidence-based practice is a problem-solving approach to clinical practice that combines the conscientious use of best evidence in combination with a clinician's expertise, patient preferences and values, and available health care resources in making decisions about patient care (Melnyk and Fineout-Overholt, 2011; Sackett et al., 2000). It incorporates quality research data into patient care.
6. Valuable non–research-based evidence may be found in
   - Performance improvement data
   - Risk management data
   - International and local clinical guidelines
   - Infection control data
   - Benchmarking
   - Retrospective or concurrent chart reviews
   - Clinicians' expertise
7. A peer-reviewed article is one submitted for publication and reviewed by a panel of experts familiar with the topic or subject matter of the article.
8. A qualitative research study focuses on trying to understand patients' experiences with health problems and the contexts of their experiences. It is descriptive rather than experimental.
9. The primary way that a nurse can integrate evidence into practice is by applying it into the plan of care for a patient. Evidence can also be incorporated into agency policies and procedures, teaching tools, clinical practice guidelines, and new assessment or documentation tools.
10. PDSA stands for: (P) Plan, (D) Do, (S) Study, and (A) Act.
11. Some examples of patient outcomes and measurements include the following:

Outcomes	Measurements
Patient will describe the signs and symptoms of hypoglycemia/hyperglycemia.	Communication with the patient
Patient's blood pressure will remain within therapeutic limits.	BP measurement every shift and as needed
Patient will be satisfied with outpatient surgery education.	Patient satisfaction survey

12. A randomized control trial (RCT) includes a, b, c, and e.
13. An evidence-based article includes a, c, d, and f.
14. Examples of competencies for evidence-based practice include
   - Demonstrate knowledge of basic scientific methods and processes
   - Describe EBP to include components of research evidence, clinical expertise, and patient/family values
   - Differentiate clinical opinion from research and evidence summaries
   - Describe reliable sources for locating evidence reports and clinical practice guidelines
   - Explain the role of evidence in determining best clinical practice
   - Describe how the strength and relevance of available evidence influences the choice of interventions in provision of patient-centered care
   - Discriminate between valid and invalid reasons for modifying evidence-based clinical practice based on clinical expertise or patient/family preferences
15. Sources for new scientific information are the standards and practice guidelines available from national agencies or organizations such as the Agency for Healthcare Research and Quality (AHRQ), the American Pain Society (APS), and the American Association of Critical-Care Nurses (AACN).
16. True
17. Examples of comprehensive databases include MEDLINE, CINAHL, and PubMed.
18. Evidence-based practice can be communicated to others through grand rounds, agency committees, professional organizations, abstracts, and posters and podium presentations at conferences.
19. Root cause analysis is a structured method used to analyze serious adverse events. A central tenet of RCA is to identify underlying problems that increase the likelihood of errors while avoiding the trap of focusing on mistakes by individuals.
20. The PICOT components for the example are
   P - Patient population of interest: patients with pressure ulcers
   I - Intervention of interest: wound healing when the ulcer is left open to air
   C - Comparison of interest: if there is a difference in healing for wounds with the typical dressings that are being used on the unit
   O - Outcome: pressure ulcers left open to air for 2 hours/day will heal faster than those that are covered all day
   T - Time: 4 months of observation
21. 4
22. 1

CHAPTER 8

Case Studies

1. a. In approaching a multiple patient assignment, you may benefit from doing the following:
   - Looking at the patients' backgrounds: diagnoses, baseline data, etc.
   - Determining the current status of each patient
   - Identifying the priority assessments and interventions
   - Making sure that what you need is available: equipment, medications, etc.
   - Organizing actions to maximize efficiency and patient safety and satisfaction
   - Writing specific notes for each patient, with the schedule for treatments and medications
   - Coordinating and communicating with patients and other staff members
   - Documenting actions as soon as possible

2. a. The nurse may choose to return to the office to obtain supplies and then make a later visit to this patient. This option is possible if the nurse has other patients to visit or if there is work to be done at the office. This option will, however, take time away from the nurse and extend visiting hours. The nurse may choose to purchase necessary items from a local pharmacy, but the nurse may not have the necessary funds or be able to be reimbursed for this purchase. It may be most appropriate for the nurse to investigate what alternative resources are available in the patient's home, such as clean cloths, boiled water, salt, and tongs (all to be used only with patient permission).

   b. The nurse should determine what resources the patient has in the home, including running water, waste disposal, and methods for heating and refrigeration. In addition, a financial screening may be needed if indicated for the determination of available funds and/or insurance coverage for supplies and equipment.

3. a. For this patient, there are a number of areas to focus on, including his
   - knowledge of the diagnosis and treatment
   - familiarity and comfort with the diet and food choices
   - support system—other family members, finances
   - need to do his own shopping and cooking
   - emotional response to the diagnosis

Chapter Review

1. e
2. d
3. b
4. c
5. a
6. Examples of critical thinking throughout the nursing process:
   a. Assessment: collecting and analyzing data
   b. Nursing diagnosis: identifying the appropriate patient problems
   c. Planning: establishing expected outcomes, prioritizing, collaborating, and delegating
   d. Implementation: performing nursing interventions safely
   e. Evaluation: determining achievement of outcomes, reassessing as indicated
7. The levels of critical thinking are
   a. Basic
   b. Complex
   c. Commitment
8. The elements of the critical thinking model are specific knowledge base, experience, competence, attitudes, and standards.
9. Examples of critical thinking attitudes:
   a. Confidence
   b. Thinking independently
   c. Discipline
   d. Creativity
   e. Integrity
10. a. Reflection allows the nurse to look back and learn from an experience and identify opportunities for improvement.
    b. Language must be used clearly and precisely to communicate effectively with patients, families, and other members of the health care team.
    c. Learning is a continuous process and necessary for nurses as the profession grows. With experience and learning, nurses get better at forming assumptions, presenting ideas, and making valid conclusions about patient care.
11. Two useful tools for developing critical thinking skills are reflective journaling and concept mapping.
12. Accurate statements regarding critical thinking attitudes are c, d, and e.

13. 4	17. 3	21. 4
14. 3	18. 4	22. 1
15. 1	19. 2	23. 2
16. 3	20. 1	

CHAPTER 9

Case Studies

1. a. The nurse should obtain additional data about the patient's medical history and current health status. The patient may be seeing a physician or other primary care provider and have medication prescribed for hypertension.
   b. A community health fair allows for general screening of large numbers of people, but it usually does not offer opportunity or space for privacy to complete health histories or physical assessments. Individuals demonstrating alterations from expected norms, such as this patient, are referred to clinics, personal physicians, or other health care delivery agencies, as appropriate.

2. a. The relevant assessment data obtained from the patient include
   - Being newly diagnosed with hypertension
   - Having a new prescription of an antihypertensive medication

- Demonstrating insecurity about the medication regimen
- Relating his father's death at age 54 from a heart attack

b. Nursing diagnoses for the patient may include
  - *Knowledge Deficit* related to unfamiliarity with the diagnosis and treatment of hypertension
  - *Knowledge Deficit* related to newly prescribed medication (as manifested by his verbalization of uncertainty as to how and when to take his medications)
  - *Fear* related to possible repeat of father's medical history and early death

3. a. Sample diagnoses, goals, and outcomes for the patient:

Nursing Diagnoses	Goals	Expected Outcome
Knowledge Deficit related to newly prescribed medication (as manifested by his verbalization of uncertainty as to how and when to take his medications)	Patient will recognize the purpose of the hypertensive medication and prepare an administration schedule by the end of the clinic visit.	Patient will restate the use of the antihypertensive medication and scheduling of administration during the visit.
Fear related to possible repeat of father's medical history and early death (as manifested by verbalization of concern over similar family history)	Patient will demonstrate effective coping mechanisms within the next month. Patient will identify reduction or elimination of feelings of fear.	Patient will discuss his concerns about his father's medical history and early death during this visit. Patient will acknowledge his fear of repeating this history during his visits.
Knowledge Deficit related to unfamiliarity with diagnosis of hypertension	Patient will make specific lifestyle alterations and participate in the treatment regimen.	Patient will identify the etiology and therapeutic regimen for hypertension after the next two clinic visits.

b. Nursing interventions should include (1) teaching the patient about his medication and frequency of administration and (2) arranging uninterrupted time to sit with the patient and allow him to discuss his feelings and concerns regarding the diagnosis and family history. (Refer to the box below for interventions based on each diagnosis.)

Knowledge Deficit	Fear
- Assess patient's willingness and readiness to learn about his diagnosis and medication regimen. - Identify and present appropriate information about hypertension and the medication regimen counseling, as indicated. - Establish an environment and strategy for teaching patient that are conducive to learning. - Provide effective learning materials, including pamphlets, videos, photos, and charts, for example.	- Assess the degree of patient's fear. - Observe nonverbal and verbal responses. - Listen to patient's concerns and feelings. - Provide information on coping mechanisms to assist in reducing his level of fear. - Offer referral to a support program/counseling, as indicated.

4. a. For his hypertension to be controlled, the patient needs to take his medication on a regular basis. The nurse should focus on the implementation method of teaching. Counseling also may be involved, especially if the patient is experiencing other difficulties at work or home that are interfering with his ability to manage his therapeutic regimen. Emphasis may be placed on the patient taking his medication along with a daily routine, such as with meals or after bathing.

   b. The nurse should look at the original goals, outcomes, and nursing interventions to determine what alterations may be necessary. The strategies for providing the information on the patient's diagnosis and medication may not have been appropriate. In addition, the patient's fear about his father's medical history may have been blocking his ability to focus and/or influencing his degree of motivation to participate in the therapeutic plan.

5. a. The patient appears to be achieving most of his goals. He states that he is exercising regularly and trying to use the relaxation techniques when he feels stressed. The patient also is expressing his method of coping with his father's medical history.

   b. Areas for reassessment may include the patient's actual medication schedule (because his blood pressure is still slightly elevated) to determine that it is within the prescribed regimen. Determination also may be made to see if the patient may benefit from additional exercise (per review with the physician), and a review of his relaxation techniques may be conducted.

6. a. It is important for you to assess the following:
   - Overall physical status of the child and how she has responded to the medical treatment
   - Emotional response of the child and her parents
   - Ability of the child and her parents to comply with the treatment regimen
   - Home environment: socioeconomic considerations
   - Child's preference for foods and activities

   b. *Knowledge deficit* related to new diagnosis and lack of familiarity with treatment regimen

Chapter Review

1. c
2. g
3. j
4. d
5. e
6. f
7. b
8. h
9. i
10. a

11. The three phases of the interview are the orientation phase, working phase, and termination phase.
12. Possible nursing diagnoses are
    a. *Diarrhea*
    b. *Activity Intolerance*
13. a. *Knowledge Deficit related to the need for postoperative care at home*
       Goal: Perform, or obtain assistance in performing, postoperative care at home
       Expected outcome:
       • State the purpose and procedure for postoperative care
       • Demonstrate postoperative care before discharge
       Nursing intervention:
       • Provide appropriate materials for patient review of postoperative care before surgery
       • Review and demonstrate the postoperative care to patient after surgery
       • Observe the patient's independent performance of postoperative care before discharge
    b. Alteration in elimination: *Constipation related to lack of physical activity*
       Goal:
       • Reestablish normal pattern of elimination
       • Participate in specified daily physical activity, to tolerance
       Expected outcome:
       • Ambulate in hallway 3 times each day
       • Perform active range-of-motion exercises twice each day
       Nursing intervention:
       • Instruct and assist patient in performance of physical activity
       • Observe tolerance to physical activity
       • Assess elimination pattern daily
       • Promote additional measures to improve elimination, such as the intake of fluids and fiber
    c. *Risk for injury*
       Goal:
       • Patient will remain free of injury throughout hospital stay
       Expected outcome:
       • Change positions slowly
       • Sit on the edge of the bed before rising
       • Request assistance before ambulating if feeling dizzy
       Nursing intervention:
       • Instruct the patient to change positions slowly
       • Monitor the patient's blood pressure and other indications that could contribute to dizziness or instability
       • Assist the patient to ambulate
14. a. Psychomotor
    b. Interpersonal
    c. Interpersonal
    d. Psychomotor
    e. Cognitive
15. Before implementing standing orders, the nurse should determine the accuracy and appropriateness of the standing orders for the patient. In addition, the nurse should have the knowledge and competency necessary to carry out each order safely.
16. The steps of the implementation phase of the nursing process are as follows: reassess, review/revise the care plan, organize resources and care delivery, and anticipate and prevent complications.
17. If a new patient need is identified, the nurse should modify the care plan.
18. Specific procedures are termed a protocol for care.
19. Indirect nursing interventions include the following: delegation, environmental safety, infection control, documentation, and collaboration.
20. Activities a, c, d, and g can usually be delegated.
21. Examples of how patient outcomes may be improved are
    a. Erythema will be reduced in area by 2 inches within 2 days.
    b. Pulse rate will be within the patient's baseline of 60 to 70 beats per minute after medication administration.
    c. Patient will have a daily increase of 50 to 100 calories at each meal until ideal weight is achieved.
22. A good interview environment is
    • Free of distractions, unnecessary noise, and interruptions
    • Private and out of earshot of other patients, visitors, and staff
    • Scheduled when no other activities are planned to avoid interruptions
    • Well lit, warm, and with the patient in a comfortable position
23. The following data are subjective: a and c. Objective data are b, d, and e.
24. The medical record is a source for the patient's medical history, laboratory and diagnostic test results, current physical findings, and the health care provider's treatment plan. Data in the records offer a baseline and ongoing information about the patient's response to illness and progress to date.
25. a. The nurse can validate the patient's statement by observing him/her to see what the tolerance is to activity.
    b. The nurse can validate that the pressure ulcer is larger by measuring the ulcer daily and keeping track of the changes in its size.
26. a. Direct care: providing hygienic care, administering medications, performing dressing changes
    b. Counseling: allowing opportunities for the patient to discuss concerns, providing emotional support
    c. Teaching: giving information about the treatment for a disease, demonstrating how to perform care or prepare medications
    d. Controlling adverse reactions: evaluating the patient's response to a medication, checking for unexpected responses to treatments (i.e., redness by tape used on a dressing)
27. The evaluation process includes five elements: (1) identifying evaluative criteria and standards, (2) collecting data to determine if you met the criteria or standards, (3) interpreting

and summarizing findings, (4) documenting findings, and (5) terminating, continuing, or revising the care plan.

28. The nurse can ask the patient about particular preferences, as well as observe the patient's practices.

29. Interventions for the nursing diagnosis *Feeding Self-Care Deficit* can include assisting with the arrangement of food on the plate for easy access, obtaining utensils that are easier to hold, providing support of the patient's hand in using the utensils, sitting the patient up and feeding the patient slowly, and observing the patient's abilities and responses.

30. 4	37. 4	44. 2
31. 1	38. 1	45. 3
32. 1	39. 2	46. 4
33. 2	40. 2	47. 3
34. 3	41. 1	48. 2
35. 4	42. 4	49. 4
36. 4	43. 4	

CHAPTER 10

Case Studies

1. a. A transfer report should include the following information:
   - Patient's name and age, name of primary physician, and medical diagnosis
   - Summary of medical progress to the time of transfer
   - Current physiological and psychological status
   - Current nursing diagnoses/plan of care
   - Critical assessments to be completed shortly after transfer
   - Any special equipment needed
   b. More specifically, the primary nurse may want to know about the surgical procedure, how it was tolerated by the patient, how the patient responded to the anesthesia, and observations made and treatments completed in the PACU.

2. Sample SOAP documentation for the patient:
   S: Patient states she is having intense pain in her right hip area and does not want to move because of the pain.
   O: Patient is grimacing and moaning in pain.
   A: There is an alteration in comfort related to new surgical incision to right hip.
   P: Reduce or eliminate discomfort by administering analgesic medication as ordered and assisting patient to more comfortable position.
   Sample DAR documentation for the patient:
   D: Patient is grimacing and moaning in pain. She states that she is having intense pain to right hip and does not want to move because it "really hurts." Dressing is dry and intact.
   A: Patient is assisted to more comfortable position, with leg supported. Analgesic administered per order.
   R: Patient expressed reduction in discomfort to tolerable level.

3. a. Documentation should include the information presented, method of instruction (e.g., discussion, demonstration, videotape, booklet), and patient response, including questions and evidence of understanding such as return demonstration or change in behavior. It would be important to note what material was presented to the patient regarding type I diabetes, including self-injection of insulin, dietary guidelines, and general care. The patient's response should be identified, such as his ability to prepare and administer the injections and specify foods to avoid in his daily diet.

Chapter Review

1. d
2. e
3. a
4. b
5. c
6. The proper guidelines for written documentation are
   a. Record all entries legibly and in black ink.
   b. Use only objective descriptions of the patient and use quotes for patient comments.
   c. Use complete, concise descriptions of patient interactions.
   d. Draw a single line through the error, write the word error above the line, initial or sign the error, and complete the correct notation.
   e. Use consecutive lines for charting and do not leave margins. Draw lines through unused space and sign your name at the end of the notation.
   f. Include only factual information in the notation.
   g. Identify that the physician was called to clarify an order for the patient.
   h. Have the other caregiver document the information, unless the individual calls with additional information. Document that the information was provided by another individual.
   i. Record pertinent information throughout the shift, signing each entry.
7. a. False
   b. False
   c. True
8. Standards are set by The Joint Commission (TJC) and National Committee for Quality Assurance (NCQA).
9. a. Communication: for continuity of care and accurate patient status
   b. Financial: for reimbursement, DRGs, insurance audits
   c. Educational: for teaching nursing and medical students
   d. Research: for statistical data and patient responses
   e. Auditing/Monitoring: for Joint Commission standards, incidence of patient falls, pain management
10. Malpractice issues related to documenting include the following: Failure to document, verbal orders, charting in advance of care, timing of events, incorrect data, and failure to report.
11. The five characteristics of quality documentation are factual, accurate, complete, current, and organized.

12. Subjective statements by the patient should be quoted and may be supported with objective findings.

13. Student nurses should sign their names, followed by either SN or NS and the school affiliation.

14. All of the notations are vague and should include more specific information. For example:
    a. Identification of the specific intake, such as "Consumed 8 ounces of hot cereal, 6 ounces of orange juice, and an 8-ounce cup of coffee for breakfast."
    b. Notation of an accurate output, such as "Voided 200 mL of clear, amber urine."
    c. Description of care, such as "10 AM Cleansed wound to left lower leg with normal saline and applied dry 4×4 dressing"; "qd" is removed, because it is not an acceptable abbreviation.

15. SBAR:
    S: Situation
    B: Background
    A: Assessment
    R: Recommendation

16. Discharge summaries should include the following: procedures that should be performed and the instructions given, medications prescribed and precautions, signs and symptoms of complications, names and phone numbers of health care providers, names of community resources, follow-up requirements, actual time of discharge, transportation used, and name of person accompanying the discharged patient.

17. Home care documentation is also completed for financial reimbursement.

18. The process of completing narrative notes only when abnormalities exist is part of "charting by exception."

19. Nursing informatics are the retrieval, storage, presentation, and sharing of data, information, and knowledge to provide quality, safe patient care. Nursing informatics facilitates the integration of data, information, and knowledge to support patients, nurses, and other providers in decision making in all roles and settings.

20. Electronic records are safeguarded through the use of passwords, firewalls, audit trails, and disaster recovery systems.

21. Four concepts included in informatics are data, information, knowledge, and wisdom.

22. The correct actions are a, c, d, and f.

23. Information available usually includes the multidisciplinary inpatient, outpatient, and emergency care provided, current health status and medical history, and medical orders and treatments, including medication administration and diagnostic test results.

24. Problem-oriented medical records include a, c, d, and f.

25. Written materials for class that are prepared based on clinical experiences should not have any patient identifiers on them, such as the patient's last name and room number, date of birth, medical record number, or other identifiable demographic information.

26. The errors in the charting example are: The word patient is not usually written in the narrative. The vital signs should be identified as BP, Pulse and Respiration and/or put in a flow sheet. The amount of weight gained should be indicated, as well as how much breakfast was eaten. Complaints about the physician should not be included in the record.

27. 3	31. 4	35. 2
28. 4	32. 4	36. 3
29. 3	33. 4	37. 1
30. 3	34. 4	

CHAPTER 11

Case Studies

1. a. The following techniques may be effective for an older individual with a moderate hearing impairment:
   - Reducing background noise
   - Checking and cleaning a hearing aid
   - Speaking slowly and clearly
   - Using a low-pitched rather than high-pitched voice
   - Avoiding shouting at the patient
   - Using short, simple sentences
   - Facing the patient to allow for lip reading
   - Not covering the mouth while talking
   - Talking toward the unaffected ear
   - Using facial expressions and gestures

   b. The following techniques may be effective for individuals who do not speak English:
   - Speaking in a normal tone of voice
   - Establishing signals or methods of nonverbal communication
   - Obtaining an interpreter familiar with the language and culture
   - Allowing time for communication to take place
   - Developing a communication board, pictures, or cards for common requests
   - Having a dictionary available for reference

   c. The following techniques may be effective for an individual who is blind:
   - Announcing yourself when entering the room
   - Communicating verbally before touching the patient
   - Orienting the patient to the environment
   - Explaining the procedure in advance
   - Having the patient handle the equipment, as appropriate
   - Informing the patient when you are done and will be leaving the room

   d. The following techniques may be effective for an individual of another culture who is experiencing an invasive procedure for the first time:
   - Explaining the procedure in advance, using an interpreter if necessary
   - Recognizing possible discomfort with exposure and maintaining privacy
   - Staying with the patient to provide emotional support

   e. If the patient is not responsive:
   - Call the patient by name during interactions.
   - Communicate both verbally and by touch.
   - Speak to the patient as though he or she could hear.
   - Explain all procedures and sensations.
   - Provide orientation to person, place, and time as needed.
   If the patient is responsive:
   - Use a communication board
   - Provide a pen/pad

2. a. For an individual who is illiterate, you should implement the following:
   - Identify the patient's reading and comprehension level so that you do not communicate above or below his ability.
   - Organize what you want to say so that the most important points come first.
   - Break complex information into smaller and more understandable parts.
   - Use simple language, avoiding jargon, and define technical terms.
   - Use the active voice instead of passive (e.g., "You will receive the discharge instructions before you leave.").

Chapter Review

1. c	4. h	7. b
2. g	5. e	8. a
3. f	6. d	

9. a. Intrapersonal level
   b. Interpersonal level
   c. Public level
10. Compassion fatigue may develop in situations where nurses observe ongoing patient distress and pain, or participate in difficult relationships with fellow staff or physicians.
11. a. Public zone
    b. Social zone
    c. Intimate zone
    d. Social zone
    e. Intimate zone
    f. Public zone
    g. Personal zone
12. Appropriate communication techniques for the older adult with impaired communication include selections a, c, and d.
13. a. Courtesy should be used. The patient should be called by his or her name, such as Mrs. Jones or Mr. Brown.
    b. Courtesy should be used. The patient should be identified by name, not by room number or diagnosis.
    c. Confidentiality should be applied. The patient should not be discussed outside of the immediate patient area where anyone not involved in the patient's care may overhear the conversation.
    d. Availability should be applied. The nurse should spend time with the patient or identify to the patient when he or she will return to be with the patient.
    e. Avoidance of medical jargon should be considered. The nurse should explain to the patient, in understandable terms, what to expect of the procedure.
14. Examples of ways in which the nurse could enhance communication with the patient include
    a. "How do you feel today?"
    b. "Do you take any medications at home?" or "What types of medication do you take at home?"
    c. "Have you noticed any areas of swelling around your arms or legs?"
    d. "Do you have any questions about the procedure that will be done today?" or "Has the physician explained the procedure to you?"
15. The communication strategies being used are
    a. Using silence
    b. Attentive listening
    c. Encouraging conversation
    d. Clarifying
    e. Focusing
16. To assist the patient who has an aphasia, the nurse may
    - Use simple gestures and statements
    - Provide visual cues, such as pictures or flash cards
    - Listen and observe attentively
    - Allow time for responses, either verbal or nonverbal
    - Have call bells within easy reach
    - Encourage the patient to interact as much as possible
17. Positive responses include answers c and d.
18. Considering the patient's culture, actions b and d are appropriate.
19. The acronym SOLER is:
    S: Sit facing the patient
    O: Offer an open posture
    L: Lean toward the patient
    E: Establish and maintain intermittent eye contact
    R: Relax
20. Actions/responses during the Orientation Phase of the Helping Relationship include d, e, and f.
21. This is an example of lateral violence in the workplace.
22. Many altered health states limit communication, including facial trauma, cancer of the larynx or trachea, aphasia after a stroke, breathing problems, Alzheimer's disease, high anxiety, pain, and heavy sedation. Certain mental illnesses cause patients to have impaired communication like pressured speech, constant verbalization of the same words or phrases, or a slow speech pattern.
23. The nurse has an odd facial expression that can create a problem with communication, as well as not looking directly at the patient. Since the nurse is holding the chart, the patient could be concerned about what has been documented.

24. 3	30. 3	36. 4
25. 2	31. 3	37. 1
26. 4	32. 3	38. 3
27. 1	33. 1	39. 1
28. 4	34. 4	40. 2
29. 1	35. 3	41. 4

CHAPTER 12

Case Studies

1. a. The patient has no prior knowledge about her diagnosis or prescribed medication. She also has a family history of coronary disease, with her father dying of a heart attack at 54 years of age.
   b. Sample teaching plan for the patient:

Learning Need	Resources	Objectives	Teaching Strategies
Knowledge deficit related to newly diagnosed hypertension and antihypertensive medication therapy	Educational media: Video and audio programs on hypertension, written materials on the diagnosis and the medication, information from the physician and other health care providers (e.g., dietitian), nurse's knowledge of diagnosis and treatment regimen	Patient will be able to describe the diagnosis, etiology, treatment, and complications; describe the actions, side effects, and time of administration for the antihypertensive; identify when to contact the physician if complications or problems occur; independently monitor and record her blood pressure daily and as necessary; develop a meal plan for a week that incorporates the therapeutic diet	Provide patient with available educational media and written information on hypertension and antihypertensive medications; use illustrations to explain the functions of the heart and circulatory system and the effects of hypertension; demonstrate the technique for monitoring blood pressure, and have the patient and/or significant other return to demonstrate the procedure; involve significant others in the educational program

2. a. The family will need to know about the following:
   - Diagnosis, along with the prognosis, complications, and precautions
   - Treatment plan: insulin, diet, exercise
   - Health care support: when to contact the physician/nurse, follow-up office or clinic visits
   b. For the 8-year-old, you would include him in learning about the disease and how to manage it, including self-injection and how to recognize problems. Age-appropriate materials should be provided, including books, comics, and videos that will get his attention.

3. a. In preparing for the presentation, you should assess for distractions, noise, physical comfort (temperature, lighting, etc.), appropriate size and location, and the availability of necessary equipment (such as a computer).

Chapter Review

1. d
2. c
3. f
4. a
5. b
6. e

7. The six aspects of the ACCESS model are
   -Assessment of the cultural norms of the patient's lifestyle, health beliefs, and health practices
   -Communication with awareness of the many variations in verbal and nonverbal responses
   -Cultural negotiation and compromise that encourages awareness of various characteristics of the patient's culture and awareness of one's own biases
   -Establishment of respect for patient's cultural beliefs and values; establishment of a caring rapport as the basis of a therapeutic relationship
   -Sensitivity of how diverse cultures perceive their care needs and of the various patterns of communication (terms, concepts, tone, and style of communication)
   -Safety that enables patients to feel culturally secure and avoids disempowerment of their cultural identity

8. True

9. Examples of health maintenance and promotion topics include selections a, d, and f.

10. Specific teaching methods that may be implemented are
    a. Infant: Maintaining consistency in routines (bathing, feeding), holding the child firmly while smiling and speaking softly, and having the infant touch different textures
    b. Toddler: Using play to teach about procedures or activities, offering picture books, and using simple words to promote understanding
    c. Preschooler: Using role-playing, imitation, and play to make it fun to learn, encouraging questions and offering explanations, using simple explanations and demonstrations, and encouraging children to learn together through pictures and short stories
    d. School-age child: Teaching psychomotor skills needed to maintain health, and offering opportunities to discuss health problems and answering questions
    e. Older adult: Teaching when the patient is alert and rested, involving the adult in the discussion or activity, focusing on wellness and the person's strengths, using approaches that enhance reception of stimuli for patients with sensory alterations, and keeping teaching sessions short

11. The presence of pain, anxiety, and distractions may make it difficult for the learner to concentrate.

12. Patients need size, strength, coordination, and sensory acuity to learn psychomotor skills.

13. A nurse should consider the following factors when selecting an environment for teaching: privacy, room temperature, lighting, noise, ventilation, furniture, and space.

14. Written materials are generally at the fifth grade reading level or below.

15. Teaching sessions should last about 20 to 30 minutes, with critical information being taught first.

16. If the patient becomes fatigued during a teaching session, you should stop teaching and resume when the patient feels rested.

17. For the nursing diagnosis *Noncompliance with medication regimen related to insufficient knowledge of purpose and actions*, possible goals/outcomes and nursing interventions include

    Goal: Take medications as prescribed
    Outcome:
    • Verbalize purpose and actions of medication regimen
    Nursing interventions:
    • Provide information about prescribed medications, including purpose and actions; give patient written information about medications and their use; use visual aids as necessary to reinforce the material
    • Allow opportunity for patient to express concerns and ask questions

18. The preferred teaching styles are
    a. Visual: written materials (linguistic style) and pictures, models, and demonstrations (spatial)
    b. Tactile: writing, drawing pictures, and manipulating models of information
    c. Auditory listening, speaking, repeating the information to themselves or to others

19. The domains of learning are
    a. Psychomotor
    b. Affective
    c. Cognitive
    d. Affective
    e. Psychomotor
    f. Cognitive

20. Recommendations for instructional techniques are
    a. Lecture, group discussion
    b. Demonstration and return demonstration
    c. Demonstration and role-playing

21. Explaining in advance is preparatory instruction.

22. a. Almost 50% of adults in the United States have difficulty reading and understanding health information.
    b. Available literacy assessment tools: Single Item Literacy Screener (SILS) and The Newest Vital Sign

23. A better way to inform the patient about the injection is to identify the brief experience that will occur, such as a pinch. This reduces the anticipatory discomfort

24. "Teach-Back" is going through the process of asking the patient/family about components of the instruction to evaluate the level of understanding.

25. A focused assessment includes
    a. Learning needs
    b. Resources
    c. Ability to learn

26. Documentation of patient teaching should include
    Assessment data and related nursing diagnoses: Provide information and support for goals and outcomes.
    Interventions planned and used: Planned education provides continuity of care. Specifically describe subject matter so that other nurses can follow up and reinforce teaching (e.g., "verbalized side effects of digoxin").
    Evaluation of learning: Document evidence of learning (e.g., a return demonstration of coughing and deep breathing). This informs staff about the patient's progress and determines material that you still need to teach. Always use the Teach-Back method.
    Ability of patient and/or family to manage care: Identify needs for outpatient or home care follow-up after discharge. Appropriate referrals better meet the patient's needs.

27. 4	31. 3	35. 4
28. 4	32. 2	36. 1
29. 3	33. 1	37. 4
30. 4	34. 2	38. 2

CHAPTER 13

Case Study

1. a. After determining what needs to be done and prioritizing your interventions, you can delegate to the nursing assistant activities such as vital sign measurements, evening hygienic care, basic procedures (catheter care), and assistance with meals. The nursing assistant may also be asked to obtain necessary supplies and equipment for patient care. You also may have the assistant check on the general status of the patients and report any immediate problems.
   b. To safely delegate activities, you must determine the level of acuity of the patients and the knowledge and ability of the aide. If some of the patients are having abnormal vital signs, such as dysrhythmias, then it would not be appropriate to delegate pulse rate measurement to the nursing assistant.
   c. Some examples of opportunities for multiple tasks are
      • determining the patient's range of motion, communication patterns, and mental status when hygienic care is provided.
      • during treatments, discussing how the procedure may be done by the patient or family at home.
      • talking about the diet, food preparation, and/or shopping at mealtimes.

Chapter Review

1. The nurse manager responsibilities include:
   • Assist staff in establishing yearly goals for the unit and the systems needed to accomplish goals.
   • Monitor professional nursing standards of practice on the unit.
   • Develop an ongoing staff development plan, including one for new employees.
   • Recruit new employees (interview and hire).
   • Conduct routine staff evaluations.
   • Establish self as a role model for positive customer service (customers include patients, families, and other health care team members).
   • Serve as an advocate for the nursing staff to the administration of the institution.

- Submit staffing schedules for the unit.
- Conduct regular patient rounds and help to solve patient or family complaints.
- Establish and implement a quality improvement (QI) plan for the unit.
- Review and recommend new equipment needs for the unit.
- Conduct regular staff meetings.
- Conduct rounds with health care provider.
- Establish and support necessary staff and interdisciplinary committees.

2. A person who is reasonably independent in decision making is demonstrating autonomy.

3. The right task, right circumstances, right person, right direction/communication, and right supervision.

4. The correct terms are
   a. Responsibility
   b. Authority
   c. Accountability

5. Case management is the coordination and linking of health care services to patients and their families with the goal of promoting quality, cost-effective outcomes.

6. Staff members can be actively involved in a decentralized decision-making environment by:
   - establishing nursing practice or problem-solving committees.
   - encouraging collaboration between nurses and health care providers.
   - promoting interdisciplinary collaboration.
   - encouraging staff communication.
   - providing staff education.

7. Team communication can be promoted by respecting one another's ideas, sharing information, keeping one another informed, setting expectations of one another, always treating colleagues with respect, listening to the ideas of other staff members, and being honest and direct in what you say.

8. For the example the SBAR is:
   S - The patient's blood sugar is elevated well beyond expected limits.
   B - The patient was admitted 2 days ago with ketoacidosis and has been taking a longer-acting insulin.
   A - The insulin and dietary management are not managing the patient's blood sugar.
   R - A different type or dosage of insulin, along with a review of the dietary intake and other patient factors, is recommended.

9. 2
10. 1
11. 1
12. 4
13. 4
14. 2
15. 4
16. 3

CHAPTER 14

Case Studies

1. a. The nurse should implement the following measures to prevent a urinary tract infection:
   - Provide personal hygiene, perineal care

- Use aseptic technique when manipulating the catheter and drainage equipment
- Keep the drainage bag unobstructed and below the level of the bladder
- Provide ample fluids, within patient's limitations

2. a. To prevent a wound infection, the nurse should
   - Maintain sterile technique during dressing changes
   - Use medical asepsis in all interactions with the patient
   - Instruct the patient in hand washing/asepsis
   - Dispose of contaminated materials appropriately and promptly
   - Assist in keeping the patient and environment clean and dry
   - Limit the number of caregivers working with the patient
   - Provide optimum nutrition and fluids, within patient's limitations
   - Administer antibiotics, if prescribed

3. a. The nurse should include the patient and family/significant others in the preparation for instituting contact isolation precautions.
   The nurse should
   - Discuss the disease process and the need for isolation precautions
   - Explain and demonstrate isolation procedures
   - Teach the patient and family how to perform hand hygiene and apply PPE
   - Maintain a friendly, understanding manner; listen to the patient's concerns
   - Provide for the patient's sensory stimulation during isolation; encourage the family to bring the patient reading materials, puzzle books, etc.
   - Explain the patient's potential risk for depression or loneliness to family members
   - Encourage visitors to avoid negative expressions or actions concerning isolation; advise family members on ways to provide meaningful stimulation
   - Carefully observe the patient's response to isolation

Chapter Review

1. k
2. f
3. j
4. c
5. b
6. g
7. d
8. h
9. a
10. e
11. l
12. m
13. i

14. Sterile technique is required for options b, c, and e.

15. Examples of outcomes for this patient are the following: Wound will decrease in diameter by 1 cm in 2 days; wound will be free of signs of infection, including edema and drainage.

16. Immunizations are available for selections a, b, c, and f.

17. The nurse should discard the item or redo the sterile field in the case of b, c, and f.

18. Nursing interventions include
    a. Control or eliminate the infectious agent: clean, disinfect, and sterilize contaminated objects
    b. Control or eliminate the reservoir: remove sources of body fluids, drainage (dressings), or solutions that harbor microorganisms; discard disposable articles contaminated with infectious material

c. Control the portals of exit: avoid talking, sneezing, or coughing directly over a wound or sterile dressing field; teach patient to protect others; and handle all body fluids carefully (hand hygiene and use of gloves)

d. Control the transmission: disinfect equipment, provide a personal set of equipment for patients, do not shake linens or allow them to come in contact with the uniform, and perform hand hygiene

e. Susceptible host: hygienic care, adequate nutritional and fluid intake

19. a. White blood cell count: elevated in an acute infection, decreased in viral/overwhelming infections

b. Erythrocyte sedimentation rate: elevated with infectious processes

c. Iron level: decreased in chronic infections

d. Neutrophils: elevated with acute, suppurative infections; decreased with overwhelming bacterial infections

e. Basophils: remain normal during infections

20. a. Health care–acquired infections can be reduced with hand hygiene and the use of aseptic technique.

b. Patients more susceptible to HAI are those who have multiple illnesses, are older adults, are poorly nourished, have a lowered resistance to infection because of underlying medical conditions, have invasive treatment devices (such as catheters), or have been treated with multiple antibiotics for long periods of time.

21. A patient's gastrointestinal defenses are altered by the administration of antacids and histamine-2 blockers.

22. Appropriate techniques for isolation precautions include selections b, d, and f.

23. Handling of biohazardous waste includes "red" bagging for incineration or special handling.

24. The order for application of PPE is mask, gown, and then gloves.

25. The first items removed when leaving the isolation room are the gloves.

26. Appropriate asepsis is demonstrated in selections b, c, f, and h.

27. For the nursing diagnosis *Impaired skin integrity, related to 2-inch-diameter pressure ulcer on sacrum*, possible patient outcomes and nursing interventions include
Patient goal: Sacral ulcer will heal within 2 to 3 weeks
Outcomes:
• Sacral ulcer will reduce in size by 1 inch (within time frame).
• Skin will remain intact over remainder of body surfaces.
• Sacral ulcer will remain free of infection.
Nursing interventions:
• Provide wound care as prescribed using aseptic technique.
• Assess condition of ulcer.
• Provide skin care: Keep clean and dry, and apply moisturizers as needed.
• Turn and reposition patient every hour.
• Assess wound for presence of infection, and obtain culture if indicated.
• Provide for patient's nutritional and fluid needs.

28. c, d or b, then a

29. Disposal of contaminated sharps includes placing all needles (safety needles and needleless systems) into punctureproof containers, which should be located at the site of use.

30. An example would be the nurse touching a nonsterile package with sterile gloves, recognizing the action as a break in technique, and then discarding the gloves and restarting the procedure.

31. To collect a urine specimen for a patient with an indwelling catheter, the nurse should obtain a sterile cup to collect 1 to 5 mL of urine, a needleless safety syringe to collect the specimen from the sampling port on the catheter, and an antiseptic wipe to clean the port (dependent upon the agency policy).

32. The correct actions for hand hygiene are b, e, and g.

33. Some patients perceive the simple procedures of proper hand hygiene as evidence of rejection. Help patients and families reduce some of these feelings by discussing the disease process, explaining the reason for the procedures, and maintaining a friendly, understanding manner.

34. The current immunization schedule can be found on the CDC website.

35. The three most common infections in long-term care are pneumonia, urinary tract infections, and pressure ulcers.

36. The organisms that are transmitted through blood are b, d, and f.

37. The correct steps for the procedure are c, e, d, a, b.

38. The nurse should use a face shield when splashing of bodily fluids is anticipated during care.

39. In the photo, the nurse has broken sterile technique by:
Photo A: The nurse is holding the sterile object below the level of the field on the table. It also appears that her gloved hand may be touching her scrubs.
Photo B: The sterile field is folded over, there is a wet spot and the dressing and instruments are sitting on the wet area.

40. 1	45. 2	50. 4
41. 1	46. 4	51. 1
42. 3	47. 2	52. 4
43. 4	48. 4	53. 2
44. 4	49. 3	54. 4

CHAPTER 15

Case Studies

1. a. Generally, an individual who has a blood pressure reading of above 120/80 mm Hg to 139/89 mm Hg on repeated assessments should be referred for medical follow-up. An average of two or more systolic readings higher than 140 mm Hg and diastolic readings higher than 90 mm Hg are usually indicative of hypertension.

b. Additional information should be noted, such as the arm used and the position (e.g., sitting, standing, lying down) of the patient during the measurement, previous blood pressure readings, known medical problems, and any medical care being received and medications being taken by the patient.

2. a. The patient's pulse rate and blood pressure reading may be obtained in the lower extremities. The pulses available include the femoral, popliteal, posterior tibial, and dorsalis pedis. The blood pressure is assessed by placing the thighsized cuff over the posterior aspect of the middle thigh region while the patient is in the prone position. The popliteal

artery is used for palpation and auscultation of the blood pressure. Measurement in the lower extremities may be 10 to 40 mm Hg higher in the systolic reading than that of the upper extremities.

3. a. A febrile patient may exhibit the following signs and symptoms:
   - Increased body temperature
   - Flushed, dry, warm skin
   - Chills
   - Feeling of malaise
   - Tachycardia

   b. Nursing interventions for febrile patients may include
   - Assessment of vital signs, especially temperature
   - Observation of patient response, including skin color and temperature, and chills
   - Promotion of patient comfort, responding to chills, thirst
   - Collection of appropriate specimens, such as blood cultures
   - Promotion of rest and reduction of activities that increase heat production
   - Promotion of heat loss by removing coverings and keeping the patient dry
   - Provision of care to meet increased metabolic demands, including oxygen, nutrition, and fluid requirements
   - Monitoring of ongoing status

4. a. You are anticipating that a patient who is brought to the emergency room with signs of heat stroke will have hypothermia blankets applied, receive intravenous (IV) fluids, and have irrigations of the stomach and lower bowel with cool solutions.

   b. To prevent future occurrences, the following information should be included in a teaching plan for the patient and family:
   - Avoid strenuous exercise in hot, humid weather.
   - Avoid exercising in areas with poor ventilation.
   - Drink fluids such as water and clear fruit juices before, during, and after exercise.
   - Wear light, loose-fitting, light-colored clothing.
   - Wear a protective covering over the head when outdoors.
   - Expose themselves to hot climates gradually.

5. a. The anticipated readings for oxygen saturation should be 95% to 100%, but at least above 90%.

   b. If the pulse oximeter does not appear to be working, there may be problems with light transmission or a reduction of the patient's arterial pulsations. The site for measurement should be checked to determine that it is clean, warm, and dry; not directly near another light source; and receiving adequate circulation. The patient also may have to be reminded to limit excessive motion of the extremity that is being used for measurement.

   c. You can assist the alert patient to increase oxygen levels by taking deep breaths, especially if he/she has had general anesthesia. This will help to remove the residual from the lungs and improve oxygenation.

Chapter Review

1. f	5. e	9. d
2. j	6. h	10. b
3. g	7. a	11. l
4. i	8. c	12. k

13. a. $(97° F − 32) \times 5/9 = 36° C$
    b. $9/5 \times (38.4° C + 32) = 101.1° F$
    c. $38.9° C$
    d. $102.9° F$

14. The nurse is alerted to temperature alterations of above 100.4° F or below 96.8° F on an oral Fahrenheit thermometer, and measurements above 38° C or below 36° C on an oral centigrade scale. Rectal temperature readings may be 0.9° F or 0.5° C higher than oral measurements, with axillary readings ranging this same number of degrees lower than oral temperatures. Temperatures above 102.2° F for an adult and 104° F for a child can be harmful.

15. The pulses should be palpated as follows:

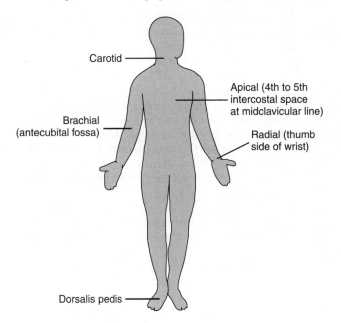

16.

17. False
18. Interventions to reduce body temperature by
    a. Conduction: ice packs, tepid baths, heated blankets
    b. Convection: fans
    c. Evaporation: loss through the skin (diaphoresis) and respiration
19. The thermometer of choice for a patient in isolation is a disposable chemical dot thermometer.
20. A pulse deficit is assessed by two nurses who synchronize their measurement of the patient's apical and radial pulses. A deficit is found if there is a difference between the two readings.
21. For a patient who has had a right mastectomy, the left arm or lower extremities should be used for blood pressure measurement.
22. Vital signs are usually recorded on a graphic or flow sheet.
23. Decreasing hemoglobin levels will increase the respiratory rate.
24. A pulse oximeter may be applied to the earlobe, finger, or bridge of the nose.
25. The pulse pressure for the BP of 150/90 is 60.
26. The correct techniques for blood pressure measurement include options a, c, e, and f.
27. The appropriate action is to wait 15 minutes before measuring the temperature if the patient has smoked, chewed gum, or ingested hot or cold liquid or food.
28. A patient's blood pressure may have to be palpated if the patient's arterial sensations are too weak to create Korotkoff sounds, such as with severe blood loss.
29. a. Temperature: Sites for measurement vary depending on the child's age and condition. For example, it is contraindicated to take a tympanic membrane temperature on a child with otitis media.
    Tympanic membrane: Used in children age 2 and older
    Axilla: Used with newborns and children of any age
    Temporal artery: Used in premature infants, newborns, and children
    b. Blood pressure: An infant or child younger than 5 years of age lies supine with the arm supported at heart level. Older children sit. It is important for the child to be relaxed and calm. Allow at least 15 minutes for children to recover from recent activity or excitement before taking a reading. It may be helpful to have a parent present. You prepare the child for the BP cuff's unusual sensation during inflation. The cuff needs to be the appropriate width: infant cuff is 2½ to 3¼ inches; child cuff is 4¾ to 5½ inches.
30. The correct techniques for a tympanic temperature measurement are a, b, and f.
31. A patient's pulse is expected to be increased with the following factors: a, d, and e.
32. The contradictions for these temperature assessments are
    a. Axillary temperature: Not recommended to detect fever in infants and young children.
    Requires exposure of thorax, which results in temperature loss, especially in newborns. Not used if skin lesions are present.
    b. Rectal temperature: Not used for patients who have had diarrhea or who have had rectal surgery, rectal disorders, bleeding tendencies, or neutropenia. Not used routinely for infants.
33. End-tidal carbon dioxide values are used for patients who are on mechanical ventilation.

34. For a blood pressure reading in the lower extremity:
    a. The patient should be in the prone position, if tolerated. If such a position is impossible, flex the knee slightly for easier access to the artery.
    b. The popliteal artery is used for the palpation and auscultation.
    c. The systolic blood pressure is expected to be higher in the lower extremity.
35. The correct order of the steps for apical pulse measurement is f, c, e, d, a, b.
36. An increased temperature in young children can lead to dehydration and febrile seizures.
37. Commonly used antipyretic medications are acetaminophen, salicylates, indomethacin, ibuprofen, and ketorolac. Corticosteroids also may be used, but be alert to the masking of infection.
38. Orthostatic hypotension is assessed by obtaining pulse and blood pressure readings with the patient supine, sitting, and standing.
39. For core temperature readings:
    a. Readings are measured through invasive means.
    b. Sites include the pulmonary artery, esophagus, and bladder.
40. The diaphragm of the stethoscope is used to auscultate bowel, lung, and heart sounds (high-pitched sounds). The bell of the stethoscope is used to auscultate heart and vascular sounds (low-pitched sounds).
41. a. Increased temperature
    b. Decreased temperature
42. The correct techniques for pulse oximetry are b and d.
43. Respiration is influenced as follows:
    a. Anxiety - increases respiration rate and depth.
    b. Analgesics - depresses respiration rate and depth.
    c. Body position - Standing or sitting erect promotes full ventilatory movement and lung expansion; stooped or slumped position impairs ventilatory movement; lying flat prevents full chest expansion.
44. Hypotension can be seen with a and d.

45. 1	54. 3	63. 4
46. 3	55. 1	64. 1
47. 3	56. 4	65. 4
48. 2	57. 2	66. 2
49. 4	58. 2	67. 1
50. 1	59. 3	68. 4
51. 4	60. 1	69. 2
52. 1	61. 4	70. 1
53. 1	62. 2	

CHAPTER 16

Case Studies

1. a. For the 4-year-old boy, you are aware that the experience may be new and frightening. You can show the child the assessment procedures on a doll or model, while giving simple, understandable information, and he may handle equipment that will be used (as appropriate). The exam should be conducted in a comfortable environment, with time allowed for the child to play. The child may be

called by his first name, and he may be asked assessment questions that he will understand.

- For a 16-year-old girl, the nurse may begin the health assessment with the parent(s) in the room with the patient. There should be time, however, when the patient is by herself with the nurse to discuss concerns. The adolescent girl should be asked if she wants a parent present during the physical assessment, but the option is provided for the patient to not be accompanied. Procedures and findings should be explained to the parent(s) and the patient.
- The older Hispanic woman may have responses to the examination that are influenced by her culture. She will need to be informed and prepared for the breast and pelvic assessments, with consideration given to her privacy. This patient may desire another woman to be present during the examination or to conduct the physical. Care should be taken to determine that this patient understands the information and instruction provided by an examiner who may speak only English. An interpreter may be obtained if the patient is conversant in Spanish. The environment should be warm and comfortable. Ample time should be allowed for the patient to answer questions and assume necessary positions for the exam. For each of the patients, opportunity should be provided to use the bathroom before, during, and after the examination.

2. a. For the patient who has expressed a difficulty in hearing, the nurse should do the following:
   - Have the patient remove any hearing aid if worn.
   - Note the patient's response to questions. Normally the patient responds without excess requests to have the questions repeated.
   - If you suspect a hearing loss, check the patient's response to the whispered voice. Test one ear at a time while the patient occludes the other ear with a finger. Ask the patient to gently move the finger up and down during the test. While standing 30 cm to 60 cm (1 to 2 feet) from the testing ear, cover your mouth so the patient is unable to read lips. After exhaling fully, whisper softly toward the unoccluded ear, reciting random numbers with equally accented syllables such as *nine-four-ten*. If necessary, gradually increase voice intensity until the patient correctly repeats the numbers. Then test the other ear for comparison.

3. a. The lesion and surrounding tissue on the abdomen should be assessed for location, size, shape, depth, and color. The drainage should be assessed for amount, color, consistency, and odor.
   b. After explaining the procedure, providing privacy, positioning the patient either dorsal recumbent or side-lying, and making sure there is adequate lighting, you should apply gloves and examine the area gently.

Chapter Review

1. f	5. h	9. e
2. c	6. g	10. i
3. b	7. d	
4. a	8. j	

11. The five skills used in physical assessment include
    - Inspection: Use of vision and hearing to detect characteristics of body parts and functions
    - Palpation: Use of the hands to touch body parts to determine temperature, texture, position, and movement
    - Percussion: Striking the body surface with the finger to produce a vibration and elicit sounds
    - Auscultation: Listening to sounds created in the body organs (use of stethoscope)
    - Olfaction: Use of smell to determine the presence of characteristic odors

12. The positions for the physical examination are
    a. Sitting
    b. Supine
    c. Dorsal recumbent
    d. Lithotomy
    e. Sims'
    f. Prone
    g. Lateral recumbent
    h. Knee-chest

13. The pulses being palpated are
    a. Ulnar
    b. Posterior tibial
    c. Femoral
    d. Brachial
    e. Dorsalis pedis

14. The skin lesions are
    a. Papule
    b. Ulcer
    c. Macule
    d. Atrophy
    e. Wheal

15. The PMI is located in the left anterior chest wall, at approximately the fourth to fifth intercostal space, at the midclavicular line.

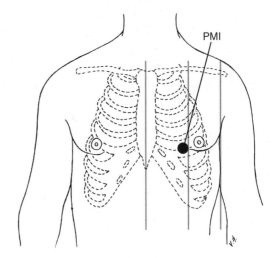

16. The following are findings that may indicate abuse:
    a. Child sexual abuse
       Physical findings:
       - Genital discharge, bleeding, pain, itching
       - Difficulty sitting or walking
       - Foreign bodies in genital tract or rectum

173

Behavioral findings:
- Problems eating or sleeping
- Fear of certain people or places
- Regressive or acting-out behavior
- Preoccupation with own genitals

b. Domestic abuse

Physical findings:
- Injuries and trauma inconsistent with reported cause
- Multiple injuries, burns, bites
- Old and new fractures

Behavioral findings:
- Eating or sleeping disorders
- Anxiety, panic attacks
- Low self-esteem
- Depression, sense of helplessness
- Attempted suicide

c. Older adult abuse

Physical findings:
- Injuries and trauma inconsistent with reported cause
- Bruises, hematomas, burns, fractures
- Prolonged interval between injury and treatment

Behavioral findings:
- Dependent on caregiver
- Physically and/or cognitively impaired
- Combative, belligerent

17. Abdominal assessment:

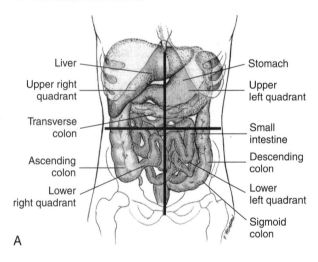

A

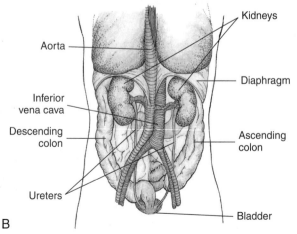

B

18.
a. Expected	v. Unexpected
b. Unexpected	w. Expected
c. Expected	x. Unexpected
d. Expected	y. Unexpected
e. Unexpected	z. Unexpected
f. Unexpected	aa. Expected
g. Expected	bb. Unexpected
h. Unexpected	cc. Expected
i. Unexpected	dd. Unexpected
j. Expected	ee. Expected
k. Expected	ff. Unexpected
l. Expected	gg. Expected
m. Unexpected	hh. Unexpected
n. Unexpected	ii. Expected
o. Unexpected	jj. Expected
p. Expected	kk. Expected
q. Expected	ll. Expected
r. Unexpected	mm. Unexpected
s. Expected	nn. Expected
t. Expected	oo. Unexpected
u. Expected	pp. Expected

19. The nurse examines the area of discomfort last (b).
20. High-pitched sounds are best heard with the diaphragm of a stethoscope (a).
21. The nurse pulls the ear up and back (a).
22. The patient is placed in lithotomy position, if possible.
23. The patient is placed in the dorsal recumbent position.
24. In a general survey, the nurse assesses the patient's
    - Primary health problems
    - Behavior and appearance
    - Hygiene, skin condition, and body image; emotional state; recent changes in weight; and developmental status
25. A weight gain of 5 lb or 2.2 kg/day indicates fluid retention.
26. The correct examination techniques are answers a, d, and e.
27. True
28. The correct techniques are c and d.
29. For the anxious patient, the nurse should stop the examination, explain what is happening, ask the patient how he/she is doing, and postpone the procedure, if indicated.
30. Tests for colorectal cancer include fecal immunochemical test (FIT), fecal occult blood test (FOBT), colonoscopy, and barium enema.
31. Positions for cardiac assessment include answers b, d, and e.
32. Signs and symptoms of cardiopulmonary disease include chest pain or discomfort, palpitations, excess fatigue, cough, dyspnea, edema of the feet, cyanosis, fainting, or orthopnea.
33. The risk factors for osteoporosis are b, d, e, and g.
34. Techniques for assessment of lymph nodes include the use of a methodical approach to avoid overlooking any single node or chain. Examples:

Neck: The patient relaxes with the neck flexed slightly forward. Inspect and palpate both sides of the neck for comparison. During palpation either face or stand to the side of the patient for easy access to all nodes. Using the pads of the middle three fingers of each hand, gently palpate in a rotary motion over the nodes.

To palpate supraclavicular nodes, ask the patient to bend the head forward and relax the shoulders. Palpate these nodes by hooking the index and third finger over the clavicle, lateral to the sternocleidomastoid muscle. Palpate the deep cervical nodes only with the fingers hooked around the sternocleidomastoid muscle.

Axilla: Palpate the axillary nodes with the fingertips gently rolling soft tissue. Normally lymph nodes are not palpable. Note the number, consistency, mobility, and size of palpable nodes.

35. Continuous dilation of the pupils is found with patients experiencing neurological pathologies, glaucoma, opioid withdrawal and trauma, or taking ophthalmic medication.

36. An expected response is that the pupils will converge and accommodate by constricting when looking at close objects. The pupil responses are equal.

37. a. Basket or platform scale
    b. A platform scale

38. Tinnitus is ringing in the ears.

39. Causes of hearing loss are working or living around loud noises, premature hearing loss from continued exposure to loud music through earbuds connected to electronic music devices or loud concerts, deterioration of the cochlea and thickening of the tympanic membrane in older adults, and ototoxicity resulting from high maintenance doses of antibiotics (e.g., aminoglycosides).

40. To assess for a pulse deficit, the nurse should auscultate the apical pulse first and then immediately assess the radial pulse (one-examiner technique). Assess the apical and radial rates at the same time when two examiners are present. When a patient has a pulse deficit, the radial pulse is slower than the apical.

41. An irregular pulse should be counted for at least 60 seconds (1 minute).

42. Risk factors for breast cancer are b, d, and e.

43. a. The sequence for the exam is inspection, auscultation, palpation, percussion.
    b. Bowel sounds usually occur 5 to 35 times/minute.
    c. A patient with ascites will have a distended abdomen, taut skin, and bulging flanks.
    d. Absent bowel sounds can occur as a result of lack of peristalsis, possibly because of a bowel obstruction, paralytic ileus (decreased or absent peristalsis), or peritonitis (inflammation of the peritoneum).

44. Signs and symptoms of prostate cancer include weak or interrupted urine flow, an inability to urinate, difficulty in starting or stopping the urine flow, polyuria, nocturia, hematuria, dysuria, or continuing pain in the lower back, pelvis, or upper thighs.

45. Recent memory can be tested by asking the patient to recall by repeating a series of numbers in the order they are presented or in reverse order. Patients normally recall five to eight digits forward or four to six digits backward. Another test for recent memory involves asking the patient to recall events occurring during the same day. To assess past memory, ask the patient to recall the maiden name of the patient's mother, a birthday, or a special date in history.

46. Findings on the skin of an individual who is suspected of substance abuse are b, d, and e.

47. 4	57. 3	67. 1
48. 2	58. 1	68. 3
49. 1	59. 1	69. 3
50. 2	60. 4	70. 1
51. 1	61. 1	71. 3
52. 4	62. 4	72. 3
53. 1	63. 1	73. 4
54. 4	64. 1	74. 2
55. 3	65. 1	75. 4
56. 4	66. 4	76. 3

CHAPTER 17

Case Studies

1. a. Your initial action is to review all of the medications prescribed for the patient and determine what he does remember about each one.

   A general teaching plan for medication administration should include
   - Adapt your approaches so that patients will understand instruction.
   - Provide information about the purpose of medications and their actions and effects.
   - Identify how to take a medication properly and what will happen if he or she fails to do so.
   - Demonstrate how to properly administer medications.
   - Teach ways to change medication schedules to fit into their lifestyles.
   - Teach family members or friends how to administer medications, if necessary.
   - Provide specially designed equipment such as syringes with enlarged calibrated scales for easier reading or Braille-labeled medication vials for patients with visual alterations.
   - Reinforce the basic guidelines for medication safety, including the proper use and storage of medications in the home.

   To assist this patient to maintain the medication regimen at home, you may create a large, colorful, easy-to-read schedule, chart, or calendar that the patient can use to check when medications have been taken. The patient's medications also may be arranged, by time of administration, in a commercially available or homemade container so that the patient also may be able to determine if the medications were taken as prescribed. (Some commercial devices "beep" when it is time for medications to be taken.)

2. a. If the prescriber's handwriting is illegible, it is unsafe to make assumptions about the medication order. To avoid errors, you should contact the prescriber as soon as possible and clarify the medication orders.

3. a. A patient without an identification band should not receive medications. To verify the identity of the patient, find another nurse or health care worker who is familiar with the patient. On verifying the name of the patient, obtain and provide the identification band for the patient. Asking the patient his or her name assists in verification but may be inaccurate if the patient is not aware or oriented to the surroundings.

4. a. When administering an injection to a child, you must be very careful to avoid injuring or severely agitating the child. An appropriate, well-developed muscle site should be selected. You also may need to have someone else assist in holding or distracting the child by talking. The injection should be given quickly and accurately. An anesthetic ointment may be applied to the site before the injection to decrease the amount of discomfort. Children should not be told that they are receiving a "shot" or that it will not hurt. A sleeping child should be awakened before being given an injection.

5. a. Expected treatment for an anaphylactic reaction includes notifying a patient's health care provider immediately; anticipating that antihistamines, epinephrine, and bronchodilators will be prescribed; and documenting medication allergies in the patient's medical record. Patients may require emergency treatment for airway constriction or obstruction, such as oxygen or intubation.

6. a. This discrepancy in the narcotic count should be reported immediately to the nurse in charge. Usually an attempt is made to determine if the missing dose can be accounted for by checking with all of the other staff members. If the missing medication cannot be tracked down, the discrepancy has to be documented on the computerized or written record. The agency's protocol for this situation then should be followed in relation to where and how the documentation is forwarded.

7. a. For the patient who requires an antipyretic but is experiencing nausea and vomiting, the nurse should contact the prescriber and have the medication order changed to a rectal suppository. For patients who have difficulty tolerating oral medications, the nurse should investigate alternative forms of the medication.

Chapter Review

1. i	5. c	9. b
2. j	6. e	10. h
3. k	7. l	11. d
4. g	8. f	12. a

13. Federal and state legislation, state Nurse Practice Acts, and agency policies and procedures control or regulate the nurse's administration of medications.

14. a. Strategies to prevent errors with look-alike medications include the following: ordering medications by the generic name, including the diagnosis on the prescription; repeating verbal orders to the prescriber; discussing the medications with the patient; reinforcing instructions with the patient; advising patients to check medication labels; and having the patient report any changes in the medication's appearance.
    b. Patient identifiers include name and patient identification number. Agencies may include other aids, such as the birth date or the bar code on the name band.

15. Factors influencing the actions of medications:
    a. Dietary factors: Drug and nutrient interactions can alter a drug's action or the effect of the nutrient; proper drug metabolism relies on good nutrition.
    b. Physiological variables: age, sex, weight, nutritional status, disease states
    c. Environmental conditions: stress, exposure to heat/cold, comfort of the setting

16. The routes for parenteral administration include intramuscular, intradermal, subcutaneous, and intravenous.

17. The components that are missing in the orders are
    a. Dosage
    b. Route
    c. Time for administration
    d. Route

18. The rights are
    1. Right drug
    2. Right dose
    3. Right patient
    4. Right route
    5. Right time
    6. Right documentation

19. The correct sequence for removing medication from a vial is e, a, g, h, j, c, f, i, b, d. Please note: air bubbles should first be dislodged while the needle is still in the vial.

20. The forms of medication are
    a. Capsule
    b. Suppository
    c. Elixir
    d. Aqueous suspension
    e. Lotion

21. Commonly abused over-the-counter medications include aspirin and cough and cold medicines.

22. a. Noncompliance or nonadherence may be related to a dislike of the side effects, the cost of the medication, or a busy lifestyle.
    b. Compliance with medication administration may be promoted by
       • Involving the patient in decisions about the schedule
       • Simplifying the schedule as much as possible
       • Clearly explaining about the medications
       • Providing aids to assist in remembering the schedule
       • Teaching patients about the medications and possible side effects
       • Encouraging patients to refill prescriptions before they run out
       • Checking the patient's medications to see that they are correct

23. MedWatch is a voluntary program for reporting when a medication causes serious harm.

24. Faster absorption or action is found with
    a. IV
    b. intramuscular
    c. acidic oral medication
    d. solutions
    e. large surface area
    f. highly lipid soluble medication
    g. nonalbumin-binding medication

25. This is the peak action of the drug.
26. Oral medications are contraindicated for the patient who has an NPO order, GI alterations, dysphagia, nausea, vomiting, gastric suction, NG tube, or received anesthesia.
27. The problem with this order is that the decimal point may be missed and the patient would receive 10 times the actual dose.
28. The equivalents are
    a. 15 gtt
    b. 2 ounces
    c. 1 L
    d. 3000 mg
    e. 250 mL
    f. 5 mL
29. The five types of medication orders are standing, prn, single (one-time), STAT, and now.
    Possible examples of the different orders:
    1. Standing: Lasix 40 mg PO daily
    2. prn: Morphine sulfate 10 mg IM q4h prn for pain
    3. Single: Versed, 6 mg IM on call to OR
    4. Give Apresoline, 10 mg IM STAT
    5. Give vancomycin 1 g IV piggyback now
30. Verbal orders are to be signed within 24 hours.
31. This number of tablets is not common, so the nurse should recheck the calculation to determine accuracy. Another nurse may be asked to verify the final calculation.
32. An adverse effect is an undesired, unintended, and often unpredictable response to a medication. A side effect is a predictable and often unavoidable adverse effect produced at a usual therapeutic dose.
33. If the patient identifies that the medication looks different, it is important for the nurse to check and make sure that the medication and the order are correct.
34. The correct responses regarding medication administration are c, f, and h.
35. The generic names are
    a. levofloxacin.
    b. furosemide.
    c. ibuprofen.
    d. haloperidol lactate.
36. When preparing medications, compare the label of the medication container with the medication administration order three times: (1) while removing the container from the drawer or shelf, (2) as you remove the amount of medication ordered from the container, and (3) at the bedside before administering the medication to the patient.
37. Techniques for administering medications to children include
    a. Oral medications: Give frozen juice bars, juice, or soft drinks after the medication is swallowed (as allowed).
    b. Injections: Wake the child before an injection, ask for assistance in holding the child, distract the child during the injection, give the medication quickly, avoid calling the injection a "shot," and inform the child that it may "pinch."

38. The discomfort of an injection may be minimized by
    • Using a sharp-beveled needle of the smallest possible size
    • Positioning the patient comfortably
    • Selecting the proper site
    • Diverting the patient's attention away from the procedure
    • Inserting the needle quickly and smoothly
    • Holding the syringe steady while injecting the solution
    • Injecting the medication slowly and steadily
    • Using the Z-track technique
    • Massaging the site, unless contraindicated
39. The Z-track technique should be used for medications that are irritating to the tissues.
40. a. Intramuscular: 90-degree angle
    b. Subcutaneous: 45-degree angle
    c. Intradermal: 5-degree to 15-degree angle
41. Medication may be administered IV via
    1. Mixtures with large volumes of IV fluids
    2. Injection (bolus) or intermittent access devices
    3. Piggyback through an existing IV line
42. A wireless barcode scanner is used to identify you (the nurse), the medication package, and the patient (armband).
43. a. ac = before meals
    b. bid = twice a day
    c. prn = as necessary
    d. q4h = every 4 hours
    e. STAT = immediately
44. Answers determined by dimensional analysis method.
    a. 150 mcg
       75 mcg × 1 tablet = 2 tablets should be given
       Conversion of 0.150 mg to mcg: multiply 0.150 by 1000
    b. 40 mg
       20 mg × 1 tablet = 2 tablets should be given
    c. 20 mg
       10 g × 1 mL = 2 mL should be given
    d. 200 mg
       50 mg × 1 mL = 4 mL/day, but this is divided into two equal doses
       4 mL divided by 2 doses = 2 mL (marked on syringe)
    e. 100 units = 1 mL
       24 units/100 units = 0.24 mL
    f. 500 mg
       250 mg × 1 tablet = 2 tablets should be given
    g. 50 mL × 60 gtts
       60 minutes 1 mL = 50 gtts/minute
       The hour time frame is converted to 60 minutes and the minidrip is 60 gtts (drops)/mL.
45. Patient assessments that should be completed before medication administration include:
    Parenteral injections: The size of the patient, condition of the injection site (integument and muscle condition), circulatory status
    For all patients, the type of medication and its effect on the patient are to be evaluated by the nurse.

46.

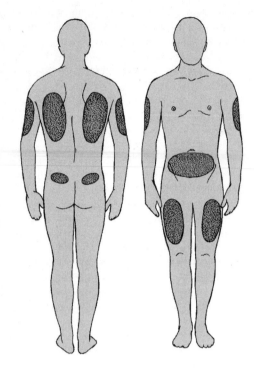

47. The correct techniques for administration of medications to patients with dysphagia are listed in answers b, c, and f.
48. a. Proper placement of the nasogastric tube is a priority assessment.
    b. The tube should be flushed with 15 to 30 mL of sterile water in between medications, with 30 to 60 mL of water given after all of the medications have been administered.
49. The nurse should apply clean gloves before administering topical medications. Sterile gloves may be indicated for medications applied to open wounds.
50. For administration of ear drops:
    a. Position the patient side-lying or sitting in a chair with the head tilted to the side.
    b. Pull the outer ear of an adult up and back.
    c. Irrigate with 50 mL of solution at room temperature.
51. For a pressured metered-dose inhaler:
    a. A spacer should be used.
    b. The patient should inhale for 3 to 5 seconds and hold breath for 10 seconds.
    c. 20 to 30 seconds should be given in between puffs of the same medication.
    d. This canister should last for 20 days (8 puffs/day, 160 total puffs in the canister).
    e. The patient should rinse out the mouth and/or brush the teeth after receiving a corticosteroid via the pMDI.
52. The patient should be placed in left Sims' position, if tolerated.
53. a. Anticoagulant: review of laboratory tests for clotting/bleeding times; assessment of the skin, mucous membranes, urine, and feces for signs of bleeding
    b. Antihypertensive: measurement of blood pressure
    c. Analgesic: completion of a pain assessment; measurement of vital signs, especially respirations and level of sedation

d. Cardiotonic: assessment of apical pulse; measurement of vital signs; determination of the presence of cardiac-related signs and symptoms
54. False
55. For pediatric medications: b, c, e are correct.
56. The correct sequence is e, b, f, a, c, d.
57. True
58. a. The medication for an IV push/bolus should be given at a rate of 0.5 mL/30 seconds.
    b. If the medication is incompatible, the nurse should stop the IV fluids, clamp the IV line, flush with 10 mL of normal saline or sterile water, give the IV bolus over the appropriate amount of time, flush with another 10 mL of normal saline or sterile water at the same rate as the medication was administered, and then restart the IV fluids at the prescribed rate. This allows you to give IV push medication through the existing line without creating potential risks associated with IV incompatibilities. If IV infusion that is currently hanging is a medication (e.g., ranitidine), disconnect IV line and administer IV push medication to avoid giving a sudden bolus of the medication in the existing IV line to the patient. Verify institutional policy regarding the stopping of IV fluids or continuous IV medications. If unable to stop IV infusion, start a new IV site and administer medication using the IV push (IV lock) method.
59. Intradermal injections are given on the inner forearm and upper back.
60. a. Tuberculin tests are read within 48 to 72 hours.
    b. A positive test for an individual with no known risk factors is 15 mm or more of induration.
61. a. Dorsal recumbent position
    b. The applicator is inserted 5 to 7.5 cm (2 to 3 inches)
62. An example of a positive synergistic effect is: antihypertensives/vasodilators and diuretics. An example of a negative synergistic effect is CNS depressants and alcohol.
63. An advantage of computerized order entry by physicians is the ability to read the orders accurately and reduce errors from misinterpretation.
64. Orders must be rewritten by the prescriber when the patient goes for surgery, is transferred to another unit, or is discharged to home or another facility.
65. Care should be taken when breaking open the neck of the ampule and a filter needle should be used to withdraw the fluid. Medication cannot be saved in the ampule after it is opened.
66. For rotation of subcutaneous sites, the same general location should be used at the same time each day, but each injection should be at least 2.5 cm apart.
67. The correct sequence for administration of an oral medication is e, g, b, d, f, a, c.
68. The four pharmacokinetic processes are absorption, distribution, metabolism, and excretion.
    a. Absorption is influenced by the route of administration, ability of a medication to dissolve, blood flow to the site of administration, body surface area, and lipid solubility of a medication.
    b. Distribution is influenced by circulation, membrane permeability, and protein binding.

c. Metabolism is primarily influenced by the ability of the liver, along with the lungs, kidneys, blood, and intestines.

d. Excretion is influenced primarily by the function of the kidneys, along with the lungs, intestines, and skin.

69. 2	77. 4	84. 1
70. 3	78. 2	85. 2
71. 2	79. 3	86. 3
72. 4	80. 1	87. 1
73. 4	81. 3	88. 4
75. 1	82. 2	89. 3
76. 2	83. 3	

CHAPTER 18

Case Studies

1. a. A patient taking both digoxin and Lasix is more susceptible to fluid volume deficit (FVD) and hypokalemia. Digoxin strengthens the contraction of the heart muscle, improving the cardiac output and circulatory volume. Lasix is a potent diuretic that does not have a potassium-sparing effect. The patient should be instructed to be alert to the signs of decreased fluid and decreased potassium levels as follows:
   • Hypokalemia: weakness, fatigue, decreased muscle tone, intestinal distention, change in pulse rate or rhythm
   • FVD: poor skin turgor, thirst, sunken eyeballs, dryness, weakness, change in pulse rate or rhythm
   The patient also should be instructed in the technique for taking her own pulse rate and on the importance of dietary replacement of potassium (e.g., bananas, oranges, potatoes) or administration of prescribed supplements.

2. a. The patient on prolonged immobility is prone to hypercalcemia as a result of calcium being released from the bones into the bloodstream. The nurse is alert to changes in the cardiac rate and rhythm (e.g., tachycardia) and increases in the BUN and serum calcium levels. If the patient is conscious, there may be anorexia, nausea, vomiting, low back pain, and a reduction in the level of consciousness.
   Alcoholic patients are more susceptible to malnutrition and hypomagnesemia. The nurse is alert to muscle tremors, hyperactive reflexes, confusion, disorientation, dysrhythmias, positive Trousseau/Chvostek signs, and a serum magnesium level less than 1.5 mEq/L.

3. a. The nurse may anticipate that this patient will have signs and symptoms of diminished oxygenation, including dyspnea, wheezing, coughing, activity intolerance, restlessness, pallor/cyanosis, and possible lack of concentration.
   b. This patient most likely will experience respiratory acidosis.

4. a. The priorities before administration of the blood include
   • If the patient has IV access already in place, assess the site for signs of infection, infiltration, and patency. Determine the gauge of the IV cannula.
   • Assess the patient to determine if he or she knows the reason for the blood transfusion and whether the patient ever had a previous transfusion or transfusion reaction.

   • Ensure the patient or representative has signed the informed consent.
   • Check the blood products and the patient, and verify the compatibility of the blood and the patient. Some hospitals use bar code technology to identify patients and verify compatible blood before beginning transfusions.
   • Obtain the patient's baseline vital signs before a transfusion begins.
   b. The safety measures to be implemented to reduce complications are
   • Before a blood transfusion, two registered nurses or one registered nurse and a licensed practical nurse (see agency policy) must simultaneously check the label on the blood product against the patient's identification number, blood group, and complete name. *If even a minor discrepancy exists, do not give the blood. Notify the blood bank immediately*.
   • Initiation of a transfusion begins slowly to allow for the early detection of a transfusion reaction.
   • Maintain the infusion rate, monitor for side effects, assess vital signs, and promptly record all findings.
   • It is important to stay with the patient during the first 15 minutes, the time when a reaction is most likely to occur. After that time period, continue to monitor the patient and obtain vital signs periodically during the transfusion as directed by agency policy. If a transfusion reaction is suspected, STOP the transfusion immediately. Disconnect the blood tubing, and connect the normal saline infusion to maintain an open IV line. Once the normal saline line is established, obtain vital signs and notify the health care provider. The unused blood product is returned to the blood bank.

Chapter Review

1. e	4. b	7. i
2. f	5. a	8. g
3. h	6. c	9. d

10. a. Extracellular fluid
    b. Interstitial fluid
    c. Intracellular fluid

11. a. Sodium: cation, extracellular—maintenance of water balance, nerve impulse transmission, regulation of acid-base balance, and participation in cellular chemical reactions
    b. Potassium: cation, intracellular—necessary for glycogen deposits in the liver and skeletal muscle, transmission and conduction of nerve impulses, cardiac rhythm, and skeletal and smooth muscle contraction
    c. Calcium: cation, intracellular—bone and teeth formation, blood clotting, hormone secretion, cell membrane integrity, cardiac conduction, transmission of nerve impulses, and muscle contraction
    d. Magnesium: cation, intracellular—enzyme activities, neurochemical activities, and cardiac and skeletal muscle excitability
    e. Chloride: anion, extracellular—follows sodium
    f. Bicarbonate: anion, both intracellular and extracellular—major chemical base buffer

12. The three types of acid-base regulators within the body are chemical, biological, and physiological.

179

13. Infants, young children, and older adults are most susceptible to fluid and acid-base disturbances.
14. a. Isotonic
    b. Hypotonic
    c. Isotonic
    d. Isotonic
    e. Hypertonic
15. The types of medications that may cause fluid, electrolyte, or acid-base disturbances include diuretics, steroids, potassium supplements, respiratory center depressants, antibiotics, and antacids.
16. Nursing diagnoses for imbalances include
    Ineffective Breathing Pattern
    Decreased Cardiac Output
    Deficient Fluid Volume
    Excess Fluid Volume
    Impaired Gas Exchange
    Impaired Skin Integrity
    Impaired Tissue Integrity
    Ineffective Tissue Perfusion
17.

18. A patient who is NPO and receiving IV fluids needs to have potassium added to the solution.
19. Signs and symptoms of phlebitis at an IV site are redness, inflammation, tenderness, and warmth.
20. A patient with a PICC line who develops a fever and increased WBCs will have the PICC line discontinued and receive an order for antibiotic therapy.
21. Based on the patient's status, the nurse should slow the rate of IV infusion, notify the health care provider, raise the head of the bed, provide supplemental oxygen as ordered, and monitor the patient's vital signs.
22. Transfusion of a patient's own blood is an autologous transfusion.
23. a. Hyponatremia
    b. Hyperkalemia
    c. Hypocalcemia
    d. Hypomagnesemia

24. a. 500 mL in 5 hours (300 minutes) with 15 gtt/mL = 25 gtt/min
    b. 1000 mL in 8 hours (480 minutes) with 10 gtt/mL = 21 gtt/min
    c. 200 mL in 4 hours (240 minutes) with 60 gtt/mL = 50 gtt/mL
    d. 2000 mL in 18 hours = 111 mL/hr
25. a. Pituitary hormone—ADH (antidiuretic hormone)
    b. Adrenal hormone—aldosterone
26. True
27. Arterial pH is an indirect measurement of the hydrogen ion concentration.
28. Oxygen moves into the lungs by diffusion.
29. An average adult's daily intake of fluid is approximately 2200 to 2700 mL.
30. The correct order for the steps is c, a, e, b, d. Note that cleansing the area and re-application of the tourniquet may be interchanged.
31. Intake = 1465; Output = 370
32. Fluid volume deficit may be the result of a, d, and f.
33. The nurse anticipates that the patient who has insufficient fluid as a result of a fever will have orders for antipyretics and oral and/or IV fluids. The nurse will also provide comfort measures, such as keeping the patient dry if there is diaphoresis.
34. The IV should be started in the most distal site.
35. INS standards specify the use of an arm board or other joint stabilization device to protect the IV site by keeping the joint extended (INS, 2011). Use padding with arm boards because they may cause skin or nerve damage from pressure. It may be more comfortable for the patient to have an infusion started in a new location rather than relying on a site that causes problems.
36. The order for the steps when removing an IV are f, a, c, g, b, e, d.
37. When preparing the IV, the nurse should look at the fluid to note the type of fluid and amount, expiration date, integrity of the container, and clarity of the solution.
38. For patient safety, follow the agency's procedure to verify three things: the blood components delivered are the ones that were ordered; the blood delivered is compatible with the patient's blood type listed in the medical record; and the right patient receives the blood. An assessment of the patient before the administration is done to establish a baseline for comparison, in the event of a transfusion reaction.
39. For a patient experiencing hypokalemia, the correct signs are a, d, f.
40. In performing an IV site dressing, the nurse should do b, c, d, and f.

41. 2	51. 4	61. 1
42. 1	52. 3	62. 4
43. 1	53. 4	63. 2
44. 2	54. 3	64. 2
45. 3	55. 2	65. 1
46. 3	56. 4	66. 4
47. 3	57. 4	67. 3
48. 1	58. 3	68. 3
49. 2	59. 4	69. 4
50. 3	60. 3	70. 3

CHAPTER 19

Case Studies

1. One of the most important things that the nurse can do for the patient's daughter and her family is to sit with them and allow them to verbalize their feelings about the situation. Listening to the family and acknowledging their emotions lets them know that their feelings and concerns are important. It also demonstrates that the nurse is responsive to their needs and is involved in the holistic care of the patient. The nurse should explain how the patient's condition has progressed and the treatments that currently are being provided for comfort and support. The nurse may provide the daughter with the opportunity to assist with or observe the physical care being given to the patient. Providing information on available resources, such as hospice, is also important in demonstrating caring and concern for the well-being of the patient and her family.

2. a. The student giving the bath to the patient is missing the caring behaviors of comforting touch, maintaining dignity, and performing care appropriately.

   b. The nurse should enter the patient's room to provide privacy immediately. With the patient covered and safe, the nurse should speak with the student outside of the room about the observations. By being a role model and performing the bath in a caring manner, the nurse can demonstrate the appropriate method and reinforce the discussion with the student.

Chapter Review

1. The theories of caring are
   a. Swanson.
   b. Watson.
   c. Benner and Wrubel.
   d. Leininger.

2. Examples of clinical interventions for the following are
   a. Providing presence: staying with the patient while waiting for a procedure or test results
   b. Touch: holding the patient's hand, giving a massage, skillfully and gently performing a procedure
   c. Listening: opening the lines of communication, attentively listening to what the patient is saying, and responding appropriately
   d. Knowing the patient: centering on the patient and providing information that is relevant to the patient's circumstances

3. The nurse demonstrates caring behaviors during an IV insertion by explaining the procedure to the patient in advance and during the intervention, using skillful and gentle technique, and maintaining eye contact.

4. Caring and spirituality are connected in the way that the nurse identifies and provides for the patient's spiritual needs. Spirituality offers intrapersonal (connected with oneself), interpersonal (connected with others and the environment), and transpersonal (connected with the unseen, God, or a higher power) connectedness.

5. Nurses can care for each other by recognizing signs of compassion fatigue, providing mentorship, assisting in patient care activities, and allowing for discussion of concerns and feelings.

6. 1
7. 3
8. 3
9. 4
10. 4
11. 3
12. 4
13. 2
14. 1
15. 4
16. 2

CHAPTER 20

Case Study

1. a. Involvement of the family is important in assisting the patient to achieve an optimal level of well-being, but there may have to be limits placed on the number of family members who may stay in the room, a reasonable time frame for visiting to allow the patient to rest and receive treatment, and the determination of where the family may gather to conduct discussions.

   b. The therapeutic diet may have to be adapted to avoid meat and meat products but still provide necessary nutrients (protein) or avoid unwanted ingredients (sodium). In an acute or restorative care setting, the dietitian should be involved in providing a menu that meets the patient's cultural preferences but is also tasteful, satisfying, and within therapeutic guidelines.

   c. A healer may provide emotional as well as health care support for the patient. The nurse should work with the health care team to integrate, as much as possible, the actions of the healer. Traditional remedies or treatments should be investigated, however, to determine if there may be any interaction with the prescribed medications or therapies.

   d. To promote communication with individuals and families who speak another language, the nurse should obtain an interpreter who is proficient in that language, use word signs or charts, refrain from speaking loudly, use appropriate titles and greetings, be attentive to nonverbal communication, and clarify uncertain areas.

Chapter Review

1. Nursing diagnoses related to cultural needs may include
   Impaired Verbal Communication
   Compromised Family Coping
   Ineffective Health Maintenance
   Impaired Social Interaction
   Noncompliance

2. a. Cultural awareness: Gain in-depth awareness of one's own background, stereotypes, biases, prejudices, and assumptions about other people.

   b. Cultural skills: Develop skills such as communication, cultural assessment, and culturally competent care.

3. A question may be, "Do you have any cultural practices or rituals that we should know about?" or "Do you use any traditional remedies?"

4. Examples of cultural patterns of communication that may influence the nurse-patient interaction:
   a. Differences in status and position, age, sex, and outsider versus insider perspectives that determine the content and process of communication
   b. Conflict seen as embarrassing or demeaning, with the use of indirect, face-saving communication

c. Awareness of a distinct linear hierarchy, with negotiation of conflict occurring between persons within the same level of position or authority

d. Nonverbal communication, including the amount of personal space that is comfortable, the degree of eye contact, the extent of touching, and how much private information is shared with others

e. Difference in language
   Interventions: use of the mnemonics (e.g., LEARN), interpreters, understanding of cultural meanings related to communication

5. Linguistic competence is the capacity of an organization and its personnel to communicate effectively and convey information in a manner easily understood by diverse audiences. Those audiences include people of limited English proficiency, those who have low literacy skills or are not literate, individuals with disabilities, and those who are deaf or hard of hearing.

6. Disadvantaged groups are those who "have systematically experienced greater obstacles to health based on their racial or ethnic group; religion; socioeconomic status; gender; age; mental health; cognitive, sensory, or physical disability; sexual orientation or gender identity; geographic location; or other characteristics historically linked to discrimination or exclusion." The challenges faced include reduced access to health care, inequality in health services, and poor outcomes (e.g., higher infant mortality rates).

7. Cultural considerations are incorporated into "teach back" by specifically determining if the information was communicated effectively and understood by the patient, especially if he/she speaks a different language.

8. Working with an interpreter
   • Provide language assistance services free of charge to all patients who speak limited English or are deaf at all points of contact.
   • Notify patients, verbally and in writing, of their rights to receive language-assistance services.
   • Take steps to provide auxiliary aids and services, defined to include qualified interpreters, note takers, computer-aided transcription services, and written materials.
   • Ensure that interpreters are competent in medical terminology and understand issues of confidentiality and impartiality.

9. L - listen
   E - explain
   A - acknowledge
   R - recommend
   N - negotiate

   R - rapport
   E - empathy
   S - support
   P - partnership
   E - explanations
   C - cultural competence
   T - trust

10. 4
11. 1
12. 4
13. 3
14. 4

CHAPTER 21

Case Study

1. a. The nurse should obtain information about the extent to which the patient practices Buddhism, including whether he or she is a vegetarian, fasts and refuses treatment on holy days, avoids alcohol, and hesitates to use medications. In addition, the patient's advance directives should be obtained because life support may be removed, if indicated.

   b. Dependent upon the degree to which the patient practices his or her faith, adaptations may have to be made as follows:
      • Special dietary request for a vegetarian diet
      • Scheduling of treatments or tests, for example, on days that are not considered holy
      • Determination of medications that may be acceptable
      • Inquiry into the patient's ability to use medications or mouthwash with alcohol
      • Providing contact with a Buddhist priest

Chapter Review

1. d	4. b	6. g
2. a	5. f	7. c
3. e		

8. General nursing interventions for promotion of spiritual health include establishing presence, supporting a healing environment, using support systems, providing diet therapy, supporting practices and rituals, and allowing opportunities for prayer and/or meditation.

9. Nursing interventions for patients who had near-death experiences include the following: promoting open communication, providing a chance for the patient to explore the experience, supporting the patient's discussion with family/significant others.

10. Possible nursing diagnoses include
    • *Readiness for Enhanced Spiritual Well-Being*
    • *Spiritual Distress*
    • *Ineffective Coping*
    • *Anxiety*
    • *Hopelessness*
    • *Powerlessness*
    • *Risk for Spiritual Distress*
    Possible patient outcomes include
       Regain spiritual comfort, affirm a purpose in life, participate in religious practices, pray and meditate daily/prn, recognize/request need for spiritual support, communicate with family and/or significant others about spiritual health

11. The acronym stands for
    F—Faith or belief
    I—Importance of spirituality
    C—Individual's spiritual **Community**
    A—Interventions to **Address** spiritual needs

12. Examples of questions to determine a patient's spiritual belief system include
    "What is most important in your life?"
    "What gives your life meaning or purpose?"

13. The patient's religious background should be checked, because a Jehovah's Witness or Christian Scientist may refuse the blood.

14. Rituals or practices associated with spirituality and religion include participating in group or private worship or prayer, having baptism or communion, fasting, singing, meditating, scripture reading, making offerings or sacrifices, requiring burial or cremation, providing special care of the deceased, and/or having male children circumcised.

15. The correct responses are b, d, and e.

16. The four dimensions of spiritual well-being are
    - Personal dimension: refers to how you relate with yourself in finding meaning and purpose in life
    - Communal dimension: relates to the quality of your interpersonal relationships
    - Environmental dimension: describes how you interact in the world, including your sense of awe with the environment
    - Transcendental dimension: refers to the relationship between you and some higher power

17. The correct statements about spirituality are b, c, and e.

18. The nurse uses *presence* by spending quality time with patients, giving attention, answering questions, listening, having a positive and encouraging (but realistic) attitude, and offering closeness with a patient physically, psychologically, and spiritually.

19. The appropriate nursing actions to promote spiritual health are c, d, and e.

20. 4	23. 1	26. 4
21. 1	24. 3	27. 3
22. 4	25. 1	28. 2

CHAPTER 22

Case Studies

1. a. Promotion of growth and development for the hospitalized infant may include the following:
     - Having the parents/guardians provide most of the care to avoid interfering with the attachment process
     - Limiting the number of caregivers and following the parents' directions for care to promote trust
     - Limiting negative experiences and providing pleasurable sensations

   Promotion of growth and development for the hospitalized 5-year-old child may include the following:
     - Creating a comfortable environment for the child and parents
     - Providing consistent and appropriate care, if the parents are not available
     - Limiting the number of caregivers
     - Providing an environment of acceptance for regressive behavior and reassuring parents that the behavior is normal for children in this situation
     - Allowing children to examine equipment that may be used and participate in procedures, as appropriate
     - Providing comfort items, such as a tape with the parents' voice, pictures of family members, and favorite toys

   - Providing opportunities for play and social interaction with other children
   - Explaining routines in understandable language
   - Incorporating activities of daily living into the hospital routine

   Promotion of growth and development for the hospitalized 16-year-old may include the following:
     - Allowing for peers to visit or have telephone/Internet access
     - Addressing the adolescent rather than the parents during assessments
     - Providing the opportunity for the patient to make choices whenever possible
     - Supporting the amount of parental contact that the adolescent needs, whether intermittent visits or longer stays

   b. A teaching plan for the new parents of an infant should include information on
     - Safety in the environment
     - Feeding: breastfeeding or formula/bottles
     - Hygiene needs
     - Elimination patterns
     - Sleep patterns ("back to sleep")
     - Cord care: immediate neonatal stages
     - Immunization and medical follow-up schedule
     - Expectations for behavior
     - Support for each other

2. a. This patient may benefit from reality orientation, which includes the following:
     - Using time, date, place, and name in conversation
     - Reinforcing reality and providing meaningful things to do
     - Encouraging participation in activities
     - Ensuring that hearing aids or glasses, for example, are working or fitted correctly
     - Providing bowel and bladder training
     - Reinforcing positive behaviors
     - Being patient and allowing sufficient time for completion of activities
     - Speaking slowly and clearly, repeating as necessary
     - Providing clear, simple directions
     - Maintaining a caring and stimulating environment

3. a. Children in this age group usually are interested in games and sports. For indoor recreation, board games, electronic games, or word games may be suggested. Hobbies and crafts are also appropriate if they stimulate and maintain the children's interest. If the children will be outdoors, supervised games such as volleyball, softball/baseball, kickball, tennis, or relay races may be organized. Some sports may have to be modified to meet the physical abilities of the age group. Swimming, bicycling, rowing/canoeing, walking, and hiking are activities that do not have to involve competition but promote exercise.

4. a. Suicide is one of the main causes of death in adolescents and young adults. Parents should be aware of the following warning signs:
     - Diminished performance in school
     - Withdrawal from social activities with family and friends
     - Substance abuse
     - Changes in personality

- Disturbances in sleep, appetite, and usual activity levels
- Talking about death or suicide
- Giving away personal items

Chapter Review

1. d   3. c   5. b
2. a   4. e

6. Teratogens include communicable diseases, alcohol and drugs, smoking, and pollutants.
7. The leading cause of death in the toddler and preschool age group is accidents.
8. The behaviors are associated with the following age groups:

    a. Toddler   j. School age
    b. Infant   k. Preschool age
    c. School age   l. Older adult
    d. Infant   m. School age
    e. Young adult   n. Adolescent
    f. Toddler   o. Young adult
    g. Adolescent   p. Older adult
    h. Middle adult   q. Middle adult
    i. Toddler   r. Preschool age

9. To promote awareness of time, place, and person, the nurse should implement reality orientation.
10. Prescription or use of more medications than indicated is called polypharmacy.
11. Safety concerns in the home environment include

    a. Toddler: access to poisons, such as cleaning supplies; electrical outlets; ability to exit the home; swimming pools; kitchen appliances; auto accidents; choking on small objects

    b. Older adult: poor lighting, slippery floors and unsecured rugs, excessive water temperature, stairs

12. The expected physical assessment findings for a middle-age adult are c, d, and e.
13. Age-appropriate topic areas for the older adult group are activity and exercise, communication with the health care provider, home and medication safety, nutrition, and skin care.
14. The nurse can reduce stress for a hospitalized child by reducing the number of different caretakers, having the parents remain with the child and bring in favorite toys/objects, limiting the amount of time that the child is restrained, providing simple explanations that the child will understand, and speaking in a soothing and comforting tone.
15. Examples of potential nursing diagnoses for adolescents include *Risk for Injury, Impaired Social Interaction,* and *Ineffective Coping.*
16. The characteristics for adolescents are b, c, and f.
17. Patients in the "Sandwich Generation" are responsible not only for themselves but for older parents and children. Multigenerational responsibilities can add stress to the patients' lives and create challenges in helping these individuals find time for their own health and medical care.
18. Concerns for toddlers and school-age children include safety, nutrition, sleep, and socialization/play.
19. The accurate statements for an older adult are b, c, d, and f.

20. 4   24. 1   28. 4
21. 2   25. 4   29. 4
22. 2   26. 3   30. 4
23. 2   27. 1   31. 1

CHAPTER 23

Case Studies

1. a. This young adult patient most likely will experience alterations in his self-concept, especially the perception of his body image and identity. Young adults may be very sensitive about their physical appearance and social status, and now the patient will have to cope with an alteration in his normal activities. In addition, the paraplegia will significantly influence his sexual functioning, an area in which he will have to adapt.

    b. Sample care plan:

Nursing Diagnosis	Expected Outcome	Nursing Interventions
Disturbed Body Image related to accidental injury and resultant lack of mobility and sensation to the lower extremities (as manifested by his verbalization of his prior social activities)	Patient will adapt to change in body image by • Discussing feelings about his injury and change in activity status • Participating in care as much as possible • Reflecting on personal strengths	Provide time for talking with the patient and discussing feelings; explore coping skills that the patient has used before, and encourage and support those skills; involve the patient in health care activities.
Ineffective Sexuality Pattern related to accidental injury and resultant lack of mobility and sensation to lower extremities	Patient will learn/use measures to attain sexual satisfaction within limitations by • Discussing feelings about sexual function and adaption • Participating in educational program on alternative measures to promote sexual response • Sharing response to measures used and suggesting possible alternatives	Provide time to talk with the patient and discuss feelings and concerns; provide information on sexual response and stimulation for patients with paraplegia; obtain a referral/consultation, if indicated, for additional support and information; have another young male paraplegic individual speak with the patient; provide for patient privacy.

2. a. The patient who you suspect may be a victim of sexual abuse may be found to have
   - Physical signs: bruises, lacerations, abrasions, burns, headaches, GI problems, eating disorders, abdominal or vaginal pain
   - Behavioral signs: sleep-pattern disturbances, nightmares, insomnia, depression, anxiety, fear, decreased self-esteem, substance abuse, frequent visits to health care providers
   b. Examples of questions that should be asked include
   - "Are you in a relationship in which someone is hurting you?"
   - "Have you ever been forced to have sex when you didn't want to?"
   - "Are you afraid of the situation that you are in?"

Chapter Review

1. b	4. d	7. c
2. f	5. h	8. g
3. e	6. a	

9. a. General positive influences on self-concept include words and actions of approval, interest, and acceptance; recognition and inclusion in decision making; trust; and support.
   b. Stressors that may influence self-concept include those that threaten body image, self-esteem, role, or identity, such as the effects of traumatic accidents, surgery, and acute or chronic diseases.
10. Behaviors that may indicate an altered self-concept include c, d, f, and h.
11. Potential concerns related to self-concept include
    a. Alteration in body image: Removal of breast can lead to questions of feminine image and sexual desirability.
    b. Alteration in body image and role: Loss of hair from chemotherapy, possible hospitalizations, and diminished strength may interfere with role as mother.
    c. Alteration in body image and identity: Physical changes in appearance and function (ability to play with others)
    d. Alteration in role and self-esteem: Possible inability to maintain current occupation, dependence on others
12. Ways in which the nurse may promote self-concept in an acute care setting include the following:
    - Arranging visits with someone who has experienced similar problems/changes
    - Listening, being sensitive to, and supporting the patient's needs
    - Being aware of nonverbal communication (e.g., reactions to the patient's mastectomy)
    - Including the patient, as much as possible, in decision making and self-care
13. Alterations in sexual health include infertility, sexual abuse, sexual dysfunction, and personal and emotional conflicts.
14. Patient teaching for the promotion of sexual health may include instruction about
    - Refraining from drinking alcohol 1 to 2 hours before sexual activity
    - Discussing behavior that provides the most sexual stimulation and satisfaction with the partner
    - Options available for contraception
    - Side effects of medications that alter sexual function and response
    - Use of usual positions and selection of times when patient feels rested (for individuals with cardiac dysfunction)
    - Safe sex practices
15. For the nursing diagnosis *Situational Low Self-Esteem related to being unable to pass a required college course*, examples are as follows:
    - Goal: increased self-esteem indicated in body image, behavior, and verbalization
    - Outcome: discusses positive aspects of self and future plans
    - Nursing interventions: spend time with the person to allow for discussion of feelings and concerns, establish sense of trust
16. False
17. False
18. False
19. Promotion of self-concept for an older adult may include
    - Clarifying what life changes mean
    - Being alert to preoccupation with physical complaints and encouraging verbalization of needs
    - Identifying positive and negative coping mechanisms and supporting effective strategies
    - Encouraging the use of storytelling
    - Communicating that the individual is worthwhile by actively listening to and accepting the person's feelings and concerns
    - Allowing additional time to complete tasks and reinforcing the person's efforts at independence
20. For tattoos and body piercings, the correct statements are b, d, and e.
21. Examples of role performance stressors include becoming parents, taking over the care of older parents, becoming a widow/widower.
22. The vaccine is Gardasil.
23. Cardiovascular disease, neurological disorders (stroke, Parkinson's), diabetes mellitus, respiratory disease, and arthritis are medical diagnoses that can interfere with sexual functioning.

24. 3	29. 2	34. 3
25. 4	30. 4	35. 4
26. 4	31. 4	36. 3
27. 1	32. 4	37. 2
28. 1	33. 2	

CHAPTER 24

Case Studies

1. a. The patient, who provides the major financial support to the family, has been hospitalized with a serious health problem. His wife has maintained a traditional role as "homemaker" while her husband has worked. The younger daughter has assumed a family life that appears to be more acceptable to her parents, whereas the older son is involved in an alternative family form. The younger daughter may be more involved in her parents' life because of her family pattern.

b. The family is apparently progressing from the "Family with young adults" to the "Family in later life" stage. There are elements of both stages within this situation.

c. The nurse may begin discussions with the father and mother initially, moving toward a total family meeting at a later date. Providing opportunities for family members to express their feelings about both the health care and the family situation may facilitate open communication about family structure and relationships. The family may need to be referred for ongoing counseling if there is a negative impact on the health/recovery of the patient.

d. The patient may have feelings about his business and family roles and his ability to resume them when he is discharged. His wife will need to be involved in the educational process to follow through with the plan of care. The patient's wife may need to assume a greater decision-making role with the patient to maintain the economic and emotional status of the family.

e. Possible family-oriented nursing diagnoses include
   • *Interrupted Family Processes*
   • *Ineffective Role Performance*
   • *Compromised Family Coping*

2. a. The visiting nurse should determine what the patient's home environment is like in regard to safety and accessibility. The nurse needs to know whether there is a ramp, stairs, or an elevator. If the patient will be using an assistive device, such as a walker or wheelchair, is there sufficient room for mobility within the home? How is the home arranged? Is it open or cluttered? Is there a shower or bath? Overall, does the patient have the necessary resources to manage post-hospital care?

   b. It is important to know whether there are family members living in the home or nearby. The patient may need assistance with household management, ADLs, or transportation to heath care agencies.

Chapter Review

1. b
2. d
3. a
4. e
5. c
6. A family is a set of interacting individuals related by blood, marriage, or adoption who usually live together and fulfill functions of socialization, division of labor, and economic provisions and cooperatively meet affective and emotional needs of the individuals within the family unit.
7. Family members may need to decide on whether or not to test for the presence of the disease and/or have children. Some families choose not to have children, whereas other families choose not to know genetic risks and have children; other families choose to know the risk and then determine whether to have children. With genetic risks for certain cancers, such as certain breast cancer, the family member may choose to have prophylactic mastectomies to reduce the risk for developing the disease.
8. a. Family hardiness is the intrafamilial system of support and structure that extends beyond the walls of the household. Through divorce, remarriages, or cohabitation new members are added to a family. In addition, an extended family also includes contact with former spouses or partners.

   b. Family resiliency is the ability of the family to cope with expected and unexpected stressors.

   c. Family diversity is the uniqueness of each family unit.

9. Current concerns or challenges that may influence the family today are: a changing family structure (which means fewer children, delayed childbirth, divorce, adolescent pregnancy, single parents, same-sex couples), changing economic status, homelessness, domestic violence, employment, and access to health care.

10. a. Caregivers may manifest the following signs and symptoms of caregiver strain:
    • Physical: fatigue, frequent illness/exacerbation of previous conditions
    • Psychological: changes in mood, anxiety, depression, anger

    b. A possible nursing diagnosis is *Caregiver Role Strain*.

11. The correct statements are b, d, f, and g.

12. Inadequate functioning can have many effects on the family, including stress, impaired cardiovascular and neuroendocrine functioning, and interference with decision making and problem solving.

13. Questions that may be asked to determine cultural influence on a family include
    a. "What types of foods do you eat?"
    b. "Who cares for sick family members?"
    c. "Have you or anyone in your family been hospitalized?"
    d. "Did family members remain at the hospital?"
    e. "Do you use some of your culture's health practices, such as acupuncture or meditation?"
    f. "What role do grandparents play in raising your children?"

14. Health promotion for a family can include healthy diets (e.g., low fat), exercise plans, safety instruction, immunizations, and regular health maintenance.

15. Factors contributing to domestic violence include stress, poverty, social isolation, psychopathology, learned family behavior, alcohol and drug abuse, pregnancy, sexual orientation, and mental illness.

16. The nurse can help the family by providing information, support, assurance, and presence (e.g., giving the family information about the dying process, helping to set up home care and obtain hospice, and offering grief support) and, if present at the time of death, being sensitive to the family's needs (e.g., by providing for privacy and allowing sufficient time for saying good-byes).

17. A family with a rigid structure is in danger of altered functioning. Rigid structures specifically dictate who accomplishes different tasks and also limits the number of persons outside the immediate family allowed to assume these tasks. For example, in a rigid family the mother is the only acceptable person to provide emotional support for the children and/or to perform all of the household chores. If something happens to the mother, the role is not easily managed by the father or other members of the family.

18. 3	22. 3	26. 4
19. 4	23. 4	27. 2
20. 3	24. 2	
21. 1	25. 3	

CHAPTER 25

Case Study

1. a. This patient may demonstrate the following:
   - Physical signs: increased heart rate, respirations, and blood pressure; headaches; fatigue; sleep disturbances; restlessness; gastrointestinal distress; weight gain or loss; backaches; amenorrhea; frequent or prolonged colds or flu
   - Psychological signs: forgetfulness, preoccupation, increased fantasizing, decreased creativity, slower reactions and thinking, confusion, decreased attention span
   - Emotional signs: crying tendencies, lack of interest, irritability, negative thinking, worrying
   - Behavioral signs: diminished activity or hyperactivity, withdrawal, suspiciousness, substance abuse, change in communication or interaction with others
   b. Possible nursing diagnoses for this patient include
   - *Anxiety*
   - *Ineffective Coping*
   c. Outcomes for these nursing diagnoses: The patient will
   - differentiate effective and ineffective coping patterns.
   - identify and express the need for help.
   - verbalize a decrease in stress.
   - work on time management.
   - recognize stressors and implement stress management techniques.
   - alter her lifestyle to reduce stress.
   - call upon her personal support system.
   d. A number of alternatives may be presented to this patient so that she may select those that are most beneficial to her. The nurse may use guided imagery, biofeedback, progressive muscle relaxation, hypnosis, music/art therapy, humor, assertiveness training, or journal/diary entry.

Chapter Review

1. Evaluating an event for its personal meaning is called primary appraisal.
2. The correct statements about stress are a, d, and e.
3. A priority nursing intervention for patient safety is to determine if the patient is suicidal or homicidal.
4. True
5. Positive benefits from exercise include increased muscle tone, decreased tension, increased relaxation, weight control, increased circulation, improved posture, and endorphin release.
6. a. Maturational
   b. Sociocultural
   c. Sociocultural
   d. Situational
   e. Maturational
   f. Situational
   g. Maturational
   h. Sociocultural
7. a. Cognitive: forgetfulness, denial, increased fantasy life, poor concentration, inattention to detail, orientation to the past, decreased creativity, slower thinking and reactions, learning difficulties, apathy, confusion, decreased attention span, calculation difficulties

   b. Cardiovascular: increased heart rate, increased blood pressure, tightness in chest
   c. Gastrointestinal: nausea, diarrhea, vomiting, weight gain or loss, change in appetite, bleeding
   d. Behavioral: change in activity level, withdrawal, suspiciousness, change in communication and interaction with others, substance abuse, excessive humor or silence, no exercise, hyperactivity
   e. Neuroendocrine: headaches/migraines, fatigue, insomnia/sleep disturbances, feeling of being uncoordinated, restlessness, tremors, profuse sweating, dry mouth
8. Stress management should include instruction about instituting positive workplace habits, avoiding excessive change, time management, relaxation techniques, exercise, and establishing support systems.
9. Kegel exercises
10. With Pender's Health Promotion theory, the nurse would discuss increasing physical activity, improving diet and nutrition, and using stress management strategies to become healthy and remain healthy.
11. a. Compassion fatigue is more likely to be seen in nurses working on oncology units or in hospice care.
    b. Signs and symptoms of compassion fatigue are feelings of hopelessness, being in a state of hypervigilance, anxiety, and emotional exhaustion.
12. Applying the QSEN competency of safety to stress and coping: the nurse is alert to overt signs of crisis, suicidal or homicidal thought processes, inattention, and physical and emotional fatigue/exhaustion.
13. Stress becomes a crisis when it overwhelms a person's usual coping mechanisms and demands mobilization of all available resources.
14. Objective signs of stress include a, c, e, and f.
15. Components of cognitive therapy are a, c, and f.

16. 3	21. 4	26. 2
17. 1	22. 3	27. 1
18. 2	23. 4	28. 3
19. 1	24. 1	
20. 3	25. 2	

CHAPTER 26

Case Studies

1. a. The patient may demonstrate the following behaviors indicative of complicated bereavement:
   - Overactivity without a sense of loss
   - Alteration in relationships with friends and family
   - Anger against particular people
   - Agitated depression: tension, guilt, feelings of worthlessness
   - Decreased participation in religious or cultural activities
   - Inability to discuss the loss without crying (a year or more after the loss)
   - False euphoria
   - Eliminating all signs of the deceased (e.g., pictures) or creating a "shrine"
   - Alterations in eating and sleeping patterns
   - Regressive behavior

b. Possible nursing diagnoses for the patient may be:
- *Dysfunctional Grieving* related to sudden loss/suicide of husband
- *Ineffective Coping* related to inability to deal with husband's loss/suicide

Possible goals may be:
- The patient will accept the reality of her husband's death.
- The patient will renew activities of daily living and complete a normal grieving process.

Nursing interventions may include:
- Using therapeutic communication to promote the patient's verbalization of feelings concerning her husband's suicide
- Demonstrating support of the patient by staying with her and using comfort measures, such as touch
- Referring the patient to support groups, clergy, and/or counseling as appropriate for her needs

2. Hospice services center around the following:
- Patient and family as the unit of care
- Coordinated home care with access to inpatient and nursing home beds when needed
- Symptom management
- Physician-directed services
- Provision of an interdisciplinary care team
- Medical and nursing services available at all times
- Bereavement follow-up after a patient's death
- Use of trained volunteers for visitation and respite support

Chapter Review

1. d
2. b
3. c
4. a
5. Special circumstances that may influence grief resolution include suicide, sudden death, miscarriage, a child's death, and certain pathologies, such as AIDS.
6. True
7. Interventions that should be implemented for a family dealing with a patient's terminal illness include involving everyone in discussions, promoting open communication, answering questions, and providing caregiver support.
8. The correct interventions are c, d, and f.
9. Nursing measures that may be implemented to facilitate the mourning process include
   - Helping the patient accept that the loss is real
   - Supporting efforts to live without the deceased person or in the face of disability
   - Encouraging establishment of new relationships
   - Allowing time to grieve
   - Interpreting "normal" grief behavior
   - Providing continuing support
   - Being alert for signs of ineffective coping
10. The nurse may prevent a sense of abandonment by:
    - Answering patients' call lights promptly and assuring them that caregivers are available throughout the day and night

- Being readily available to answer questions or interpret changes in the patient's condition; offering a calm, comforting presence
- Avoiding placing patients in a private room
- Reassuring family members that their presence is important
- Allowing visitors to remain at all times with patients who are dying and relaxing other visiting restrictions

11. Federal and state legislation require that health care agencies formulate policies and procedures based on current laws to validate death, identify potential organ or tissue donors, request autopsy, and provide postmortem care.

12. a. Questions that may be asked about the nature of a loss:
    "How is the loss affecting your daily life?"
    "What past experiences have you had with loss?"
    "Tell me how you usually cope with disappointment or loss."
    b. Cultural beliefs about loss:
    "What do you believe about death?"
    "Who makes health care decisions in your family/culture?"
    "Tell me about your family's/culture's end-of-life and funeral practices."
    c. Coping strategies:
    "How are you managing with the care?"
    "What are you doing about your work and home responsibilities?"
    "Do you have plans for hospice care at home?"
    "Are you able to talk about your needs and feelings as a family?"

13. Signs of impending death include
    - Minimal intake of food or water
    - Increased sleeping and decreased consciousness
    - Disorientation and restlessness
    - Decreased urinary output and/or incontinence
    - Cool hands and feet
    - Noisy breathing
    - Irregular breathing patterns with long pauses
    At the time of death, you will note:
    - Absence of breathing and heartbeat
    - Bowel and bladder release
    - Unresponsiveness
    - Eyes fixed on a certain spot
    - Dilated pupils

14. Moving through Worden's four tasks can vary, but typically the process takes at least 1 year.

15. The Rs in Rando's R Process Model are recognizing the loss, reacting to the pain of separation, reminiscence, relinquishing old attachments, and readjusting to life after loss.

16. The correct actions for postmortem care are b, d, and e.

17. Nursing interventions include
    a. Fatigue: Help patient to identify valued or desired tasks; conserve energy for only those tasks. Assist with activities of daily living. Plan frequent rest periods in a quiet environment, and pace nursing care activities.
    b. Decreased appetite: Give patient whatever food or fluids patient enjoys. Offer frequent small meals and/or snacks rather than large meals. Do not force people to eat. Offer small portions of desired foods or home-cooked meals, per patient preference.

18. Delayed grief is seen when the survivor(s) attempts to return quickly to normal activities, pretending that everything is fine and then having a reaction at a later time.

19. An autopsy is performed in accordance with state legislation, usually in circumstances when death may have resulted from accident, homicide, or suicide.

20. Documentation should include information about the time and date of death, the name of the health care provider who pronounces the death, organ or tissue donation status, preparation of the body, medical devices left in or on the body, valuables or belongings left with the patient or given to the family, the time of discharge, and destination of the body.

21. Physical signs and symptoms associated with grieving include
    - Hollowness in the stomach
    - Tightness in the chest
    - Tightness in the throat
    - Oversensitivity to noise
    - Sense of depersonalization ("nothing seems real")
    - Feeling short of breath
    - Muscle weakness
    - Lack of energy
    - Dry mouth

22. 3	27. 3	32. 4
23. 2	28. 2	33. 4
24. 3	29. 1	34. 3
25. 4	30. 3	35. 3
26. 4	31. 1	

CHAPTER 27

Case Study

1. a. The patient should be assessed for her ability to move independently, including her posture, muscle strength, range of motion, gait (if able), balance, activity tolerance, and cognitive status. If the patient is able to bear weight on both legs and maintain an erect position, the nurse must determine if she is capable of ambulating safely. Initial assessment of the patient's transfer out of bed should be accomplished with assistance in the event that the patient is unable to maintain a standing position.

   b. If the patient is not able to ambulate independently, she may be able to use an assistive device, such as a cane or walker. If possible, one or more nurses may use a gait belt to assist the patient in ambulating. Should the patient not be able to ambulate safely, even with assistance, a wheelchair may be necessary. To assist the patient in gaining muscle strength, a program of exercise may be implemented.

Chapter Review

1. i	4. f	7. d
2. g	5. b	9. c
3. h	6. e	

10. Assessment of a patient's mobility includes range of joint motion, gait, exercise, balance, posture, and body alignment.

11. The correct principles of body mechanics are options b, d, and f.

12. False

13. a. Before ambulation, the patient should be placed in a sitting position with the legs dangled over the side of the bed.

    b. Care should be taken in making position changes slowly because orthostatic hypotension could occur.

14. Pathological influences on alignment, exercise, and activity include congenital defects; disorders of bones, joints, and muscles; central nervous system damage; and musculoskeletal trauma.

15. True

16. Examples of physiological factors that may influence activity tolerance are musculoskeletal abnormalities, diminished cardiovascular function, and diminished respiratory function.

17. Possible nursing diagnoses associated with a change in a patient's ability to maintain physical activity include
    - *Activity Intolerance*
    - *Disturbed Body Image*
    - *Risk for Injury*
    - *Impaired Physical Mobility*
    - *Impaired Skin Integrity*
    - *Acute* or *Chronic Pain*

18. The priority for this patient is pain relief.

19. The patient should be in Fowler's position—(head of the bed elevated 45 to 60 degrees) or semi-Fowler's position (head of bed elevated 30 degrees)

20. a. The general "rule of thumb" for transfers is to GET HELP to transfer a patient.

    b. Safety during transfers is the priority.

21. a. Supine
    b. Prone
    c. Lateral

22. Expected findings are answers a, e, and g.

23. The correct techniques are answers b, d, and e.

24. Patients should be repositioned at least every 2 hours.

25. a. The chair should be positioned on the patient's strong side at a 45-degree angle to the bed.

    b. More than one nurse is needed for this transfer. The correct sequence of steps for the use of a mechanical lift is the following:
    - Position the chair near the bed.
    - Raise the bed to working height with the mattress flat (as tolerated).
    - Roll the patient away from you (side rail is up on the far side).
    - Place the sling under the patient.
    - Roll the patient toward you.
    - Pull the sling through so that it is under the patient from the upper torso.
    - Check the position of the sling.
    - Move the lift under the bed and attach the sling to the lift.
    - Have the patient fold the arms over the chest.
    - Slowly lift the patient and maneuver the sling over the chair.

- Lower the patient into the chair and disconnect the lift.
- Position the patient for comfort and safety.

26. Logrolling requires at least three caregivers to perform.
27. Limited range of motion can be the result of inflammation, such as arthritis, fluid in the joint, altered nerve supply, or contractures.
28. The patient who is able to assist in positioning can be instructed to bend the knees and lift the hips and/or push up with the hands and arms. A draw sheet may also be used to move the patient up in bed.
29. Half of all back pain is associated with manual lifting tasks.
30. Improper positioning of patients in bed can lead to pressure ulcers and contractures.
31. A patient who is overweight or has a respiratory condition would not be placed in a prone position.
32. A mechanical device for repetitive motion is a continuous passive motion (CPM) machine.

33. 3	38. 2	43. 2
34. 2	39. 4	44. 4
35. 4	40. 4	45. 4
36. 1	41. 2	46. 2
37. 1	42. 4	47. 4

CHAPTER 28

Case Studies

1. a. You should assess some of the following areas regarding home safety:
   - Location of the home in the community
   - Security measures within the home
   - Environmental conditions: lighting, temperature, sanitation, stairways, floors/carpeting
   - Fire and electrical safety measures/hazards
   - Exposure to pollutants/pathogens
   b. With a toddler and a preschool child in the home, safety measures are extremely important. Accidents are one of the major problems for children, including falls and poisoning. If there are stairs in the home, gates should be in use or doors to the outside should be locked. For upper-level apartments or rooms, child-safety devices should be in place on the windows. Any household chemicals or medications should be out of reach and/or in a locked compartment. There also may be locks on other kitchen cabinets, drawers, and the refrigerator to prevent access. Electrical outlets should have covers, and plugs should be out of sight of the children. The family should have a fire safety plan, fire extinguishers, and smoke/fire alarms. Items that may be swallowed or broken should be out of reach. Additional safety measures may be in place in the kitchen and bathroom, such as faucet covers.
2. a. For the patient in the home who has diabetes mellitus and requires insulin injections, the following precautions should be taken:
   - Perform hand hygiene and maintain sterile asepsis for the injections.
   - Store the insulin properly.

- Maintain an adequate supply of insulin and injection supplies.
- Dispose of used needles and syringes appropriately; do not reuse the injection supplies (unless an insulin pen is used).
- Have adequate light for preparation and administration of the injection.
- Wear eyeglasses, if needed.

3. a. Guidelines that should be used to establish a safe, restraint-free environment include the following:
   - Involving patients and families in planning care; explaining all procedures and treatments to them
   - Encouraging family and friends to stay or using sitters
   - Using calm, simple statements and physical cues as needed
   - Using a knee band such as the Ambularm or an alarming seat belt to alert caregivers
   - Eliminating full side rails; using low beds with a floor mat at bedside
   - Assigning confused or disoriented patients to rooms near the nurses' station; observing these patients frequently and instituting regular patient checks
   - Providing appropriate visual and auditory stimuli
   - Providing ongoing pain assessment and nonpharmacological interventions
   - Using diversional activities appropriate for the patient
   - Instituting exercise and ambulation schedules as the patient's condition allows
   - Providing scheduled toileting, especially during peak fall times
   - Consulting with physical and occupational therapists to enhance strength, mobility, and exercise
   - Using protective devices such as hip pads, helmet, skid-proof slippers, and nonskid strips near bed
   - Providing prompt treatment and ongoing evaluation of medical problems

Chapter Review

1. Basic human needs in a safe environment and examples of what may affect them are
   - Oxygen: carbon monoxide, improper ventilation, pollutants
   - Degree of humidity: excessive dryness
   - Nutrition: improper storage/refrigeration, inadequate cleaning of cooking surfaces
   - Optimal temperature: excessive heat or cold
2. Inadequate lighting, clutter, lack of security, fire/electrical hazards, and temperature extremes are examples of physical hazards in the home.
3. a. Diminished vision, hearing, mobility, reflexes, and circulation are some of the reasons that older adults are predisposed to accidents.
   b. (1) Driving safety:
      Advise older adults to drive only short distances and in the daylight; avoid driving in inclement weather; use side and rear view mirrors carefully; look behind them toward their blind spot before changing lanes; and keep a window rolled down to hear sirens and horns.

(2) Home environment safety:
- Because of visual impairments in older adults, teach patients to keep living areas well lighted and free of clutter and to keep eyeglasses in good condition.
- Older adults have musculoskeletal changes that make movement difficult and increase the risk for falling. Teach patients to keep assistive devices in proper working order (canes, hand rails in tub and bathroom, and elevated seats) and to use nonskid strips in bathtubs.
- Advise older adults to avoid smoking in bed, to lower thermostats on water heaters, to avoid overloading electrical outlets, and to install and maintain smoke and carbon monoxide detectors in the house.

4. The following are examples of how the nurse may prevent health care agency risks:
   a. Falls: Complete a risk assessment, provide supervision, place the patient close to the nurses' station, orient the patient to the surroundings, use physical restraints if absolutely necessary.
   b. Patient-inherent accidents: Institute seizure precautions, remove foreign substances or hazardous items (sharps), provide supervision of the patient's activities.
   c. Procedure-related risks: Follow policies and procedures carefully, use appropriate technique for performing procedures.
   d. Equipment-related risks: Learn how to operate the equipment, have it checked regularly for proper functioning.
5. The "never events" are a, c, e, and f.
6. Active immunity is obtained through the injection of weakened or dead organisms and modified toxins.
7. Potential hazards include
   a. Infant, toddler, preschool: injuries, accidents, poisoning
   b. School-age child: sports, after-school activities, bicycle accidents, school bus injuries
   c. Adolescent: smoking, substance abuse, motor vehicle accidents, stress, sexual activity
   d. Adult: alcohol/substance abuse, motor vehicle accidents, stress-related activities
   e. Older adult: falls, medication misuse
8. Patients experiencing impaired mobility, diminished sensation and/or cognition, and decreased safety awareness are a high risk for injury.
9. Potential agents that may be used are
   a. Biological: anthrax, smallpox, typhoid, plague, botulism
   b. Chemical: cyanide, mustard gas, chlorine, nerve agents
   c. Radiological: nuclear device, "dirty bomb"
10. True
11. Teaching areas for a school-age child include crossing the street, stranger safety, bicycle safety, sport/activity safety, and personal hygiene.
12. The primary goal of restraints (safety reminder devices) is to prevent falls.
13. The correct actions for using restraints are b, c, d, and e.
14. False
15. An older adult having difficulty with medication administration in the home may benefit from the use of a medication organizer device or system.

16. In a health care agency, medication safety is promoted by properly identifying the patient, administering medicine correctly, maintaining accurate labeling and storage, and documenting promptly.
17. Environmental adjustments include
    a. Tactile deficit: Check/adjust the water heater temperature, clearly label the settings on the stove/oven, obtain easy-open medication containers.
    b. Visual deficit: Maintain adequate lighting, use stair treads and handrails, decrease clutter, use distinct colors, have large print on labels.
18. The following alternative measures may be implemented:
    - Orienting patients/families to the surroundings
    - Explaining routines and procedures
    - Encouraging family and friends to stay with the patient
    - Providing adequate stimulation, diversional activity
    - Using relaxation techniques
    - Instituting exercise and activity plans
    - Eliminating bothersome therapies as soon as possible
    - Maintaining toileting routines
    - Evaluating the effect of medications
    - Performing regular assessments of the patient's status
    - Using electronic bed and chair alarm devices
    - Placing the patient in a room near the nurses' station
19. Possible nursing diagnoses include the following:
    - *Risk for Imbalanced Body Temperature*
    - *Impaired Home Maintenance*
    - *Risk for Injury*
    - *Deficient Knowledge*
    - *Risk for Poisoning*
    - *Risk for Suffocation*
    - *Risk for Trauma*
20. a. Signs and symptoms of low concentration carbon monoxide poisoning are nausea, dizziness, headache, and fatigue. Higher concentrations are often fatal.
    b. There must be carbon monoxide detectors in the home.
21. The "Speak Up" campaign is designed to encourage patients to take a role in preventing health care errors by becoming active, involved, and informed participants in their health care (TJC, 2013b). For example, patients are encouraged to ask health care workers if they have washed their hands before providing care.
22. Resources/agencies that are available for patient safety include The Joint Commission, QSEN, CMS, OSHA, the Institute for Healthcare Improvement, the Agency for Healthcare Research and Quality, and the U.S. Department of Veterans Affairs.
23. (a) Most falls occur within the home, specifically in the bedroom, bathroom, and kitchen. Environmental factors such as broken stairs, icy sidewalks, inadequate lighting, throw rugs, and exposed electrical cords cause many accidents. Older adults typically fall while transferring from beds, chairs, and toilets; getting into or out of bathtubs; tripping over carpet edges or doorway thresholds; and slipping on wet surfaces or descending stairs.
    (b) Falls in the health care agency are usually the result of multiple factors:
    - *Intrinsic factors* are patient related and include physiological conditions such as vision disturbances,

urinary/stool frequency or incontinence, mental impairment, gait and balance disorders, polypharmacy, and older age.

  - *Extrinsic factors* are environmentally related and include room clutter, loose electrical cords, and spills.

24. Information about chemical substances in the workplace can be found on *Material Safety Data Sheets* (MSDS).

25. Signs, symptoms, and behaviors that are indicative of substance abuse are the presence of drug-oriented magazines, beer and liquor bottles, drug paraphernalia, blood spots on clothing, and the continual wearing of long-sleeved shirts in hot weather and dark glasses indoors. Psychosocial clues include failing grades, change in dress, increased absenteeism from school, isolation, increased aggressiveness, and changes in interpersonal relationships.

26. Hospitals are required to have an emergency management plan that addresses identifying possible emergency situations and their probable impact, maintaining an adequate amount of supplies, and having a formal response plan.

27. True

28. R – Rescue and remove all patients in immediate danger
A – Activate the alarm. Always do this before trying to extinguish even a minor fire.
C – Confine a fire by closing doors and windows and turning off oxygen and electrical equipment.
E – Extinguish a fire using an appropriate extinguisher.
Pull the pin. Hold the extinguisher with the nozzle pointing away from you, and release the locking mechanism.
Aim low. Point the extinguisher at the base of the fire.
Squeeze the lever slowly and evenly.
Sweep the nozzle from side to side.

29. a. Type B
    b. Type C
    c. Type A

30. The nurse should report any equipment that does not appear to be working properly to the agency's maintenance, safety, or facilities department.

31. a. Hospitals
    - Identify patients correctly
    - Improve staff communication
    - Use medicines safely
    - Use alarms safely
    - Prevent infection
    - Identify patient safety risks (e.g., suicide)
    - Prevent mistakes in surgery
    b. Home care
    - Identifies patients correctly
    - Uses medicines safely
    - Prevents infection
    - Prevents patients from falling
    - Identifies patient safety risks (e.g., patients on oxygen, risk of fire)

32. The correct order for the steps of the Timed Get Up and Go Test is e, a, c, g, f, d, and b.
An abnormal result is when a person takes more than 20 seconds to complete the test.

33. a. Use of home oxygen
    - Post "No Smoking" and "Oxygen in Use" signs.
    - Do not use oxygen around electrical equipment or flammable products.
    - Store oxygen tanks upright in carts or stands to prevent tipping or falling over.
    - Make sure that there is a sufficient supply on hand of oxygen and spare tubing.
    b. Food preparation
    - Proper refrigeration, storage, and preparation of food decrease risk of foodborne illnesses. Store perishable foods in refrigerators to maintain freshness.
    - Refrigerate foods at 40° F within 2 hours of cooking.
    - Thaw frozen foods in the refrigerator.
    - Wash hands for at least 15 seconds before preparing food.
    - Rinse fruits and vegetables thoroughly.
    - Avoid cross-contamination of one food with another during preparation, especially with poultry.
    - Use a separate cutting board for vegetables, meat, and poultry.
    - Cook foods adequately to kill any residual organisms.
    - Refrigerate leftovers promptly and label the date when leftovers are saved.

34. Based on the scenario, the following bold assessment findings require follow-up to prevent patient injuries:
Upon entering the patient's home, the visiting nurse observed that the patient was wearing **slippers with no back**. The patient stated that she seemed to **always leave her glasses somewhere**. There were **piles of newspapers and other items cluttering the floor around the living room chairs**. The **lighting in the stairway was less than 60 watts** and there were **throw rugs on the wood floors** in the halls. When looking through the medicine cabinet with the patient, the nurse noted that some **medications were expired**. The patient **admitted to falling** once **when getting up during the night to go to the bathroom.**
The patient should be wearing slippers that fit well and will not slide off and cause the patient to trip. The patient's glasses should be kept close by in a case or on a necklace, so that there is better vision. Clutter around chairs, poor lighting, and throw rugs can cause the patient to fall. Expired medications can be ineffective and dangerous to keep around. Nocturia is a concern, as is the admission of a prior fall.

35. 1	39. 3	43. 4
36. 3	40. 2	44. 3
37. 2	41. 3	
38. 1	42. 3	

CHAPTER 29

Case Studies

1. a. For the patient with diabetes mellitus, you should include the following instructions:
    - Carefully inspect the skin surfaces, particularly the extremities.
    - Perform daily foot care using lukewarm water, with no soaking; dry the feet well, especially between the toes.
    - Do not cut corns or calluses.
    - Apply bland powder if the feet perspire.
    - File the toenails straight across; no cutting.
    - Wear clean, dry socks daily.
    - Do not walk barefoot.

192

- Wear properly fitting, flexible shoes.
- Exercise regularly.
- Avoid application of hot water bottles or heating pads to the extremities.
- Clean minor cuts immediately and apply only mild antiseptics, if necessary.
- Avoid wearing elastic stockings, tight hose, or noncotton socks.
- Avoid crossing the legs.
- Avoid the use of commercial preparations for corn/callus removal, athlete's foot, or ingrown toenails.
- Consult a podiatrist as needed for foot problems.

2. a. The older adult patient may be experiencing changes in skin integrity. The skin is more fragile, so hot water and strong cleansing agents should be avoided. Older adults usually perspire less, so bathing need not be as frequent (unless personally desired). There may be an increased sensitivity or itching that may be relieved with the use of hydrocortisone cream, moisturizing soaps, lotions, or petrolatum. Humidity should be higher in the environment to alleviate skin dryness. The room temperature may have to be warmer. Care should be taken to avoid injury to the skin as wound healing is slower in this population. Range of motion should be assessed while assisting the patient. A shower or bath chair may be needed for the patient with reduced mobility.

Chapter Review

1. e	5. f	9. g
2. i	6. c	10. d
3. h	7. j	
4. a	8. b	

11. Factors that contribute to a hygiene self-care deficit are diminished mobility, chronic illness, pain, cognitive impairment, mental illness, and socioeconomic status.

12. For a patient with dementia, the nurse should use the towel bath technique. This is a person-centered in-bed approach in which a nurse uses a large towel, one or two regular-size towels, washcloths, a bath blanket, and no-rinse soap and water. This technique has been shown to produce a marked reduction in behavioral symptoms when comparing the in-bed approach to showering (Rader, 2006).

13. Appropriate techniques are answers d, e, g, and h.

14. A nurse-initiated treatment for a rash is a warm soak.

15. Plain water is used on the patient's eyes.

16. The accurate statements about the skin are a, c, d, and f.

17. The nurse should have the patient do as much of the hygienic care as possible, as well as participate in the decision making regarding his/her care.

18. A standing shower is contraindicated for a patient who is unable to safely stand, has a history of falls, and demonstrates fatigue, weakness, or unsteadiness.

19. A patient with the nursing diagnosis of *Activity Intolerance* would become easily fatigued and require rest periods and/or repositioning during the care.

20. Healthy skin can be promoted by inspecting the skin for changes in color or texture and reporting changes or abnormalities to the health care provider. Instruct patients to handle the skin gently, avoiding excessive or rough rubbing. Advise against use of hot water for bathing as well as too lengthy bathing sessions to prevent loss of oils and excessive drying of skin. Also encourage patients to consume a balanced diet including foods rich in antioxidants, vitamins, and minerals, and to consume adequate fluids. Stress safety concerns in the home such as failure to adjust the water temperature when bathing or showering or slipping on wet surfaces in the bathroom.

21. a. False
    b. True

22. The recommendations to make are b and c.

23. Chlorhexidene gluconate 4% is most useful.

24. Eyeglasses should be kept in a case on top of the bedside table or in a drawer of the bedside table when not in use.

25. Ear irrigation is contraindicated in the presence of a perforated tympanic membrane (eardrum).

26. Asepsis is maintained during linen changes by
- Keeping soiled linen away from the uniform and off the floor
- Placing soiled linen in the proper container
- Avoiding fanning or shaking of linens
- Discarding clean items that fall on the floor

27. The nurse prepares a comfortable environment for the patient by controlling the room temperature, providing for adequate ventilation and lighting, limiting noise, reducing odors, and keeping the room neat.

28. Conditions that may place the patient at risk include those that are associated with reduced sensation, vascular insufficiency, impaired cognition, incontinence, and/or decreased mobility (e.g., diabetes mellitus, cerebrovascular accident (CVA/stroke), spinal cord injury, and arterial insufficiency).

29. A commercial "bag bath" usually contains 8 to 10 premoistened towels. A single towel is used for each general body part cleansed. The towels may be microwaved for warmth.

30. When providing a tub bath for a patient, safety measures include
- Assessing the patient's mobility
- Placing rubber mat on tub or shower bottom and a disposable bath mat or towel on floor in front of tub or shower
- Helping the patient to bathroom if necessary
- Having the patient wear slippers to bathroom
- Demonstrating how to use the call signal for assistance
- Checking the temperature of the bathwater
- Instructing the patient to use safety bars when getting in and out of tub or shower
- Cautioning the patient against the use of bath oil in tub water
- Instructing the patient not to remain in the tub longer than 10 to 15 minutes
- Staying with the patient or checking on the patient every 5 minutes
- Draining the tub of water before the patient attempts to get out of it

31. The patient's cultural background may influence hygienic care as follows:
- Privacy may be a large concern, especially for women from cultures that value female modesty.
- Exposure of the lower torso and the arms of Middle Eastern and East Asian women is not appropriate.

- Family members may want to participate in the care.
- Gender-congruent care may be needed or requested.
- In some cultures (e.g., Hindu, Orthodox Jewish, Muslim, Amish), touching between unrelated males and females is forbidden.
- The frequency of bathing may differ, as well as the products that are used.
- Many Asians (Chinese, Japanese, Koreans, and Hindus) consider the top parts of the body cleaner than the lower parts.
- Hindus and Muslims often use the left hand for cleaning, whereas the right hand is reserved for eating and praying.

32. Care for the patient's acne: Wash hair and skin each day with soap and warm water to remove oil. Use oil-free cosmetics because oily cosmetics or creams accumulate in pores and make acne worse. Eliminate foods from diet that aggravate condition. Use prescribed topical antibiotics for severe acne.

33. Guidelines for patient bathing and skin care include
- Clean the skin at the time of soiling and at routine intervals. Individualize frequency of cleansing according to patient need and preference.
- Avoid hot water and use a mild cleansing agent to minimize irritation.
- Avoid the use of force and friction.
- Minimize environmental factors that lead to skin drying.
- Protect patients from injury by assessing and controlling the bathwater temperature.
- Use assistive devices when indicated.
- Use bathing as a time to interact with and assess a patient.
- Assist patients through joint range-of-motion exercises to promote circulation and joint integrity.
- For patients who fatigue easily, consider administering a partial instead of a complete bed bath.

34. Special oral hygiene will usually be required by patients who are unconscious or have artificial airways.

35. The correct order for the bath is c, b, g, d, e, f, a.

36. Safety measures for oral care of the unconscious patient include checking for the gag reflex, positioning and suctioning to prevent aspiration, checking for bleeding/anticoagulant therapy, and avoiding dislodging an E/T tube.

37. To irrigate the ear, have a patient sit or lie on the side with the affected ear up. Place a curved emesis basin under the affected ear. For adults and children over 3 years of age, gently pull the pinna up and back. In children 3 years of age or younger, the pinna should be pulled down and back. Using a bulb irrigating syringe, gently wash the ear canal with warm solution (37° C or 98.6° F), being careful to not occlude the canal, which results in pressure on the tympanic membrane. Direct the fluid slowly and gently toward the superior aspect of the ear canal, maintaining the flow in a steady stream. Periodically during the irrigation ask if the patient is experiencing pain, nausea, or vertigo. These symptoms indicate the solution is too hot or too cold or is being instilled with too much pressure. After the canal is clear, wipe off any moisture from the ear with cotton balls and inspect the canal for remaining earwax.

38. The hands and feet should be soaked for 10 minutes before nail care, unless the patient is diabetic.

39. Vascular insufficiency is indicated in the presence of decreased hair growth, absent or diminished pulses, foot infection, poor wound healing, thickened nails, shiny appearance of the skin, and blanching of the skin upon elevation.

40. For the older adult: The skin is more fragile, so hot water and strong cleansing agents should be avoided. Older adults usually perspire less, so bathing need not be as frequent (unless personally desired). There may be an increased sensitivity or itching that may be relieved with the use of hydrocortisone cream, moisturizing soaps, lotions, or petrolatum. Humidity should be higher in the environment to alleviate skin dryness. The room temperature may have to be warmer. Care should be taken to avoid injury to the skin because wound healing is slower in this population. Range of motion should be assessed while assisting the patient. A shower or bath chair may be needed for the patient with reduced mobility.

41. For the patient with a hearing aid, the correct instructions include a and f.

42. 3	46. 3	50. 3
43. 1	47. 2	51. 1
44. 4	48. 1	52. 4
45. 4	49. 3	

CHAPTER 30

Case Study

1. a. To gather further information from the patient about her current respiratory status, the nurse should ask the following questions:
- "When do you experience shortness of breath/difficulty breathing?"
- "What activities bring on the shortness of breath?"
- "Does the shortness of breath interfere with your activities of daily living?"
- "Do you find that it is hard to inhale or exhale?"
- "Do you sleep with extra pillows at night?"
- "Are you more tired than usual?"
- "Do you smoke?"
- "Are you exposed to smokers or other environmental hazards at home or at work?"
- "When does the cough start?"
- "Are there times when your breathing/coughing is better or worse?"
- "What are you bringing up when you cough?"
- "Have you been exposed to anyone with a respiratory infection?"
- "Have you recently had an upper respiratory infection?"
- "Have you had pain in your chest when you breathe?"
- "Are you currently taking any medications?"
   b. Based on additional information from the patient, possible nursing diagnoses for this patient may be
- *Activity Intolerance*
- *Ineffective Airway Clearance*
- *Impaired Gas Exchange*
- *Risk for Infection*
   c. Nurse-initiated actions may include measurement of vital signs, auscultation of lung sounds, inspection of sputum, positioning for optimum respiratory function and comfort, and preparation of oxygen and suctioning equipment in case severe respiratory distress develops.

194

Answer Key

d. General teaching for health promotion should include the importance of
- Receiving the pneumococcal and influenza vaccines (if she has not had them)
- Limiting exposure to crowds and environmental pollutants
- Avoiding smoking or secondhand smoke
- Covering the mouth and nose if exposed to cold air
- Determining and improving activity and exercise tolerance
- Taking medications regularly
- Performing breathing/coughing exercises

Chapter Review

1. c	5. i	9. h
2. d	6. a	10. j
3. e	7. g	
4. b	8. f	

11. The average resting heart rate for an adult is 60 to 80 beats per minute.
12. Conditions that may affect chest wall movement include pregnancy, obesity, musculoskeletal abnormalities, abnormal structural configuration, trauma, muscle diseases, and nervous system diseases.
13. a. Right ventricular heart failure
    b. Right ventricular heart failure
    c. Left ventricular heart failure
    d. Left ventricular heart failure
14. Hyperventilation may be caused by answers a, b, and d.
15. a. Decreased oxygen-carrying capacity: anemia, inhalation of toxic substances (carbon monoxide)
    b. Decreased inspired oxygen concentration: airway obstruction, higher altitudes
    c. Hypovolemia: fluid loss, dehydration, shock
    d. Increased metabolic rate: fever, pregnancy, hyperthyroidism
16. A premature infant may have a deficiency of surfactant.
17. Controllable risk factors include smoking, substance abuse, poor nutrition, lack of exercise, and stress.
18. Changes that occur in the cardiopulmonary system as a result of aging include answers b, e, and g.
19. This condition is noted by the nurse as paroxysmal nocturnal dyspnea (PND).
20. Wheezing is a high-pitched, musical lung sound that is heard on inspiration and/or expiration.
21. a. Ventricular fibrillation
    b. Ventricular tachycardia
22. a. Retraction is the visible sinking in of the soft tissues of the chest between and around firmer tissue and ribs, often seen in the intercostal spaces.
    b. Paradoxical breathing is asymmetrical or asynchronous breathing in which the chest contracts during inspiration and expands during expiration.
23. Surgical asepsis or sterile technique is used to suction the trachea.
24. Continuous bubbling in the chest tube water-seal chamber indicates an air leak.
25. Nursing interventions to achieve the following include
    a. Dyspnea management: administration of medications (e.g., bronchodilators), supervision of oxygen therapy, and instruction in breathing and coughing techniques and relaxation measures
    b. Patent airway: instruction in coughing techniques, suctioning, and airway placement
    c. Lung expansion: positioning, administering chest physiotherapy, instruction in the use of incentive spirometry, and management of chest tubes
    d. Mobilization of secretions: hydration of the patient, humidification/nebulization of oxygen therapy, and administration of chest physiotherapy
26. a. Simple face mask: 40% to 60% (5 to 8 L/min)
    b. Venturi mask: 24% to 60% (4 to 12 L/min)
27. For tuberculin (Mantoux) testing:
    a. Forearm
    b. 48 to 72 hours
    c. Negative reaction
    d. Positive
28. For chest percussion, vibration, and postural drainage:
    a. Bleeding disorders, osteoporosis, fractured ribs
    b. Exhalation
    c. Positioned on the nurse's/parent's lap
29. For CPAP:
    a. Sleep apnea, and improvement of ventilation for heart, neuromuscular, and pulmonary diseases
    b. 5 to 20 cm H_2O
    c. Hypercapnea, gastric distention, discomfort, risk for skin irritation, noise
    d. BiPAP (Bilevel positive airway pressure) works by providing assistance during inspiration and preventing airway closure during expiration. It provides two levels of pressure: inspiratory positive airway pressure (IPAP) and a lower expiratory positive airway pressure.
30. a. An indication for home oxygen therapy is an SaO_2 of 88% or less.
    b. Safety measures for home oxygen use include
    - Place "No smoking" signs on the patient's room door and over the bed. Inform the patient, visitors, roommates, and all personnel that smoking is not permitted in areas where oxygen is in use.
    - Determine that all electrical equipment in the room is functioning correctly and is properly grounded.
    - Know the fire procedures and the location of the closest fire extinguisher.
    - Check the oxygen level of portable tanks before transporting to ensure there is enough oxygen in the tank.
    - Have an alternative source of oxygen in case of a power failure.
31. The steps of CPR:
    C: Circulation
    A: Airway
    B: Breathing
32. Defibrillation is recommended within 5 minutes outside of a hospital/medical center and 3 minutes for an in-hospital victim.
33. a. True
    b. False
34. For the patient with a nasal cannula:
    - Verify setting on flowmeter and oxygen source for proper setup and prescribed flow rate.

- Monitor patient's response to changes in oxygen flow rate with pulse oximetry.
- Observe patient's external ears, bridge of nose, nares, and nasal mucous membranes for evidence of skin breakdown.
- Check cannula/mask every 8 hours.
- Keep humidification container filled at all times.

35. For the nursing diagnosis *Ineffective Airway Clearance related to the presence of tracheobronchial secretions*, possible patient outcomes and nursing interventions are the following:
Patient outcomes:
- Sputum clear within 24 to 36 hours
- No adventitious lung sounds auscultated
- Respiratory rate of 16 to 24 breaths per minute
- Coughing and clearing airway within 24 hours
Nursing interventions:
- Instruct patient on coughing and deep breathing
- Assist with position changes and ambulation
- Provide 2000 to 2500 mL of fluid, if not contraindicated
- Monitor vital signs
- Suction prn
- Provide chest physiotherapy, if indicated

36. The appropriate interventions for suctioning are b and e.

37. Cardiac output is the result of stroke volume × heart rate.

38. a. Signs and symptoms of hypoxia include tachycardia, peripheral vasoconstriction, dizziness, and mental confusion.
b. Treatment may include cardiac and respiratory stimulant drugs, oxygen therapy, mechanical ventilation, and frequent analysis of blood gases.

39. Possible nursing diagnoses for a patient with anemia include *Activity Intolerance* and *Fatigue.*

40. Cardiopulmonary status may be influenced by the intake of a diet high in fat, cholesterol, salt, and calories, and low in iron and essential nutrients.

41. The most effective positioning for a patient is 45-degree semi-Fowler's.

42. An incentive spirometer will encourage the postoperative patient to breathe deeply.

43. Hazards include
Environmental: air pollution, smog, and allergens (e.g., pollen)
Occupational: exposure to asbestos, talcum powder, dust, and airborne fibers

44. Cardiac dysrhythmias may be caused by ischemia, valvular abnormality, anxiety, drug toxicity, caffeine, alcohol, or tobacco use, cardiothoracic surgery, or a complication of acid-base or electrolyte imbalance.

45. Atrial fibrillation is treated with synchronized cardioversion, rate control medication therapy, such as diltiazem or beta-blockers, interventions based on the underlying cause, and blood thinners such as warfarin (Coumadin).

46. To prevent the incidence of VAP, the nurse should
- Monitor cuff pressure frequently to ensure there is an adequate seal to prevent aspiration of secretions.
- Provide daily oral care with chlorhexidine.
- Always drain ventilator circuit condensation away from the patient and into the appropriate receptacle. Drain the tubing hourly to prevent accumulation.
- Keep the head of the patient's bed raised between 30 and 45 degrees unless other medical conditions do not allow this to occur.

47. Treatment for hyperventilation involves treating the underlying cause, improving tissue oxygenation, restoring ventilation, reducing respiratory rate, and achieving acid-base balance.

48. The sequence for in-line suctioning is c, f, b, d, a, e.

49. The areas on the chest tube drainage system are

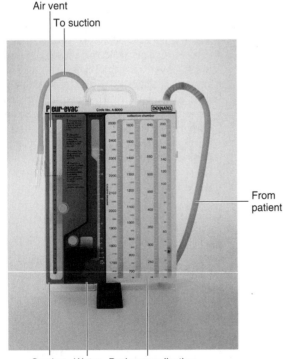

Suction control   Water seal   Drainage collection chamber

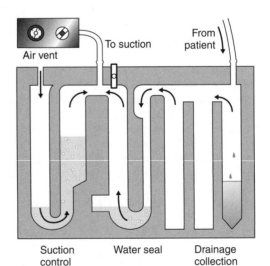

Suction control   Water seal   Drainage collection

50. The correct responses for chest tube care are b, d, and e. Appropriate care for the patient with a chest tube includes
    • Assessment of respiratory status and system integrity:
      • Observation for air leaks, kinked tubes
    • Proper positioning of the patient with chest tubes to facilitate chest tube drainage and optimal functioning of the system
    • Careful ambulation and transfers
    • Identifying and reporting any changes in vital signs, level of comfort, SpO$_2$, or excessive bubbling in water-seal chamber
    • Immediately managing/reporting if there is a disconnection of the system, change in type and amount of drainage, bleeding, or sudden cessation of bubbling
    • Determining if milking/stripping is agency policy
51. Examples of pathologies that can reduce chest wall expansion are
    • Musculoskeletal abnormalities, such as pectus excavatum and kyphosis
    • Muscle diseases, such as muscular dystrophy
    • Nervous system diseases, such as myasthenia gravis, Guillain-Barré syndrome, and poliomyelitis
    • Disease or trauma involving the medulla oblongata and spinal cord
    • Trauma to the chest wall: multiple rib fractures, chest wall or upper abdominal incisions
52. The following signs and symptoms are indicative of cardiac pain in women: epigastric pain, complaints of indigestion, nausea or vomiting, or a choking feeling and dyspnea.
53. Factors contributing to respiratory problems in infants and children are prematurity (surfactant deficiency, respiratory syncytial virus [RSV] infection), frequent exposure to other children, exposure to secondhand smoke, nasal congestion from teething, and airway obstruction from foreign objects.
54. The lifestyle factors that contribute to poor cardiopulmonary outcomes are a, c, d, and e.
55. Fatigue is an early sign.
56. The nurse should complete the assessment in short sections to allow the patient to rest and recover. If the patient is breathless or fatigued, ask closed-ended questions, with yes or no answers. Focus the initial assessment on the patient's immediate problems.
57. Nebulization is used for the administration of bronchodilators and mucolytic agents.
58. A Yankauer suction catheter is used for oropharyngeal suctioning.
59. The patient should be positioned with the right side up, so he/she would be laying on the left side.
60. Bronchodilators and other ephedrine-containing products are contraindicated for patients with asthma.
61. Caution is used when administering oxygen to a patient with chronic lung disease because patients with COPD and hypercapnia (high carbon dioxide levels) have adapted to the higher carbon dioxide level. The carbon dioxide–sensitive chemoreceptors are no longer sensitive to increased carbon dioxide as a stimulus to breathe. Their stimulus to breathe is a decreased PaO$_2$.

When you administer excessive oxygen to patients with COPD, this satisfies the body's oxygen requirement and negates the stimulus to breathe.

62. The patients who should receive the flu vaccination are d and e.

63. 3	69. 2	75. 3
64. 3	70. 3	76. 1
65. 4	71. 3	77. 3
66. 1	72. 4	78. 2
67. 2	73. 1	79. 2
68. 4	74. 1	

CHAPTER 31

Case Studies

1. a. A possible nursing diagnosis for this patient is *Disturbed Sleep Pattern related to current life situation: stress at home and work*. Goal includes
    • Patient will achieve an adequate amount of nightly sleep within 1 month.
    Outcomes include
    • Patient will identify and verbalize about current life stressors.
    • Patient will practice stress reduction/relaxation techniques as needed.
  b. The nurse may implement the following:
    • Sit with the patient and offer an opportunity for her to vent about her feelings and concerns.
    • Instruct the patient on stress reduction/relaxation techniques.
    • Advise about the value of exercise and activity before sleep.
    • Discuss manipulation of the environment to provide maximum comfort and minimum distraction.
    • Instruct the patient on the avoidance of heavy meals before bedtime and excessive caffeine or alcohol intake.
    • Have the patient maintain a log of sleep/rest patterns.
2. a. To assist the nurse to obtain sufficient sleep while adapting to the change in his work schedule, you should
    • complete an assessment of the nurse's sleep patterns and general health.
    • have the nurse complete a sleep diary to determine routines and previous success in getting to sleep.
    • suggest methods to promote a restful environment: reduce noise and light, adjust the temperature, have a comfortable bed/mattress and covering, turn off phones and other devices.
    • suggest methods to promote sleep: take a warm bath or shower, eat a nutritious snack, perform relaxation exercises, read for a little while.
    • for chronic insomnia, the nurse may need to be evaluated at a sleep center or request a change in schedule.

Chapter Review

1. f	4. a	7. d
2. b	5. g	8. i
3. h	6. c	9. e

10. Sleep may be affected by physical illness, medications/substances, lifestyle changes, sleep pattern alterations, emotional stress, environmental variations, exercise, fatigue, and food and caloric intake.
11. The correct responses are c, f, and h.
12. The nurse may promote a restful environment by checking that the:
    - patient's bed is clean and dry.
    - lights are lowered and not directed at patient's eyes.
    - temperature and ventilation in the room are at comfortable levels.
    - amount of noise is decreased.
    - number of distractions is decreased.
13. True
14. False
15. Sleep cycles usually last 90 to 110 minutes, followed by REM sleep.
16. a. Comfort measures for the patient:
    - Having loose-fitting nightwear
    - Having the patient void before bedtime
    - Giving a relaxing back rub
    - Removing minor irritants, such as changing wet dressings or diapers
    - Providing an extra blanket to prevent chilling
    - Applying dry or moist heat
    - Providing proper positioning
    - Administering pain medications 30 to 60 minutes before the patient goes to bed
    b. Safety measures for the patient:
    - Setting beds lower to the floor
    - Removing clutter and moving equipment from the path a patient uses
    - Assisting the patient to ambulate, if necessary
    - Making sure the call light is within the patient's reach
    - Positioning patients so that they will not fall out of the chair when sleeping; elevating the feet on an ottoman or small bench
17. A sleep diary usually includes information on waking and sleeping activities, such as exercise, work, mealtimes, alcohol and caffeine intake, the time and length of naps, evening and bedtime routines, the time the patient tries to fall asleep, time and number of awakenings, and the time of morning awakening.
18. The best type of bedtime snack is one containing protein and carbohydrates, such as cereal and milk or cheese and crackers, which contain L-tryptophan and help promote sleep.
19. Infants should be placed on their backs or sides for sleep.
20. Examples of possible outcomes:
    - Patient will fall asleep within ½ hour of planned time.
    - Patient will have less than two awakenings during the night.
    - Patient will identify factors that interrupt sleep patterns.
21. a. Physical and behavioral problems include fatigue, irritability, mood changes, blurred vision, decreased reflexes, slow response time, confusion, and alterations in motor performance, memory, and equilibrium. Sleep deprivation affects immune functioning, metabolism, nitrogen balance, protein catabolism, and quality of life. A loss of REM sleep often leads to confusion and suspicion.

b. Safety considerations include instruction about the need for caution during activities, because attention is diminished and accidents are more prevalent.
22. True
23. REM sleep appears to be important for early brain development, cognition, and memory (Hobson, 2009). Researchers associate REM sleep with changes in cerebral blood flow, increased cortical activity, increased oxygen consumption, and epinephrine release. This association assists with memory storage and learning.
24. Central sleep apnea is associated with stroke, degeneration of the cervical spine, obesity, and encephalitis, and frequently is seen in patients with congestive heart failure.
25. Examples of questions to ask about sleep habits include
    - Tell me what you do just before going to bed.
    - Have you recently had any changes at work, school, or home?
    - How long does it take you to fall asleep?
    - How often during the week do you have trouble falling asleep or staying asleep?
26. For a patient with chronic insomnia, the nurse should refer the patient for medical follow-up and treatment and/or a sleep center for evaluation.
27. Recommendations for health promotion are a and e.

28. 3	35. 2	42. 1
29. 4	36. 3	43. 4
30. 1	37. 1	44. 1
31. 2	38. 4	45. 3
32. 2	39. 1	46. 3
33. 3	40. 1	47. 4
34. 2	41. 4	

CHAPTER 32

Case Studies

1. a. To successfully use a PCA pump, the patient must understand the purpose and use of the medication and pump, as well as be able to locate and push the button on the pump that controls the administration of the medication. The nurse should assess the IV site to ensure it is patent and without complications. The baseline blood pressure and respiratory rates should be recorded before the infusion begins. After the infusion starts, the vital signs are monitored as often as every 15 to 30 minutes for the first few hours until the patient gains relief at a constant dosage. If the patient's blood pressure or respirations decrease, the infusion rate is reduced according to the physician's or health care provider's order or agency policy. For severe respiratory depression, small doses of the opioid antagonist naloxone (Narcan) IV are administered, according to policy, to increase respiratory rate and depth.
   b. Usual medications for the PCA pump include opioids, such as morphine, hydromorphone, and fentanyl.
   c. Teaching for this patient should include
   - Use of the equipment
   - Purpose of PCA, action(s) of the medication, expected pain relief, precautions, and potential side effects of the medication (CNS depression)

- General precautions for an IV infusion
- Caution against family members/visitors operating the device for the patient

2. a. The patient may have an expectation that this labor and delivery experience will also be "horrible," which could predetermine her responses. She could be very fearful of repeating the severe pain and not getting any relief.

   b. Patient-centered care should include assessing the patient carefully, and providing the patient with explanations about her status and the procedures that are implemented. Demonstrating support and concern for her comfort is critical, so that she knows you will be her advocate and respond to her pain. Encouraging the presence of a family member or significant other can also assist in creating a supportive environment.

Chapter Review

1. h
2. a
3. d
4. g
5. e
6. c
7. b
8. f

9. The four physiological processes of pain are transduction, transmission, perception, and modulation.
   Transduction: Transduction converts energy produced by these stimuli into electrical energy. The process begins in the periphery when a pain-producing stimulus sends an impulse across a sensory peripheral pain nerve fiber (nociceptor) initiating an action potential.
   Transmission: Pain-sensitizing substances surround the pain fibers in the extracellular fluid, spreading the pain message and causing an inflammatory response. Nerve impulses travel along afferent peripheral nerve fibers. Two types of peripheral nerve fibers conduct painful stimuli: the fast, myelinated A-delta fibers and the small, slow unmyelinated C fibers. The A fibers send sharp, localized, and distinct sensations that specify the source of the pain and detect its intensity. The small C fibers relay slower impulses that are poorly localized, visceral, and persistent.
   Perception: The pain impulse ascends to the brain and the central nervous system extracts information, such as location, duration, and quality of the pain impulse.
   Modulation: The brain releases inhibitory neurotransmitters such as endogenous opioids, serotonin, norepinephrine, and gamma aminobutyric acid (GABA). The neurotransmitters hinder the transmission of pain to help produce an analgesic effect.

10. The gate control theory suggests that heat, cold, transcutaneous electrical nerve stimulation (TENS), and pharmacological interventions will reduce pain.

11. The physiological responses to pain as a result of sympathetic stimulation include b, d, and e.

12. a. Associated symptoms of chronic pain include fatigue, insomnia, anorexia, weight loss, apathy, hopelessness, and anger.

   b. The influence of chronic pain on an individual's lifestyle can include the following: change of sleep patterns, inability to perform hygienic care, sexual dysfunction, alteration in home or work management, and interruption of social activities.

13. An infant may respond to pain by crying and by exhibiting changes in vital signs, facial expressions, or extremity movement. A child may respond to pain with crying, irritability, loss of appetite, quietness or restlessness, disturbed sleep patterns, or rigid body posture.

14. The single most reliable indicator of pain is the patient's self-report.

15. For the PQRSTU assessment:
   a. Quality: Suggest a change in medications if the quality of pain changes.
   b. Region: Position the patient so that body weight is shifted away from area of pain; apply heat/cold directly to the site.
   c. Timing: Administer medication so that the peak effect occurs when pain is most acute.

16. a. Toddler: Use of words that the child can understand ("boo-boo"), pictures ("Oucher" scale), and dolls to act out with, and pointing to areas of discomfort
   b. Person who speaks English as second language: Use of an interpreter, pictures (pain scale), and gestures, and pointing to areas of discomfort
   c. For the person with dementia, note their vocal response, facial movements, body movements, and inactivity.

17. a. In determining the location of the pain, the nurse should ask the patient to point to the area, or draw or trace the extent of the pain.
   b. Sample documentation: *Stating that pain is located on the R lower abdominal quadrant. Reports that the pain radiates upward slightly, with an intensity of 4 on a scale of 1-10.*

18. A pain rating of 7 or higher on a scale of 0 to 10 is an emergency.

19. The nurse should administer the pain medication about 30 minutes before painful activities.

20. Individualizing a patient's pain management may include
   - Using different types of pain relief measures
   - Providing pain relief measures before the pain becomes severe
   - Using measures that the patient believes are effective
   - Using the patient's ideas for pain relief and scheduling
   - Suggesting measures that are within the patient's capability
   - Choosing pain relief measures on the basis of the patient's responses
   - Encouraging the patient to try measures more than once to see if they may work
   - Keeping an open mind about nontraditional measures
   - Protecting the patient from more pain
   - Educating the patient about the pain

21. The correct statements regarding TENS are b, c, and e.

22. Medications used for mild to moderate pain include a and e.

23. Nonpharmacological interventions for pain relief include reduction/removal of painful stimuli, cutaneous stimulation, distraction, relaxation, guided imagery, anticipatory guidance, biofeedback, and hypnosis.

24. Adjuvant medications that may be used in conjunction with analgesics to manage pain are sedatives, anticonvulsants, steroids, antidepressants, antianxiety agents, and muscle relaxants.

25. The usual dosage of on-demand morphine for PCA is 1 mg every 10 minutes.
26. a. Priority nursing interventions for the patient with an epidural infusion include assessment of the site and patency of the tube along with maintenance of aseptic technique in site care.
    b. Priority assessment before and during administration of all analgesics is the patient's response to the medication, including respiratory status and degree of pain relief.
27. The nurse may adapt/alter the patient's environment to increase comfort by
    • Straightening wrinkled bed linen
    • Repositioning the patient
    • Loosening tight clothing or bandages (unless contraindicated)
    • Changing wet dressings or bed linens
    • Checking the temperature of hot/cold applications and bathwater
    • Lifting the patient up in bed, not pulling
    • Positioning the patient correctly on the bedpan
    • Avoiding exposure of the skin or mucous membranes to irritants (e.g., urine)
    • Preventing urinary retention by keeping the catheter patent
    • Preventing constipation by use of fluids, diet, and exercise
    • Reducing lighting that glares/shines directly on the patient
    • Checking the temperature of the room and the sensation of the patient
    • Reducing the level of noise and traffic
28. Phantom pain is seen in patients who have lost limbs or had strokes with paralysis.
29. Patient-controlled oral analgesia is Medication on Demand or MOD.
30. The best way to evaluate the effectiveness of pain management is to ask patients about their level of pain and/or observe their behavior.
31. The ABCDE approach is
    A: *Ask* about pain regularly. *Assess* pain systematically.
    B: *Believe* the patient and family in their report of pain and what relieves it.
    C: *Choose* pain control options appropriate for the patient, family, and setting.
    D: *Deliver* interventions in a timely, logical, and coordinated fashion.
    E: *Empower* patients and their families. *Enable* them to control their course to the greatest extent possible.
32. Concomitant symptoms associated with pain are nausea, headache, dizziness, urinary frequency, constipation, depression, restlessness, and anxiety.
33. a. True
    b. True
    c. False
    d. False
    e. True
    f. False
    g. False
    h. True
    i. True
    j. False
    k. True
    l. True

34. 3	39. 4	44. 4
35. 3	40. 3	45. 4
36. 4	41. 1	46. 2
37. 3	42. 1	47. 3
38. 2	43. 3	48. 4

CHAPTER 33

Case Studies

1. a. To assist this patient and the family with dietary planning, it is important to find out the following information:
    • Who prepares the food in the home?
    • Who buys the food, and where is the food purchased?
    • What foods are regularly eaten? Are there special foods for holidays or family occasions?
    • What are the patient's food preferences?
      In addition, the patient should keep a record of dietary intake (usually recorded for 3 to 7 days).
   b. Teaching about foods that are high in sodium and saturated fat is an important part of the plan for this patient. Reading labels and menus (if the patient eats out) will help in the selection of appropriate foods. The patient and family also may be informed about possible substitutions for foods, spices, and oils that are high in sodium and fat. Alternatives, such as polyunsaturated oils, lean meats, and egg substitutes, may be incorporated into meal preparation. A separate meal plan for the patient is usually not necessary because flavorings, such as lemon, can make foods attractive (as well as healthy) for the entire family. The most difficult times are often during holidays and special occasions, when food plays a central role in the family's activities. Low-salt and low-fat substitutions, wherever appropriate, should be used. Fresh or frozen fruits and vegetables, without sodium or fat-based sauces or additives, may be more flavorful than low-sodium canned foods. The patient also may be able to eat traditional foods, in moderation, on these occasions. Realistic expectations may work best for the patient rather than offering harsh, uncompromising restrictions.
2. Nutritional recommendations for a pregnant patient include
    • An increase of an additional 30 to 60 g protein daily
    • Calcium intake, especially critical in the third trimester
    • Supplemental iron
    • Folic acid intake increasing to 600 mcg daily during pregnancy
3. Nutritional considerations for an older adult patient include
    • Eating a balanced diet that contains a variety of foods; avoiding too much fat, cholesterol, sugar, and sodium or salt
    • Eating foods that have adequate amounts of starch and fiber, such as fruits and vegetables and whole-grain cereals and breads
    • Avoiding grapefruit and grapefruit juice
    • Drinking adequate fluids

- Consuming cream soups and meat-based vegetable soups as nutrient-dense sources of protein, with cheese, eggs, and peanut butter as useful high-protein alternatives
- Drinking milk for calcium and vitamin D; providing calcium supplements if lactose intolerance is present
- Taking vitamin and nutrient supplements, if necessary, for nutritional deficits

4. a. *Imbalanced Nutrition: More Than Body Requirements*
   General goals: safely achieve weight reduction, correct poor dietary patterns, achieve calorie or nutrient targets on a daily or weekly basis
   - Patient loses ½ to 1 lb per week.
   - Patient's daily fat intake is less than 30%.
   - Patient eliminates sugared beverages from diet.
   - Patient increases fruit and vegetable servings in diet to five servings per day.
   b. The teaching plan for these employees should include
   - Guidelines for nutrients and calories
   - Avoidance of foods high in fat, cholesterol, sugar, and sodium
   - Avoidance of "fast foods" and eating out too frequently
   - Label reading
   - Integration of exercise
   - Realistic weight loss goals
   - Avoidance of rapid weight loss plans or pills
   - Maintenance of the diet within the work environment and schedule

Chapter Review

1. i	5. j	9. b
2. c	6. g	10. d
3. a	7. f	
4. h	8. e	

11. The *Healthy People 2020* nutritional objectives are for individuals to decrease saturated fat intake in population 2 years and older; increase the variety of vegetable and fruit intake in the population 2 years and older; increase grain products intake and consumption of calcium in the population 2 years and older; reduce daily intake of sodium in the population 2 years and older.
12. a Vitamin K is synthesized by the body.
    b. Vitamins A, D, E, and K are fat soluble.
    c. Antioxidant vitamins are beta-carotene and vitamins A, C, and E.
13. a. Carbohydrates
    b. Proteins
    c. Fats
    d. Carbohydrates
    e. Fats
    f. Proteins
    g. Carbohydrates
14. Prevention of diarrhea: soluble fiber
    Prevention of constipation: insoluble fiber
15. Some general nutritional guidelines to share are
    - Eat a variety of foods; consume plenty of grains, fruits, and vegetables.
    - Balance the intake of food with the amount of physical activity.
    - Reduce the intake of sugar, sodium, fat/saturated fat, and cholesterol.
    - Moderate the intake of alcoholic beverages.
    - A copy of the ChooseMyPlate program may be provided and discussed with the patient.
16. Examples of alternative dietary patterns include vegetarians, ovolactovegetarians, and lactovegetarians. In addition, patients from diverse sociocultural backgrounds may have dietary patterns that are unique.
17. Minerals are inorganic elements that catalyze biochemical reactions. Macrominerals help to balance the pH of the body.
18. The roles of water in the body include transportation of nutrients and waste products; providing structure to large molecules (protein, glycogen); participation in metabolic reactions; serving as solvent, lubricant, and cushion; regulating body temperature; and maintaining blood volume.
19. a. Food and nutrient intake: 24-hour recall, percentage of meals consumed, food preferences, allergies, dislikes, and physical barriers to eating (oral discomfort, dysphagia)
    b. Physical examination: signs and symptoms of nutrient deficiencies, fat deposits, and poor muscle tone and skin turgor
    c. Anthropometric measurements: height, weight, and any changes in height or weight
20. Indicators of malnutrition include a, d, e, f, h, i, k, m, n, and p.
21. The nurse calculates this individual's BMI as 24.5, within the expected range of 18.5 to 24.9. The weight in pounds is rounded to 82 kg and the 6-foot height is 3.34 m^2.
22. Neurogenic causes of dysphagia include stroke, cerebral palsy, Guillain-Barré syndrome, multiple sclerosis, ALS, diabetic neuropathy, and Parkinson's disease.
    Myogenic causes include myasthenia gravis, aging, muscular dystrophy, polymyositis, and dermatomyositis.
23. A common sign of food-borne illnesses is diarrhea, often accompanied by cramping, nausea, and vomiting.
24. a. Stressors in the acute care environment include diagnostic testing (NPO, scheduling), pathologies, unit schedules, cafeteria food served, and medication administered.
    b. To promote a patient's appetite in the acute care setting, the nurse should
    - Enhance food presentation
    - Remove food covers from the patient's food tray
    - Clean the area and remove odors
    - Provide oral care
    - Provide for the best temperature and seasoning of the food
    - Include food preferences, as appropriate, within the diet
25. The patient with dysphagia should be
    - Provided with a rest period before eating
    - Positioned upright, with support as necessary, with the head flexed to a chin down position
    - Fed or taught to eat to the stronger side of the mouth
    - Given thicker fluids
    - Evaluated for the best level of diet
    - Fed slowly, provided smaller size bites, and allowed to chew thoroughly and swallow the bite before taking another
    - Allowed time to empty the mouth after each spoonful

26. Advantages of enteral nutrition include the following: decreased prevalence of hypoglycemia and electrolyte imbalances, increased use of nutrients, maintenance of structure and function of the GI tract, safer and less costly than parenteral nutrition.

27. a. Contraindications to N/G tubes are recent nasal surgery, basilar skull fractures, facial traumas, nosebleeds, and receiving anticoagulation.
    b. The most serious complication associated with tube feedings is aspiration.
    c. Aspiration can be avoided by positioning the patient upright (head of bed elevated at least 30 degrees).
    d. Displacement of the jejunostomy tube can lead to infusion of fluid into the peritoneal space, which can lead to serious complications.
    e. If the N/G tube becomes clogged, the nurse should
       • Verify that the tube is not misplaced or kinked.
       • Flush with warm water.
       • Flush the tube with water after checking the residual volume and periodically as ordered or per institutional protocol to avoid clogging.
       To prevent clogging:
       • Administer medications into the tube in liquid form whenever possible. If medications are appropriate to crush, ensure they are finely crushed and adequately diluted before administration.
       • Administer water before and after the administration of *each* medication.
       • Shake the formula in the feeding container periodically to reduce the settling of formula as sediment. Sediment at the bottom of the delivery container may clog the tube.
    f. Intermittent feeding tubes are clamped/closed to prevent air from entering the stomach.
    g. Gastrostomy tubes are preferred for enteral feeding longer than 3 weeks.

28. The label indicates that there are a fairly significant number of calories for only ½ cup. In addition, almost half of the calories are based on the fat content, with a significant percent being saturated fat. There is also more than ¼ of the recommended sodium, no fiber, and small amounts of vitamins and minerals.

29. Foods that could cause toddlers to choke are hot dogs, candy, nuts, grapes, raw vegetables, and popcorn.

30. Factors contributing to adolescent obesity and nutritional deficits include skipping meals or eating meals with wrong choices of calories, nutrients, and snacks.

31. The pH of gastric aspirate for a fasting patient is usually between 1 and 4.

32. A central venous line is used for a hyperosmolar solution.

33. a. PN is used because the patient is unable to ingest or digest enteral feedings.
    b. Nursing goals for PN are to prevent infection, maintain the PN system, prevent complications, and promote the patient's well-being.
    c. Nursing interventions to prevent complications of PN therapy include weighing the patient daily, monitoring I&O and caloric intake, testing urine or blood for glucose, obtaining blood samples for nutritional assessment, observing for fluid and electrolyte balance, and maintaining the correct infusion rate.

    d. The recommended infusion rate for lipids is 1 mL/min. Solutions should not be used if there is a separation of contents (oil/creamy layer on top) or if the solution is more than 12 hours old.

34. For patients without teeth or with ill-fitting dentures, a soft diet may be ordered. Patient preferences for foods should be taken into account, as well as consistencies, flavors, and colors.

35. The correct information for the Mini Nutritional Assessment (MNA) is found in a, c, d, and e.

36. a. True
    b. True
    c. True

37. ChooseMyPlate is directed at helping the obese and overweight population choose healthier foods and confront the obesity epidemic by providing a basic, visual guide for making food choices for a healthy lifestyle.

38. The correct interventions for the patient receiving enteral feedings are a, c, and e.

39. To decrease cholesterol, the best type of fatty acid intake is monounsaturated.

40. There will be slight variations to the documentation, depending on the record format, but the following should be indicated:
    10 Fr N/G tube inserted into left nare. Procedure tolerated without distress or complications. Placement verified via bedside X-ray.

41. The correct order to the enteral feeding is b, e, d, f, c, a, g.

42. The Subjective Global Assessment (SGA) includes a patient history, measurement of weight, and physical assessment.

43. 1	52. 4	61. 2
44. 1	53. 1	62. 1
45. 2	54. 4	63. 3
46. 2	55. 3	64. 2
47. 4	56. 1	65. 3
48. 1	57. 1	66. 2
49. 2	58. 4	67. 4
50. 2	59. 4	68. 4
51. 2	60. 1	

CHAPTER 34

Case Studies

1. a. Before the IVP, the patient should be assessed for
      • Allergies to shellfish, iodine, or contrast dyes.
      • Fluid status (avoid dehydration from bowel preparation because this may increase the potential toxicity of the contrast dye).
      • Medical conditions that increase risk (e.g., renal insufficiency).
      • Recent barium studies (tests within 2 to 3 days of the IVP will obscure findings).
      The patient should be instructed to
      • Take the cathartic the evening before the IVP.
      • Remain NPO after midnight.
      • Expect an IV infusion to be started for the injection of the dye.

- Expect a flushing sensation and a feeling of warmth, dizziness, or nausea when the dye is injected.
- Expect that a number of x-rays will be taken during the test and that voiding will be done near the end of the test.

   b. After the IVP, the nurse will monitor I&O and report decreased or absent urination. The patient is informed that a normal diet may be resumed, fluid intake is encouraged, and any signs of an allergic reaction (e.g., itching or hives) should be reported.

2. a. The nurse may safely delegate the following urinary care measures: Assisting the patient with the use of the bedpan/urinal, monitoring I&O, maintaining aseptic technique, and promoting patient privacy and dignity. In some institutions, the established policy may allow for additional measures to be delegated, such as routine catheter care and specimen collection. Delegation to unlicensed assistive personnel requires that the nurse evaluate their ability to safely and accurately perform the specified measures.

3. a. The action proposed by the primary nurse is unsafe because it could result in serious damage to the patient's urethra. The correct procedure requires that you prepare a clean disposable towel, gloves, and a sterile syringe (same volume as the fluid in the catheter balloon). The patient is positioned in the same way as for catheter insertion, the syringe is attached to the balloon port, and the entire amount of fluid is aspirated. The catheter then is pulled out slowly and smoothly. If resistance is encountered, an additional attempt is made to remove fluid from the balloon. The catheter then is wrapped in a waterproof pad and disposed of in an appropriate container, along with the drainage tubing and bag (after emptying and measuring the remaining amount of urine). Perineal care then is provided to the patient, and the nurse will monitor the urinary output carefully.

4. a. The patient is provided with a sterile specimen cup, sterile disinfectant wipes, and clean gloves. He is instructed to apply the gloves and wipe the urinary meatus in a circular motion, moving up from the meatus to the glans penis. He also is cautioned against using the contaminated wipe repeatedly. After cleansing, the patient should discard the initial urination and begin collection in the sterile cup at the midstream portion of voiding. The cover of the specimen cup then is replaced, and the specimen is sent to the lab within 1 hour of the collection. If necessary to promote patient understanding, the use of more understandable terms, other than meatus and voiding, may be more effective.

5. a. With an incontinent urinary diversion, the urine drains continuously and the patient has no sensation or control over urinary output. This requires the application of a collection pouch at all times. The pouch will contain the urine and protect the skin from local irritation and skin breakdown as well as provide a barrier against odor. The pouch should be changed every 3 to 7 days, being cut to fit or a precut size. Each pouch may be connected to a bedside drainage bag for use at night. Consideration must be given to skin care to prevent breakdown. The patient may benefit from a referral to an ostomy support group.

Chapter Review

1. d   5. a   9. f
2. g   6. j   10. c
3. i   7. e
4. h   8. b

11. Noninvasive procedures for examination of urinary function include abdominal roentgenogram (radiograph of kidneys, ureters, and bladder [KUB]), intravenous pyelogram (IVP), renal scan, and computed tomography (CT).

12. Intermittent catheterization is used for immediate relief of bladder distention, long-term management of patients with incompetent bladders, sterile urine specimen collection, assessment of residual urine, and instillation of medication. Indwelling catheters are used for urinary outflow obstructions, patients having surgery of the urinary tract or surrounding structures, prevention of obstruction from blood clots, accurate monitoring of I&O and prevention of skin breakdown in critically ill or comatose patients, and provision of bladder irrigations.

13. A female patient may be placed in the lithotomy or Sims' position for catheterization.

14. a. The recommended daily fluid intake is 2000 to 2500 mL.
    b. The minimum urinary output for an adult is 30 mL per hour.

15. a. Sociocultural: Privacy needs for urination and schedule expectations (e.g., intermissions/recesses)
    b. Fluid intake: Increased intake will increase output (if fluid/electrolyte balance exists); alcohol, caffeine, and foods with high fluid content promote urination.
    c. Pathological conditions: Diabetes mellitus and multiple sclerosis cause neuropathies that alter bladder function, arthritis and joint diseases interfere with activity, renal disease influences amount and characteristics of urine, fevers reduce urinary output, and spinal cord injuries disrupt voluntary bladder emptying.
    d. Medications: Diuretics promote excretion of fluid and selected electrolytes, some drugs change the color of the urine, and some medications influence the ability of the bladder to relax and empty.

16. a. Arthritis can interfere with timely access to a toilet.
    b. Diabetes is associated with voiding frequently and the possibility of absent or weak bladder contractility.
    c. Prostate enlargement can result in hesitancy and interference with the ability to empty the bladder completely.

17. a. Stress incontinence
    b. Treatment for stress incontinence may include conditioning (Kegel) exercises, estrogen replacement, alpha-adrenergic agonists, intravaginal electrical stimulation, bladder neck suspension surgery, an artificial sphincter, or penile clamp.

18. Normal characteristics of urine are b and e.

19. The condom catheter should be changed every day, with the skin checked for signs of irritation and breakdown. Perineal care is provided with each catheter change. The tubing must be checked frequently to ensure that there are no kinks or other obstructions.

20. To maintain the patient's dignity when assisting with urinary elimination, the nurse should
    a. Provide comfort, privacy, time, access, and appropriate positioning.
    b. Provide gender-congruent care.
    c. Recognize cultural practices.
    d. Explain procedures.
21. Manual compression of the bladder is called Credé method.
22. Correct statements about urinary diversions are answers b and c.
23. For strict I&O measurement, the nurse should provide the patient with a urinal, bedpan, or urinary hat for the toilet.
24. To stimulate the patient to void, the nurse should run water near the patient, place the patient's hand in warm water, or stroke the inner thigh of a female patient.
25. To assist the patient to strengthen the pelvic floor muscles, the nurse teaches the patient Kegel exercises.
26. The length of catheter insertion is
    a. Female adult patient: 2 to 3 inches (5 to 7.5 cm)
    b. Male adult patient: 7 to 9 inches (17.5 to 22.5 cm)
27. Correct indwelling catheter care techniques are listed in options a, f, and g.
28. To prevent nocturia, the nurse instructs the patient to avoid drinking fluids at least 2 hours before bedtime. If the patient is taking a diuretic, the medication should be given early in the day.
29. An older adult may need to have an assistive device for ambulation to the bathroom, such as a walker. There may also be difficulty in removing clothes or getting on and off of the toilet.
30. For acute onset urinary retention, the correct items are a, c, d, and f.
31. Urinary tract infections may be prevented in patients with indwelling catheters by
    • Following good hand hygiene techniques
    • Not allowing the spigot on the drainage bag to touch a contaminated surface
    • Not opening the drainage system at connection points to obtain specimens or measure urine
    • Wiping the ends of the tube with antiseptic solution, if reconnection is necessary
    • Having a separate receptacle to measure urine for each patient
    • Not raising the drainage bag above the level of the bladder
    • Not allowing any dependent loops of tubing
    • Draining all urine from tubing into bag before the patient exercises or ambulates
    • Avoiding prolonged clamping or kinking of the tubing
    • Emptying the drainage bag at least every 8 hours
    • Removing the catheter as soon as possible upon health care provider order
    • Securing the catheter in place
    • Performing routine perineal hygiene every 8-hour shift and after defecation
32. With regard to a cystoscopy, answers a, c, e, g, h, and i are correct.
33. During a physical assessment:
    a. Presence of a kidney infection is determined by gently percussing the costovertebral angle (the angle formed by the spine and twelfth rib)

b. The bladder is assessed by inspecting and observing a swelling or convex curvature of the lower abdomen. Upon gentle palpation of the lower abdomen, a full bladder is palpated as smooth and rounded. When a full bladder is palpated, patients will report a sensation of urinary urge tenderness or even pain. Percussion is an excellent technique to identify a full bladder. Gently tap the abdomen along the midline starting just above the umbilicus. The edge of the bladder is identified when the percussion note changes to a dull note.
34. a. The bladder scanner is used to determine the amount of residual urine.
    b. Measure post-void residual volumes 10 minutes after assisting the patient to void.
35. a. The urine for a patient taking Lasix will appear dilute.
    b. An individual with liver disease will have urine that is dark amber in color.
    c. With a urinary tract infection, the urine may be thick and cloudy with a foul odor.
36. Urinary specimens should be sent to the lab within 2 hours.
37. The correct order of steps is b, d, a, e, and c.
38. For the patient having a CT scan:
    a. Preparation before the test includes
       • Bowel cleansing (see agency or health care provider protocol)
       • Assessment for allergy to shellfish (iodine) or previous reaction to contrast media (if contrast is ordered)
       • Food and fluid restriction up to 4 hours prior to test (see agency or health care provider protocol)
       • Explain that they will be placed on a special bed that will move through a tunnel-like imaging chamber. They will need to lie still when instructed by the technician; some patients may feel claustrophobic.
    b. After the test:
       • Encourage fluids to promote dye excretion.
       • Assess for delayed hypersensitivity reaction to the contrast media.
39. To prevent a UTI, the nurse teaches the patient about hand hygiene and perineal care.
40. a. Triple lumen catheter
    b. Single lumen catheter
    c. Double lumen
41. After removal of a urinary catheter, the patient should have voiding monitored by using a voiding record or bladder diary. The bladder diary should record the time and amount of each voiding, including any incontinence. A bladder scan can be used to monitor bladder functioning by measuring post void residual (PVR). Careful monitoring should be done to observe for signs of a urinary tract infection.
42. For a suprapubic catheter:
    a. Suprapubic catheters are placed when there is blockage of the urethra (e.g., enlarged prostate, urethral stricture, after urological surgery) and in situations when a long-term urethral catheter causes irritation or discomfort or interferes with sexual functioning.
    b. Care of a suprapubic catheter involves daily cleansing of the insertion site and catheter. The same care for tubing and drainage bag as a urethral catheter applies

for a suprapubic catheter. The insertion site should be assessed for signs of inflammation and for the growth of over-granulation tissue. Site care applies principles of applying a dry dressing and institutional policy will indicate if aseptic or sterile technique is required.

43. The correct order for care of the stoma is b, d, e, c, a.
44. The medications used for urgency urinary incontinence are antimuscarinics, such as darifenacin, oxybutynin, and solifenacin.
45. Foods that can irritate the bladder include a, d, and f.
46. True
47. True
48. Urinary tract infections (UTIs) can be prevented by b, d, and f.
49. Measures to reduce the incidence of CAUTI are appropriate use, proper insertion and maintenance techniques, quality improvement programs, and ongoing surveillance for CAUTI and related causative factors.
50. Examples of possible questions are
    - Are you experiencing urgency, burning or painful urination, frequency, hesitancy, excessive urination, nocturia, dribbling, blood in the urine, straining to void, leaking urine on the way to the bathroom, leaking urine when you cough or sneeze?
    - Do you feel like you have completely emptied your bladder after you have urinated?
    - When did you last urinate?
    - Do you use a product to contain urine leakage? (adult brief, undergarment, pad)
    - How many containment products do you use during the day? At night?
51. The catheter tubing needs to be checked to make sure it is correctly anchored to the patient, as well as being hung above the floor on a part of the bed that does not move.
52. The lumen marked #3 is the one that would be used to inflate the balloon.

53. 3	62. 3	71. 4
54. 2	63. 1	72. 3
55. 3	64. 4	73. 2
56. 1	65. 4	74. 3
57. 3	66. 2	75. 2
58. 1	67. 3	76. 3
59. 2	68. 4	77. 1
60. 4	69. 2	78. 2
61. 2	70. 4	

CHAPTER 35

Case Studies

1. a. Nursing diagnosis: *Constipation related to overuse of laxatives/enemas and inadequate dietary fiber* (as manifested by patient's statement that she is having difficulty with bowel elimination)

   Goal: Patient will establish a regular defecation pattern within 1 to 2 months.

   Outcomes:
   - Patient will have a regular bowel movement within 3 days.
   - Patient's abdomen will be nondistended and nontender.
   - Patient will pass soft, formed stools at least every 2 to 3 days.

   Goal: Patient will maintain a diet that incorporates an adequate amount of fiber and fluids.

   Outcome:
   - Patient will identify and eat foods that are high in fiber and drink an adequate amount of fluid on a daily basis.

   Nursing interventions:
   - Providing instruction about foods high in fiber
   - Providing instruction on the importance of an adequate fluid intake
   - Allowing ample/regular time for defecation
   - Providing instruction on the adverse effects of reliance on laxatives/enemas
   - Investigating family and social contacts for stimulation of appetite
   - Identifying that daily bowel movements are not absolutely necessary

2. a. Before the colonoscopy, the patient should be instructed to
   - Drink clear liquids the day before.
   - Take some form of bowel cleanser (e.g., GoLYTELY).
   - Take enemas until clear, if ordered.

Chapter Review

1. c
2. e
3. a
4. b
5. d
6. Constipation in the older adult is usually the result of decreased fiber and fluid in the diet.
7. Patients should be cautioned against straining (Valsalva maneuver) on defecation if they have cardiovascular disease, glaucoma, increased intracranial pressure, or a new surgical wound.
8. a. *Clostridium difficile* is a common contributor to diarrhea in health care facilities.
   b. This occurrence may be prevented through proper hand hygiene and cautious use of antibiotics.
   c. As a result of diarrhea, the patient is at risk for fluid and electrolyte disturbances and anal irritation.
9. The most frequent complaints are related to functional bowel disorders.
10. Fecal incontinence can create skin breakdown, embarrassment, a change in body image, social isolation, depression, and diminished sexuality.
11. The following factors decrease peristalsis: a, c, d, f, g, j, and k.
12. Individuals from diverse cultural backgrounds may try to avoid exposure of the lower torso, refuse care from persons of the opposite gender, or not communicate issues related to bowel elimination.
13. Risk factors for colon cancer include
    - Age older than 50 years
    - Family history of colorectal cancer

- Ethnocultural background
- Personal history of inflammatory bowel disease
- High dietary intake of fats, with low fruit and vegetable intake

14. Examples of nursing interventions include
    a. Constipation: Increase intake of fiber (vegetables, fruits, whole grain cereals) and fluids, reduce caffeine intake, elevate the toilet seat, establish a routine, promote exercise, allow for privacy and time, provide chopped foods, rather than pureed (for poor dentition), provide mashed foods with fruit juices and hot tea (for difficulty swallowing).
    b. Diarrhea: Increase intake of low-fiber foods, replace fluids and electrolytes, reduce intake of milk/milk products and spicy foods, and provide perineal/perianal care.

15. a. Positioning: Squatting or sitting allows for intraabdominal pressure to be exerted and thigh muscles to be contracted to aid in defecation.
    b. Pregnancy: Constipation commonly occurs because of pressure of the fetus on the rectum.
    c. Diagnostic tests: Some tests require NPO or enemas in advance, and barium can harden and cause constipation if not eliminated after the test.
    d. Diet: Intake of fruits, vegetables, whole grain foods, and adequate fluid will promote bowel elimination.
    e. Personal habits: Failing to respond to the need to defecate and lack of privacy interfere with normal elimination patterns and lead to constipation. Hospitalized patients often share toilet facilities or use bedpans or bedside commodes. The resulting embarrassment causes them to ignore the urge to defecate.

16. The nurse may provide local application of heat, sitz baths, or topical medications (as prescribed) to promote comfort for the patient with hemorrhoids.

17. A GI assessment should include
    - Usual diet, fluid intake, and elimination patterns
    - Characteristics of the stool and recent changes, such as diarrhea
    - Health history: medications, illnesses, mobility, pain, surgery
    - Emotional status
    - Changes in appetite
    - Management of alterations: constipation, diarrhea, indigestion

18. a. The correct position for an adult patient is left Sims' position.
    b. 3 to 4 inches/7.5 to 10 cm for an adult and 2 to 3 inches/5 to 7.5 cm for a child.
    c. The height of the bag should be 12 inches or 30 cm.
    d. Kayexalate enema
    e. A hypertonic enema works by exerting osmotic pressure, pulling fluid from the interstitial spaces, and filling the colon with fluid. The distention in the colon promotes defecation.
    f. Fleet enema
    g. Castile soap
    h. "Enemas until clear" means that you repeat enemas until patient passes fluid that is clear of fecal matter. Check agency policy, but usually patients receive no more than three consecutive enemas, to avoid disruption of fluid

and electrolyte balance. It is essential to observe contents of solution passed. Consider the results "clear" when no solid fecal material exists, but the solution is sometimes colored.
    i. The nurse assesses or delegates the assessment of the results of the enema, including the amount and color of the stool, and the patient's response.

19. The osmotic laxatives are a, c, and f.

20. The QSEN competency of patient-centered care is applied when the patient's needs and preferences are incorporated into the care.

21. The hyperosmolarity of enteral solutions draws fluid into the intestine and promotes defecation.

22. A focused assessment of a patient's bowel function should include
    - Chewing: Check the condition of teeth, gums, and mouth and ability to eat.
    - Mobility: Observe the gait, ability to assist with transfer, positioning, activity, and use of toilet facilities.
    - Anal sphincter function: Check for abdominal distention, impaction.
    - Abdominal muscle contractility: Observe muscle contraction (bearing down) while palpating lower abdomen.

23. a. Colorectal cancer: End colostomy
    b. Diverticulitis: Temporary end colostomy with pouch

24. The teaching plan for a patient with an ostomy should include b, g, h, and i.

25. The expected characteristics are a, e, and f.

26. Before giving a patient a bedpan, the nurse should position the patient with the head of the bed elevated at least 30 degrees, warm a metal bedpan, and provide privacy.

27. Skills b and d may be delegated to assistive personnel, if indicated in agency policy.

28. The gastric pH should be 5 or less.

29. a. *C. difficile* is transmitted by contact and factors that stimulate overgrowth (e.g., antibiotic use).
    b. Transmission of *C. difficile* can be reduced or prevented by employing hand hygiene with soap and water.

30. Examples of positive outcomes for a patient with a colostomy are
    - Skin surrounding the stoma will remain intact.
    - Patient will demonstrate proper peristomal skin care.
    - Patient will recognize and report complications.

31. Normal defecation can be promoted with a high-fiber diet, fluids, exercise/activity, and proper positioning and by allowing time and privacy.

32. Nasogastric tube irrigation is done with 30 mL of saline. Low intermittent suction should be applied.

33. The steps are completed as follows: b, c, e, h, i, b, f, j, d, a, and g. There are other interventions that are also done before and during these steps. These are some of the main actions related to the skill.

34. 2	40. 1	46. 1
35. 3	41. 2	47. 2
36. 3	42. 1	48. 2
37. 4	43. 2	49. 3
38. 3	44. 4	50. 3
39. 4	45. 1	

CHAPTER 36

Case Studies

1. a. The patient may benefit the most from discussing her feelings, needs, and concerns with the nurse, and being involved, as much as possible, in the decision-making process for her plan of care. In addition, she may benefit from the following interventions:
   - Orienting her to the environment, routine/schedule, and staff members
   - Placing her with mobile patients who can interact with her
   - Encouraging frequent visits from family members and friends
   - Providing her with materials she enjoys, such as books and magazines
   - Providing stimulating diversional activity for her, such as music and games
   - Engaging in conversation with her during meals and implementation of nursing actions
   - Encouraging her to use any necessary assistive aids, such as glasses
   - Encouraging and assisting her (as necessary) to attend to daily grooming
   - Providing a stimulating physical environment, such as changing her view or decorating with personal objects

2. a. For the patient, there are safety considerations associated with the first time he will be getting out of bed. He could be prone to orthostatic hypotension, which is the drop in blood pressure from lying down or sitting to a standing position. When transferring from a supine position into a chair, move the patient gradually. First, obtain a baseline blood pressure and pulse with the patient in the supine position. Then raise the patient to a high-Fowler's position, and measure blood pressure and pulse again to detect decreases in blood pressure or elevations in pulse. Leave the patient in this position for 2 minutes to allow the body to adapt. Monitor the patient for dizziness or lightheadedness. The patient is now ready to sit at the side of the bed with the feet on the floor (dangling). If the patient experiences no dizziness, assist the patient to a chair. When transferring an immobile patient for the first time, make sure that assistance is available, if necessary.

3. a. Older adult patients are especially prone to the hazards of immobility. It is important to make sure that the following interventions are included in the patients' care:
   - Assess overall physiological and psychological status regularly
   - Skin: provide moisture, be gentle in moving and positioning
   - Respiratory: encourage deep breathing, coughing, moving
   - Musculoskeletal: incorporate range of motion into daily activities
   - Diet: make sure that sufficient fluids, vitamins and proteins are included
   - Elimination: assist in positioning, dietary intake of fluids and roughage

- Cognitive/psychological: provide diversionary activities/stimulation, reality orientation, emotional support, explanations before care
- Work with other members of the health care team to provide safe care and prevention of complications

Chapter Review

1. i
2. e
3. d
4. j
5. c
6. b
7. f
8. h
9. a
10. g

11. The objectives of bed rest are to decrease physical activity and oxygen needs, allow the ill/debilitated patient to rest, and prevent further injury.
12. Pathological influences on mobility include muscle and postural abnormalities, damage to the central nervous or musculoskeletal system.
13. The pathophysiological changes that occur with immobility include answers b, c, f, h, i, and k.
14. Fluid and electrolyte imbalances that occur with immobility include hypercalcemia and hypovolemia (initial phases).
15. An immobilized patient may react to the experience by exhibiting hostility, belligerence, inappropriate moods, altered sleeping patterns, withdrawal, confusion, anxiety, sadness, hopelessness, and depression.
16. The heart rate of an immobilized patient is generally 15% faster.
17. Virchow's triad refers to thrombus formation, and the three associated problems are (1) loss of integrity of the vessel wall, (2) abnormal blood flow, and (3) altered blood cells and clotting factors.
18. The nurse's focus for an immobilized child is on providing physical and psychosocial stimulation in order to keep pace with motor and intellectual development.
19. To maintain the patient's autonomy, the nurse encourages the patient to do as much as possible, demonstrate activities, and participate in goal setting and decision making.
20. The changes and interventions are
    - Cardiovascular system:
      - Orthostatic hypotension: Move the patient slowly from one position to another.
      - Increased cardiac workload: Place the patient in an upright position (if possible), provide regular exercise and adequate fluid intake.
      - Thrombus formation: Provide regular exercise, adequate fluid intake, and antiembolic stockings.
    - Respiratory system:
      - Hypostatic pneumonia and atelectasis: Encourage coughing and deep breathing, adequate fluid intake, and exercise; turning; upright positioning; and chest physiotherapy.
    - Integumentary:
      - Pressure ulcers: Assess the skin, use supportive devices, provide adequate nutrition and hydration, change position every 1 to 2 hours, and give meticulous skin care.

- Gastrointestinal:
  - Reduced appetite, inadequate/imbalanced nutrition, decreased peristalsis: Provide adequate nutrition (fruits, vegetables, fiber) and hydration, measure I&O, administer prescribed cathartics, promote activity or movement, and institute a bowel program.
- Urinary:
  - Urinary stasis resulting in greater risk for infection and calculi: Provide adequate hydration and promote activity and movement.
- Musculoskeletal:
  - Loss of strength and endurance, reduced muscle mass, decreased stability and balance, with possible contractures and disuse osteoporosis: Provide or encourage range-of-joint-motion exercises, turn every 1 to 2 hours, change position, and refer to physical therapy.
21. With the algorithm, a transfer aid should be selected for use.
22. Focused assessment of the patient's mobility includes range of joint motion (ROJM), pain, endurance, and activity.
23. a. Rotation of the neck
    b. Abduction of the arm
    c. Supination of the forearm
    d. Circumduction of the arm
    e. Hyperextension of the hip
24. To evaluate muscle atrophy, the nurse should perform anthropometric measurements—height, weight, and triceps skin folds.
25. The nurse checks for edema in the immobilized patient at the sacrum, hips, legs, and feet.
26. Assessment frequency (unless indicated by agency policy or changes in patient status):
    a. Respiratory status: every 2 hours
    b. Anorexia: at meals
    c. Urinary elimination: at the beginning or end of every shift
    d. Intake and output: every shift for daily measurement
    e. Anthropometic measurements: every 2 to 4 weeks
27. Specific exercises to prevent thrombus formation include ankle pumps, foot circles, knee flexion, and hip rotation.
28. For antiembolic stockings:
    a. Contraindications for use include dermatitis, open skin lesions, new skin grafts, and decreased circulation.
    b. The stockings are removed every shift.
    c. The stockings should not be partially rolled down or wrinkled, and the toes should not be uncovered.
    d. True
29. For a sequential compression device, options a and d are correct.
30. Newer Low Molecular Weight (LMW) heparins (anticoagulant) are usually given every 12 hours by the subcutaneous route.
31. For the immobilized patient with a suspected pulmonary emboli, actions b and e are correct.
32. The Morse Fall Scale should be used to assess the patient's probability of falling.
33. The patient can perform passive range of motion to the right side and active range of motion with the left side. Participation in ADLs, to the extent the patient is able, will also provide joint mobility.
34. The best ways to prevent pressure ulcers are to change the patient's position at least every 1 to 2 hours, assess the skin frequently, promote mobility, and provide moisture and hygienic care.
35. The following are examples of possible nursing diagnoses:
    - *Ineffective Airway Clearance*
    - *Risk for Constipation*
    - *Risk for Disuse Syndrome*
    - *Risk for Falls*
    - *Impaired Physical Mobility*
    - *Risk for Impaired Skin Integrity*
    - *Risk for Deficient Fluid Volume*
    - *Impaired Urinary Elimination*

36. 4	42. 3	48. 4
37. 3	43. 4	49. 2
38. 2	44. 2	50. 2
39. 3	45. 3	51. 3
40. 2	46. 1	52. 2
41. 4	47. 4	53. 4

CHAPTER 37

Case Study

1. a. Nursing diagnosis: *Risk for Impaired Skin Integrity related to prolonged pressure on bony prominences* (as manifested by reddened areas [reactive hyperemia] on sacrum, elbows, and heels)
   Goal: Integrity of skin and underlying tissues will be maintained.
   Outcomes:
   - Reactive hyperemia will subside and patient's normal skin coloration will return within 2 days.
   - Patient will assist, as possible, with turning and positioning every 1 to 2 hours.
   Nursing interventions:
   - Reposition or assist with repositioning every 1 to 2 hours.
   - Encourage the patient to shift weight when out of bed and in a chair.
   - Assess skin and underlying tissues with each position change.
   - Use supportive devices: padding for mattress and bony prominences.
   - Keep sacral area clean and dry.
   - Measure, document, and report reddened areas.

Chapter Review

1. g	5. j	9. e
2. h	6. a	10. f
3. b	7. i	
4. c	8. d	

11. Sites marked should include occipital bone (1), scapula (2), spine (3), elbow (4), iliac crest (5), sacrum (6), ischium (7), Achilles tendon (8), heel (9), and sole (10).

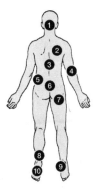

12. a. Stage I
    b. Stage III
13. External factors that contribute to pressure ulcers include shear, friction, and moisture on the skin.
    Internal factors include nutrition, infection, impaired peripheral circulation, obesity, and advanced age.
14. Infants, young children, and older adults are most susceptible to sensitivity to heat and cold therapy.
15. Dryness of the older adult's skin makes it less tolerant to pressure, friction, and shearing forces.
16. a. Primary intention
    b. Secondary intention
17. a. True
    b. True
18. a. Dehiscence
    b. Hematoma/bleeding
    c. Infection
    d. Infection
    e. Bleeding/shock
    f. Evisceration
    g. Infection
19. a. Assessment includes the location, extent of tissue damage, size (dimensions and depth of wound), tissue type (viable or nonviable) and percentage of wound tissue (e.g., viable versus nonviable), amount and color of wound exudate, and condition of surrounding skin.
    b. For darkly pigmented skin:
       • Look for changes in skin texture, temperature, and warmth.
       • Examine skin when pressure is applied and removed because the color can remain unchanged when pressure is applied.
       • Assess for color changes at the site of pressure that differ from patients with light skin color.
       • With a gloved finger, feel the area of potential skin damage as the skin in the injured area may feel cool to touch, indicating potential skin damage. Circumscribed area of intact skin is often warm to touch. As tissue changes color, intact skin feels cool to the touch.

• If a patient previously had a pressure ulcer, that location maybe lighter in skin color.
• Localized area of involved skin may be purple/blue or violet (eggplant) instead of red.
• Edema may occur with induration and may appear shiny and taunt.
• Patient may complain of discomfort at a site that is predisposed to pressure ulcer development.

20. a. Age: Infants and older adults may have decreased circulation, oxygen delivery, clotting, and inflammatory responses, with an increased risk of infection. Older adults have slower cell growth and differentiation, and scar tissue is less pliable.
    b. Obesity: Obese individuals have a decreased supply of blood vessels in fatty tissue (impaired delivery of nutrients to the site), and suturing of adipose tissue is more difficult.
    c. Diabetes: Individuals with this condition have small blood vessel disease (reduced oxygen delivery), and elevated glucose levels impair macrophage function.
    d. Immunosuppression: A reduced immune response leads to poor healing. Steroids also mask signs of inflammation/infection, and chemotherapeutic agents interfere with leukocyte production.
21. a. 3, serous
    b. 4, sanguineous
    c. 1, serosanguineous
    d. 2, purulent
22. a. Pressure reduction: Use of a supportive surface, regular and frequent turning and repositioning in the bed (q2h) and chair (q1h)
    b. Skin care: Keep skin clean and dry after incontinence, use skin barriers/protectants, turn or lift sheets to reduce friction and shear, maintain head of the bed at 30 degrees or lower, avoid vigorous massage of bony prominences or areas of redness
23. To obtain a wound culture, the steps are e, c, d, a, and b.
24. The patient who has a dirty, penetrating wound may require a tetanus toxoid injection.
25. The nurse determines wound healing by measuring the wound diameter and depth, assessing the wound tissue, checking the skin condition around the wound, and observing for exudate.
26. A patient who is out of bed in a chair should be limited to 2 hours sitting and repositioned at least every 1 hour.
27. The nurse reduces friction or shear by using a draw sheet, trapeze bar, and/or support when moving the patient and by providing skin care to maintain integrity.
28. Care of an abrasion or laceration includes control of any bleeding, rinsing of the wound under running water, gentle cleansing with mild soap, application of a prescribed or over-the-counter antiseptic, and protection with a bandage.
29. For a negative pressure wound therapy system:
    a. The purpose is to remove excess fluid, stimulate granulation tissue growth, and reduce wound bacteria.
    b. The tube is attached to suction to provide negative pressure.
    c. The dressing that is used is either black or white foam cut to fit the wound. The transparent dressing should cover

the wound, extend 3 to 5 cm beyond the wound edges, provide an occlusive seal, and be free of wrinkles.

d. If there is an increase in discomfort and using black foam, switch to white foam. Notify the supervisor and/or provider.

30. For wound irrigation:
    a. Syringe size: 35 mL
    b. Needle size: 19 gauge
    c. psi: 8
    d. The syringe is held 1 inch (2.5 cm) above the wound.
    e. Reduce the irrigating pressure and notify the health care provider.
    f. Use more fluid or pressure.

31. a. Wound closed with staples
    b. Jackson-Pratt wound drainage system

32. The correct nursing interventions are statements a and d.

33. The steps in caring for a traumatic wound are
    • Stabilize the patient's cardiopulmonary function.
    • Promote hemostasis (stop any bleeding).
    • Cleanse the wound.
    • Protect the site from further injury.

34. a. Cold (C)
    b. Heat (H)
    c. Heat (H)
    d. Heat and cold (H and C)
    e. Heat (H)

35. a. Application of heat is contraindicated in the presence of active bleeding or acute inflammation, and for patients with cardiovascular disease.
    b. Application of cold is contraindicated in the presence of edema at the site, decreased circulation, and shivering.

36. Heat and cold are usually applied for about 20 to 30 minutes.

37. The correct interventions for application of heat and cold are a and g.

38. Total score = 13 points
    Patient risk = "at risk" status

39. The correct actions for a moist dressing are a, c, and e.

40. a. Nonblanchable hyperemia is redness that persists after palpation and indicates tissue damage.
    b. This signifies that deep tissue damage is present and is commonly the first stage of pressure ulcer development.
    c. True: Damage can be reversed with the removal of pressure.

41. For a postoperative dressing, the correct actions are b, c, and e.

42. Before the patient is discharged, the nurse will want to assess/evaluate the patient's
    • Wound and overall health status
    • Ability to perform the dressing independently
    • Concerns over the care and the appearance of the wound
    • Recognition of signs and symptoms that will require notification of the physician
    • Ability to obtain necessary supplies

43. Topical skin care should include b, c, and e.

44. False. It is usually clean technique.

45. 1. c; 2. a; 3. b

46. The correct way to remove old tape is to apply pressure against the skin away from the tape. It may be necessary to moisten the tape with normal saline, if it is very sticky.

47. Discomfort may be reduced during dressing changes by administering analgesics 30 minutes before, allowing "time-outs" during painful procedures, planning dressing changes when a patient is feeling best, soaking dried dressings before removal, avoiding aggressive packing, positioning and supporting the wound area, and using low adhesive or nonadhesive dressings.

48. A sling is correctly applied by having the patient sit or lie supine for a sling application. Instruct the patient to bend the affected arm, bringing the forearm straight across the chest. The open sling fits under the patient's arm and over the chest, with the base of the triangle under the wrist and the triangle's point at the elbow. One end of the sling fits around the back of the neck. Bring the other end up over the affected arm while supporting the extremity. Tie the two ends at the side of the neck so that the knot does not press against the cervical spine. You can fold the loose fold at the elbow evenly around the elbow and pin it. To prevent the formation of dependent edema, make sure the lower arm is always supported at a level above the elbow.

49. The desired temperature for a cold soak is 59° F or 15° C.

50. 1	57. 3	64. 1
51. 3	58. 2	65. 2
52. 3	59. 2	66. 3
53. 4	60. 3	67. 2
54. 2	61. 4	68. 4
55. 4	62. 1	
56. 3	63. 3	

CHAPTER 38

Case Studies

1. a. For this patient, you may implement the following interventions to maintain sensory stimulation:
    • Referring the patient to community agencies (e.g., Foundation for the Blind)
    • Recommending/assisting in obtaining books with larger print, audiotape books, and music
    • Recommending the introduction of brighter colors (e.g., red, orange, yellow) into the home environment (which also helps for him to better differentiate between surfaces and room objects)
    • Investigating family and social contacts
    • Allowing time for discussion of feelings, needs, and concerns

    b. To promote safety, you should
    • Assist in arranging the environment so that the patient knows where everything is and that clutter is out of the way
    • Instruct/assist in improvement of lighting in halls and stairways and use of color-coding (e.g., edges of stairs, medication bottles, and appliance dials)
    • Instruct about importance of follow-up visits to the ophthalmologist

2. a. A patient in an intensive care unit (ICU) may experience sensory overload from the intensity of sounds and activity and/or sensory deprivation from restricted visits of family and friends.

b. The nurse should try to organize care so that the patient is allowed opportunity for uninterrupted rest, whenever possible. Monitors at patient's bedside may have volume controls so that they can be turned down to a lower level. The nurse also should take time to sit with the patient, either quietly or for verbal stimulation. Visits from family members and friends should be encouraged but not to the point of patient fatigue. The environment may be arranged so that the patient has a different or more pleasant view, and personal items (e.g., photos) may be placed within the patient's field of vision. It may be a challenge for the nurse in this setting to adapt the patient's sensory input, so creativity, within realistic limits, is recommended.

Chapter Review

1. a. Visual
   b. Auditory
   c. Gustatory
   d. Olfactory
   e. Tactile
   f. Kinesthetic
2. Diseases that may lead to visual impairment include age-related macular degeneration, glaucoma, cataracts, and diabetic retinopathy.
3. a. Cerumen accumulation
   b. Presbycusis
   c. Cataract
   d. Xerostomia
   e. Ménière's disease
4. a. Age, older adulthood:
   • Decreased hearing acuity, speech intelligibility, and pitch discrimination
   • Increased dryness of cerumen, with obstruction of the auditory canal
   • Reduced visual fields; increased glare sensitivity; impaired night vision; reduced accommodation, depth perception, and color discrimination
   • Reduced sensitivity to odors and diminished taste discrimination
   • Difficulty with balance, spatial orientation, and coordination
   • Diminished sensitivity to pain, pressure, and temperature
   b. Medications: may cause ototoxicity or optic nerve irritation (chloramphenicol) or may reduce sensory perception (analgesics, sedatives, antidepressants)
   c. Smoking: may cause atrophy of taste buds and interference with olfactory function
   d. Environment: excessive stimuli, frequent activities, noise, TV, bright lights, pain, confinement
5. Assessment of vision and hearing:
   • Ask the patient to read.
   • Observe the performance of ADLs (activities of daily living).
   • Observe the patient's use of glasses, magnifiers, or hearing aids.
   • Observe patient's conversation/interaction with others.
6. a. Trauma is the leading cause of blindness in children, usually as the result of flying objects or penetrating wounds.
   b. Child eyesight safety includes avoiding toys with long, pointed handles or sharp edges; keeping the child from running with a pointed object; and keeping pointed objects and tools out of reach.
   c. Chronic middle ear infections and exposure to loud noise contribute to hearing loss in children.
7. Orientation to the environment should include
   • Keeping your name tag visible, addressing the patient by name, explaining the patient's location, and frequently identifying the time and date in conversations
   • Offering short and simple, repeated explanations and reassurance
   • Encouraging family and friends not to argue with or contradict a confused patient but to explain calmly their location, identity, and time of day
   • Walking the patient through a room to feel the walls and establish a sense of direction
   • Approaching a visually impaired patient from the front
   • Explaining the location of objects within the room, such as chairs or equipment
   • Keeping all objects in the same place and position and describing the location of key items
   • Placing necessary objects such as the call light, patient-controlled analgesia (PCA) button, glasses, water, or facial tissue in front of patients
   • Asking the patient how to arrange objects so ambulation is easier
   • Removing clutter and unnecessary equipment and keeping the path to the bathroom clear
8. Sensory stimulation may be modified in the acute care environment by
   • Increasing the patient's view outside and within the room
   • Arranging decorations, plants, photos, greeting cards, and the patient's personal items
   • Providing audio books and large-print reading material
   • Spending time with the patient; listening to and conversing with the patient
   • Playing pleasant music or turning on television shows that the patient enjoys
   • Providing attractive meals at the correct temperature
   • Providing a variety of textures and aromas to enhance the patient's appetite
9. The nurse may communicate with a hearing-impaired patient by
   • Making sure that a hearing aid, if needed, is in place and in working order
   • Approaching the patient from the front to get his or her attention
   • Facing the patient on the same level, with adequate lighting
   • Making sure that glasses, if needed, are worn and are clean
   • Speaking slowly and articulating clearly, using a normal tone of voice
   • Rephrasing, rather than repeating information that is not heard
   • Using visible expressions and gestures
   • Talking toward the patient's better ear
   • Using written information to reinforce spoken words
   • Not restricting the hands of deaf patients

- Avoiding eating, chewing, or smoking while speaking with the patient
- Avoiding speaking while walking away, in another room, or from behind the patient

10. Patients with cataracts exhibit a, c, e, and f.
11. a. Hearing deficit: Amplify low-pitch sounds, use lamps with sound activation, use assistive devices for telephones, and obtain closed captioning for the television.
    b. Diminished sense of smell: Use smoke and carbon monoxide detectors, take special care with disposal of matches and cigarettes, and check the expiration dates on foods.
    c. Diminished sense of touch: Lower the temperature of the water heater and use caution when checking the bath or shower water.
12. Nursing diagnoses for a patient with a sensory deficit include
    - *Disturbed Body Image*
    - *Fear*
    - *Hopelessness*
    - *Risk for Injury*
    - *Powerlessness*
    - *Self-Care Deficit, Bathing*
    - *Self-Care Deficit, Dressing*
    - *Risk for Situational Low Self-Esteem*
    - *Impaired Social Interaction*
    - *Social Isolation*
    Possible goals/outcomes include the following: The patient will manage self-care, ambulate safely, verbalize feelings, remain oriented to surroundings, communicate/interact with others, participate in planning care, identify community resources.
13. a. General screenings include examinations for congenital blindness and visual impairment in infants and young children, routine vision and hearing tests of school-age and adolescent children, regular medical eye/ear examinations every 2 to 4 years for individuals older than age 40 and every 1 to 2 years for those older than age 65.
    b. The specific recommendation for hearing screenings is for at least once every decade through age 50, and then once every 3 years.
14. The appropriate actions for promotion of sensory stimulation in the home are a, d, and e.
15. Drugs that may cause ototoxicity are a, d, and f.
16. A patient may not use his/her hearing aid because of its appearance, a denial of its need, fit, the difficulty in manipulating a small object, cost, or a lack of understanding of its use.
17. A patient with diminished tactile sense may be helped with the use of Velcro and zippers, and providing assistance with or encouragement for grooming (e.g., hairbrushing) of the affected side.
18. Ménière's disease is characterized by progressive low-frequency hearing loss, vertigo, tinnitus, and a full feeling or pressure in the affected ear.
19. Care for a hearing aid includes
    - Making sure your fingers are dry and clean before handling hearing aids
    - Inserting and removing the hearing aid over a soft surface

- Placing the battery in hearing aid when it is turned off
- Removing the hearing aid battery when not in use and storing it in a marked container in a safe place
- Protecting hearing aids from water and excessive heat or cold
- Using a soft dry cloth to wipe hearing aids and a soft brush to clean difficult to reach areas

20. Specific adult behaviors include a, c, and e.
21. Examples of available community resources are the American Foundation for the Blind, American Red Cross, Canine Companions, Lions Club, and public health/visiting nurse services.
22. The occupational health nurse reinforces the use of protective devices, such as eye goggles and earplugs, as well as participates in safety policy development and environmental and employee screening.
23. Patients who are more prone to sensory deprivation are those in medical isolation/private rooms, alone in the home, immobilized in hospitals or other facilities, separated from family and friends, and experiencing disabilities that restrict mobility and/or sensory function.

24. 2	28. 4	32. 1
25. 2	29. 4	33. 2
26. 3	30. 2	34. 3
27. 1	31. 3	35. 1

CHAPTER 39

Case Studies

1. a. Explain and demonstrate coughing and deep-breathing exercises with splinting of the abdominal incision. Assist in and encourage turning and positioning every 2 hours. Reinforce the use of the incentive spirometer. Explain and demonstrate range-of-motion exercises. Provide prescribed analgesia before activities, keeping in mind the action and dosage of the medication and its possible effect on the patient.

2. a. Preoperative teaching for the patient who is having ambulatory surgery may occur when the patient comes for preoperative tests and physical assessment. There also may be telephone contact with the patient on the evening before the surgery, as well as a 24-hour resource line for the patient to use for questions. Additional teaching may be conducted immediately before the procedure and before the patient's discharge. Information provided to the patient usually includes instructions specific to the surgery and anesthesia (e.g., dressings, activity and dietary restrictions), signs and symptoms of complications, and time frame for follow-up visits.

   b. If the patient does not appear to understand about the surgery or possible complications, then you should contact the surgeon, so that he or she can meet with the patient and review the procedure. It is not the nurse's responsibility or appropriate for the nurse to explain the procedure. The alert and oriented patient must have an understanding of the surgery that will be performed to sign the consent.

3. a. Any significant change in the patient's status should be reported to the surgeon and/or anesthesiologist immediately. Because of the effects of general anesthesia, temperature alterations are especially critical before surgical procedures. Surgery may be postponed until the patient's temperature has returned to normal.

4. a. The patient should be informed that, under usual circumstances, all loose items are removed before surgery. If the patient will be adversely affected by the removal of his "lucky" medallion, it may be pinned inside of the patient's gown or surgical cap, depending on the type of surgery. It is important, however, that the operating room personnel be informed that the patient has the medallion in place before the surgery. It may be the policy of the agency that the patient will have to sign a form stating that he has kept the medallion (or other jewelry) on his person in case of a loss.

   b. The other items that you will remove or account for before surgery are wigs, dentures, partial plates, caps/loose caps, and all removable prosthetics (eyes, limbs, etc.). If a patient has a brace or splint, check with the surgeon to determine whether it should remain with the patient, to be reapplied after surgery. Although patients must remove hearing aids, eyeglasses, and contact lenses, do not have them do this until just before the surgery.

5. a. Before the patient's discharge, it is important to know the following:
   • Degree of mobility that the patient should have and the prescription for exercise and rest
   • Pain relief measures
   • Wound care requirements
   • Patient and family expectations for recovery, including concerns about restrictions and length of time for convalescing
   • Schedule for medical follow-up
   • Recognition of the signs and symptoms indicating the need to seek medical follow-up
   • Nutritional needs
   • Other medical conditions that may have an impact upon the patient's recovery
   • Financial concerns

6. a. For the patient in the PACU, you will need to monitor his vital signs every 15 minutes or more frequently, especially the oxygen saturation. He will have to be aroused more often and reminded to breathe deeply. In addition, the abdomen and dressing will have to be assessed to make sure that there are no signs of internal hemorrhage.

   b. For this patient, you will want to palpate or use a scanner to see if his bladder is distended. If the patient is able, you can stand him up to urinate and provide oral fluid intake. Taking the patient to the bathroom, where there is privacy and the ability to run the water, may help to stimulate urination. In the event that the patient is unable to urinate after more than 8 hours, an order for catheterization may be required.

Chapter Review

1. g	4. f	7. d
2. c	5. h	8. b
3. a	6. e	

9. a. The patient who smokes cigarettes is at a greater risk for bronchospasm or laryngospasm.

   b. Aggressive pulmonary hygiene should be instituted for this patient, including frequent turning, coughing and deep breathing, incentive spirometry, and chest physiotherapy.

10. a. The following medical conditions may increase a patient's surgical risk: bleeding disorders, diabetes mellitus, heart disease, upper respiratory tract infection, cancer, liver disease, fever, chronic respiratory disease, immunological disorders, and abuse of street drugs.

    b. Malignant hyperthermia is an inherited disorder that is associated with general anesthesia.

    c. Pregnant patients are at greater surgical risk because:
    • Cardiac output and respiratory tidal volume increase to keep up with the increase in metabolism and blood pressure decreases, making interpretation of vital signs and recognition of hypovolemic shock more difficult.
    • The high level of progesterone relaxes the lower esophageal sphincter (LES) and decreases gastrointestinal motility, which slows gastric emptying, resulting in an increased risk for aspiration of stomach contents.
    • Near term there is an increase in white blood cells beyond the normal range for that of non-pregnant women who have no infection.
    • There is an increased risk for deep vein thrombosis as a result of increased fibrinogen levels and decreased clotting time.
    • In addition, a pregnant patient and her family experience increased psychological stress because of fear of fetal loss or deformity.

11. a. Cardiovascular: Changes in structure and function reduce cardiac reserve and predispose the patient to postoperative hemorrhage, increased blood pressure, and clot formation.

    b. Pulmonary: Changes in structure and function reduce vital capacity, increase the volume of residual air left in the lungs, and reduce blood oxygenation.

    c. Renal: Changes in structure and function increase the possibility of shock with blood loss, limit the ability to metabolize drugs/toxic substances, increase the frequency of urination and the amount of residual urine, and reduce the sensation of the need to void.

    d. Neurological: Changes in function reduce the ability to respond to warning signs of complications and may lead to confusion after anesthesia.

12. Obesity places a patient at greater risk as a result of diminished ventilatory capacity and higher risk of aspiration. There may also be other issues relating to circulation, endocrine function, and musculoskeletal integrity.

13. a. Insulin: For a patient with diabetes, the need for insulin is reduced preoperatively because of NPO status. Dose requirements may increase postoperatively because of stress response and IV administration of glucose solutions.
    b. Antibiotics: Potentiation of anesthetics, possible respiratory depression from depressed neuromuscular transmission
    c. NSAIDs: Inhibited platelet aggregation and prolonged bleeding time
14. General information in preoperative teaching includes
    • Preoperative and postoperative routines
    • Expected sensations
    • Pain relief measures available (e.g., PCA)
    • Postoperative exercises
    • Activity and dietary restrictions
15. Routine preoperative screening tests include complete blood count, serum electrolyte analysis, coagulation studies, serum creatinine test, urinalysis, 12-lead electrocardiogram, and a chest x-ray.
16. Commonly used preoperative medications include
    • Sedatives: used for relaxation and decrease in nausea
    • Tranquilizers: used to decrease anxiety and relax skeletal muscles
    • Narcotic analgesics: used to sedate, decrease pain and anxiety, and reduce the amount of anesthesia needed
    • Anticholinergics: used to decrease mucous secretions in the oral and respiratory passages and prevent laryngospasm
17. Nursing diagnoses that may be formulated include
    • *Anxiety:* achieving emotional and physiological comfort and rest
    • *Deficient Knowledge:* understanding the physiological and psychological responses to surgery; understanding intraoperative and postoperative events
18. NPO criteria:
    a. 2 hours before
    b. 8 to 12 hours before
19. The uses and side effects of the types of anesthesia are
    a. General anesthesia: used for major procedures that require extensive tissue manipulation. Side effects include cardiovascular depression or irritability, respiratory depression, and liver and kidney damage.
    b. Regional anesthesia: used when operating on a specific body area. Side effects include a sudden decrease in blood pressure and respiratory paralysis.
    c. Local anesthesia: used for minor procedures, especially in ambulatory surgery, and after general anesthesia for postoperative pain relief. Side effects include local irritation and inflammation.
    d. Conscious sedation: used for procedures that do not require complete anesthesia. Respiration is maintained and the patient can respond to stimuli. Side effects include respiratory depression and decreased level of consciousness.
20. Appropriate preoperative interventions include a, c, d, and f.
21. Verification in the PSCU and OR includes
    a. Right patient: Ask patient to state name; inspect patient identification band for patient name and date of birth and compare with medical record.
    b. Right frame of mind: observe for signs of fear and anxiety, monitor vital signs for indications of excessive anxiety, and compare vital signs to baseline.
    c. Preparation for surgery: determine and mark the body area for the procedure, establish or verify IV, insert urinary catheter (if ordered), check that preoperative checklist and medications are done, and remove glasses and other prostheses.
22. a. Circulating nurse (C)
    b. Scrub nurse (S)
    c. Circulating nurse (C)
    d. Circulating nurse (C)
    e. Scrub nurse (S)
    f. Circulating nurse (C)
    g. Scrub nurse (S)
23. For intraoperative patient care:
    a. To prevent injury: sterile drapes, sponge and instrument counts, careful positioning, eye protection, grounding of electrical devices, availability of emergency equipment
    b. To maintain body temperature: warm room, warm irrigating solutions, warm blanket after surgery
    c. To prevent infection: standard precautions, sterile asepsis, skin scrubs
24. a. Pulmonary stasis: turning every 1 to 2 hours, coughing, deep breathing, incentive spirometry, chest physiotherapy
    b. Venous stasis: range-of-joint-motion (ROJM) exercises, turning, antiembolitic stockings, sequential compression device, adequate fluids
    c. Wound infection: sterile technique for dressing changes, standard precautions, adequate nutrition (proteins for wound healing)
    d. GI stasis: a gradual progression in dietary intake, promotion of ambulation and exercise, provision of an adequate fluid intake, administration of fiber supplements, stool softeners, enemas, and rectal suppositories as ordered, assisting with proper positioning, and stimulation of the patient's appetite; frequent oral hygiene and meals when the patient is rested and free from pain
25. The patient is qualified to be discharged based on options a, d, f, h, and i.
26. The patient should void within 8 hours of the procedure. For the patient who has not voided, the nurse should palpate the area above the symphysis pubis to determine the presence of bladder distention. A bladder scanner may be used to see if residual urine is present. The surgeon should be notified of the patient's inability to void.
27. The first oral intake is usually a clear liquid diet.
28. Appropriate care for an operative incision includes answers b, c, and f.
29. a. The patient in the illustration is demonstrating the use of an incentive spirometer.
    b. This device is used to prevent atelectasis and promote respiratory function.
30. For the patient who will remain alert during a surgical procedure, the nurse should explain the procedure, encourage questions, and warn the patient when unpleasant sensations will be experienced. Some settings provide music to mask unpleasant sounds and to promote relaxation.

31. Routine postoperative assessment includes
    - Monitoring vital signs and pulse oximetry
    - Respiratory assessment: monitoring respiratory rate, rhythm, and depth every 15 min $\times$ 4 or until stable, then every 30 min $\times$ 2, and then every hour $\times$ 4; comparing with baseline findings
    - Auscultating lung and heart sounds
    - Performing pain assessment with pain tool, including severity, location, description, measures used to relieve; assessing for any side effects of pain medication (altered mental status, depressed respirations, bradycardia, orthostatic hypotension, nausea or vomiting, urinary retention, constipation); observing patient's expressions, body position, ability to rest, or sleep
    - Wound assessment: observing surgical wound for redness, edema, warmth, drainage, and dehiscence; inspecting for amount of bleeding on dressing, in drainage systems, and underneath patient
    - Assessing level of consciousness and symptoms of restlessness or altered mental status
    - Observing skin, nail beds, and mucous membranes for color and hydration
    - Palpating peripheral pulses distal to surgical site, tight dressing, or cast if present
    - Inspecting any urine output; note color, consistency, and odor
    - GI assessment: inspecting for abdominal distention; auscultating for bowel sounds in all four quadrants at least every shift until discharge; palpating abdomen for firmness
    - Monitoring NG tube for patency and NG tube output for color and amount of drainage if present
    - Observing patient's ability and willingness to tolerate fluids and food
    - Monitoring laboratory values for signs of complications
32. A latex allergy is evident with the patient who has contact dermatitis with redness, inflammation, and blisters; has contact urticaria with pruritus, redness, and swelling; or has hay fever–like symptoms and anaphylaxis.
33. The recommendation is for systemic, around-the-clock analgesia.

34. The correct interventions are a, c, e, and f.
35. Interventions to decrease postoperative wound infection include the clipping of hair (vs. shaving), disinfection of the skin with an antiseptic agent such as chlorhexidene immediately before the incisional cut, administration of a prophylactic antibiotic, delay of dressing change until 48 hours after surgery, and adherence to principles of asepsis.
36. The hand-off communication is:
    A - **A**dministrative data, N - **N**ew clinical information must be updated, T - **T**asks to be performed by the covering provider must be clearly explained, I - **I**llness severity must be communicated, C - **C**ontingency plans for changes in clinical status must be outlined
37. Examples of postoperative nursing diagnoses are
    Ineffective Airway Clearance
    Anxiety
    Disturbed Body Image
    Ineffective Breathing Pattern
    Risk for Deficient Fluid Volume
    Risk for Infection
    Impaired Physical Mobility
    Nausea
    Acute Pain
    Delayed Surgical Recovery
    Examples of postoperative patient outcomes are stable vital signs, reduction in incisional pain, oxygen saturation above 92%, able to ambulate with assistance, and incision clean, dry, and infection free.

38. 3	46. 3	54. 4
39. 1	47. 3	55. 2
40. 3	48. 2	56. 3
41. 1	49. 1	57. 4
42. 2	50. 3	58. 3
43. 2	51. 4	59. 2
44. 2	52. 2	60. 3
45. 4	53. 2	61. 2